DATE DUE

OCT 10 1995	
BRODART	Cat. No. 23-221

THE SEXUAL VICTIMOLOGY OF YOUTH

Edited by

LEROY G. SCHULTZ

Professor, School of Social Work
West Virginia University
Morgantown, West Virginia

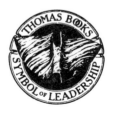

CHARLES C THOMAS • PUBLISHER
Springfield • Illinois • U.S.A.

Published and Distributed Throughout the World by

CHARLES C THOMAS ● PUBLISHER
Bannerstone House
301-327 East Lawrence Avenue, Springfield, Illinois, U.S.A.

ISBN 0-398-03925-9

Library of Congress Catalog Card Number: 79-15613

With THOMAS BOOKS careful attention is given to all details of manu-
facturing and design. It is the Publisher's desire to present books that are
satisfactory as to their physical qualities and artistic possibilities and appro-
priate for their particular use. THOMAS BOOKS will be true to those laws
of quality that assure a good name and good will.

Library of Congress Cataloging in Publication Data
Main entry under title:
Schultz
The Sexual victimology of youth.

   Bibliography: p. 376
   Includes index.
   1. Child molesting—Addresses, essays, lectures. 2. Youth—Crimes against—
Addresses, essays, lectures. 3. Sex crimes—Addresses, essays, lectures. 4. Child
abuse—Addresses, essays, lectures. I. Schultz, LeRoy G.
HQ71.S413   364.1′53   79-15613
ISBN 0-398-03925-9

Printed in the United States of America

OK - 1

CONTRIBUTORS

Robert Sam Anson
Senior Writer
New Times Publishing Co.
New York, New York

C. David Baker, J.D.
Editor-in-Chief
Pepperdine Law Review
Malibu, California

Lucy Berliner, M.S.W.
Social Worker
Sexual Assault Center
Harborview Medical Center
Clinical Assistant Professor of Social Work
University of Washington
Seattle, Washington

Renee S. T. Brant, M.D.
Staff
Beth Israel Hospital
Boston, Massachusetts

Heinz Brunold, M.D.
Senior Physician and Assistant Director
Konigsfelden Clinic
Konigsfelden, Germany

Ann Wolbert Burgess, D.N. Sc.
Professor of Nursing
Graduate School of Arts and Sciences
Boston College
Chestnut Hill, Massachusetts

M. A. Flammang
Professor of Police Science
Police Training Institute
University of Illinois
Champaign, Illinois

Henry Giarretto, Ph.D.
Director
Child Sexual Abuse Treatment Program
Santa Clara County Juvenile Probation Department
San Jose, California

Judith Herman, M.D.
Staff
Somerville Women's Mental Health Collective
Somerville, Massachusetts

Lisa Hirschman, M.A.
Staff
Cambridgeport Problem Center
Psychology Department
University of Montreal
Montreal, Canada

Lynda Lytle Holstrom, Ph.D.
Associate Professor and Chairperson
Department of Sociology
Boston College
Chestnut Hill, Massachusetts

John P. Kemph, M.D.
Associate Professor and Clinical Director
Children's Psychiatric Hospital
University of Michigan
Ann Arbor, Michigan

Anna Laszlo, M.A.
Chief Victim Specialist
Suffolk County District Attorney's Office
Boston, Massachusetts

David Libai, J.D.
Lecturer in Criminal Law and Procedure
Bar Ilan University
Ramat Gan, Israel

Parker Rossman, Ph.D.
Associate Professor of Religion in Higher Education
Yale University
New Haven, Connecticut

Sexual Assault Center Staff
Harborview Medical Center
Seattle, Washington

Suzanne M. Sgroi, M.D.
Project Internist
Connecticut Child Abuse and Neglect Demonstration Center
Hartford, Connecticut

Doris Stevens, M.S., ACSW
Chief Social Worker
Sexual Assault Center
Harborview Medical Center
Clinical Assistant Professor of Social Work
University of Washington
Seattle, Washington

Carolyn Swift, Ph.D.
Staff
Wyandotte County Association for Mental Health
Kansas City, Kansas

Veronica B. Tisza, M.D.
Staff
The Children's Hospital Medical Center
Boston, Massachusetts

Atalay Yorukoglu, M.D.
Child Psychiatrist
Children's Psychiatric Hospital
University of Michigan
Ann Arbor, Michigan

PREFACE

It has been some twenty-five years since I encountered my first sexually abused child, beside myself. A survey of the literature suggests we have gained little useful knowledge during this period. As Rousseau in 1780 (Emile) stated, "We know nothing of children; and with our mistaken notions the further we advance the further we go astray." The professional helper has little more to go on than I did twenty-five years ago. Sexuality and children, by themselves, have not gained their share of research or policy resources, but when combined have produced a national avoidance-reaction. This is no longer defensible, if it ever was. Admittedly, the control, treatment, and prevention of the sexual abuse of minors, as a problem, must compete for attention, priority, and resources with all other social problems. This does not fare well in a world where the odds are against children; where children cannot vote or influence their own policy, and where the government that claims to represent them is paralyzed by indecision over "parent right" versus "child right," or "state intervention" versus "family privacy" dilemmas.

My intent is not to speak for the child but to present a series of responsible selections of materials that best address the problem today. The material presents a diversity and variety that it would not have had it been written by a single author. My intent is to correct overgeneralization, inaccuracy, and insensitive stereotyping of both victims and offenses. The material will give the interested reader the total post-offense process the minor victim passes through. Each professional will see his own role and that of others. Each professional involved should know what the victim has gone through up to his intervention, and to anticipate what process lies ahead.

In the International Year of the Child
L.G.S.

INTRODUCTION

The literature dealing with the sexual abuse of minors is scant, unintegrated, and ambiguous. Books on the topic are rare. Articles are scattered and hidden among a wide range of journals, many in nonaccessible medical and legal journals. Keeping up with the field, while a professional and ethical obligation, is increasingly difficult for the busy practitioner, who needs the literature as the cases come in. The student in graduate and undergraduate studies in the small college or university may lack access to special journals in the small library. These articles should prove valuable for these groups as acquaintance with the sexual abuse problem becomes more democratized. While some of the articles may overlap and some contradict, such is the state of the art the reader must address.

The readings begin with a historical introduction to society's effort at control of the problem. It highlights a two-pronged approach: society as child-protector and society as oppressor of children's/minors' normal sexual development. Each section is introduced by the editor with aspects that are usually not included in the selection of articles. Two chapters deal with an appraisal of the problem today, followed by four chapters dealing with diagnosis and treatment. Regrettably, these four center on the "medical-model" only, but they are all we have to build upon at present. Then, the emotional issue of incest is taken up with a widely divergent series of articles highlighting the multi-valued nature of this kind of behavior.

One of the most neglected areas in professional literature for those addressing child sexual abuse involves that of law and legal roles. This is a critically important part of the problem because professionals are in fact practicing law through their roles as interpreters of state law and agency policy; as implementors of state law, policy, and practice involving children's rights; as reporters of offenses, expert witnesses, and preparers of various documents that may be used in hearings and legal disposition.

Lastly, included are a series of chapters dealing with the newly discovered problem of the use of children and minors in making movies, a view of minor boys as sexual love objects from the eyes of some adults, and a call to re-evaluate the age of sexual consent for those over age fourteen years.

Concluding is a bibliography divided into topical headings for those interested in pursuing further the topic of sexual abuse.

Intended Audiences

As an anthology of the best available literature on child sexual abuse, this book should prove useful to those interested in viewing victimology in an integrated sense, i.e. the manner in which social institutions react to the victim. *The National Analysis of Official Child Neglect and Abuse Reporting* 1978 revealed the following sources of reporting in 99,071 cases:

Friends, Relatives, and Parents	37.7%
Law Enforcement	11.8%
Social Welfare Agencies	9.1%
Medical Agencies	11.0%
Education Institutions	11.3%
Victim	1.4%
Child Care Agencies	1.2%

The list above indicates those professions on the front line to whom these readings are addressed.

The readings aim at both a problem focus as well as practical information. While the vocabulary of some of the readings may prove difficult for laymen, the material should prove meaningful to the 37.7 percent who report child abuse and, hopefully, to all the friends of children and minors.

Lastly, the readings will be of value to those university courses dealing with child welfare, children's rights, criminology, victimology, police science and child development.

What is Sexual Abuse?

There is an unusual condemnation of the sexual abuse of
children below the age of fourteen years. When asking what
specific behaviors are defined as sexual abuse, one receives a
confusing vague array of sexual interactions with hundreds of
private meanings. There seems little disagreement on those
sexual interactions where physical force is involved, or where
victim-offender age disparity is great. Thus, forcible rape brings
wholesale outrage, but statutory rape involving similar aged
participants brings hedging and a lot of "ifs." Phrases such as
"child-molestation," "sexual exploitation," "corruption of morals," "contributing to the delinquency of a minor," or "lewd
behavior" when defined by state, church, or adults results in a
jumble of prohibited behavior. These include french-kissing,
touching during bathing of children, allowing children to see
parents make love, parental withholding of sex education,
children and parents swimming nude, and allowing children to
see adults in their underwear, at one end of the scale, to sexual
intercourse, oral sex, and "kiddie-porn" at the other end. Incest is
considered different depending not just on force used or age of
participants, but also whether siblings or distant relatives are
involved.

Even more problematical is drawing the line between appropriate affection between people and sexual abuse, in a highly
differentiated society of ethnic groups, social classes, youth
cultures, and emerging life-styles. Behavior between adults and
children or adolescents can be expressive of nonsexual motives in
the actors, but social control agencies or neighbors may read their
own sexual definitions into such behavior. Well-meaning adults
can convert an ambiguous complaint by a child or adolescent
into a sexual offense.

Our stiff age-graded law on nonsexual freedom for children
and adolescents cannot accommodate a variety of sexual developmental stages between ages ten to sixteen years, where some at
twelve years show adult secondary sexual characteristics and
feeling, and where some sixteen year olds look and act like

children. Today's fourteen year olds may simply be the first to combine a biological fact with a sense of individual style.

There is no agreed-upon definition of sexual abuse by the state, parents, or adolescents. Professionals in social control and law enforcement agencies are handicapped by the lack of a working definition. New realistic definitions are required for "sexual abuse" as a crime and for criteria for determining parents as "unfit" or the home as "unsuitable" on the basis of sexual interaction in the home. Until uniform definitions that can be practically implemented are agreed upon by minors, parents, professionals, and law enforcement, children's rights are at risk.

Incidence and Frequency

There is a noticeable lack of reliable data on the incidence or frequency of sexual victimization of minors. There is marked confusion as to what ages to cover in defining "minor," "child," "adolescent," or "juvenile," what sexual acts to include and how to define them in ways professionals, parents, and youth can understand. There is no centralized national or state recording system or index for sexual offenses against youth. Even what little data exist, be it that of law enforcement or social science, are confusing in that police jurisdictions and researchers use different crime definitions for the same type of sex event or use broad-brush methods of including every type of reported offense under "sexual abuse;" also, statutory differences make comparisons across state lines difficult. The lack of reliable incidence and frequency data make it difficult to honestly appraise the public of the problem or to influence policymakers, budget bureaus, law enforcement, and social service agencies in determining resources of manpower and program implementation costs. The reader is cautioned as to the reliability of the figures being cited here.

Estimates of number of cases of sexual abuse range from 4,000 cases per year in large urban areas (1) to 5,000 cases of incest per year nationally (2) to approximately 200,000 to 500,000 cases of "sexual molestation" per year nationally (3). Kinsey's classic research involved a finding that 24 percent of *all* females are molested as children (4). In urban areas, one Washington, D.C., hospital reported that 24 percent of sex abuse cases were of children under fourteen years, including thirty boys (5); a Philadelphia hospital indicated that 10 percent of rape cases each year involved children under the age of fourteen years (6). A recent write-in survey of 1,070 self-defined rapes revealed that 22 percent occurred to girls under age fifteen years (7). A Minneapolis study of police records for one year indicated 291 cases of sexual abuse, of which 85 percent consisted of "indecent exposure or indecent liberties" (8).

The most reliable study to date on sexual abuse incidence was completed in 1978 and published by three organizations: National Center on Child Abuse and Neglect of H.E.W., the American Humane Association, and the Denver Research Institute. The project collected data from thirty-one states and three territories using a uniform reporting system in 1976 (9). Table I indicates their findings. The table clearly implies that "sexual molestation" and "unspecified sexual abuse" are the major offenses against girls, with the clearly dangerous years being the beginning of puberty (12 to 14 years). In the case of males, who represented but 15.7 percent of the total sample, the offenses and ages show little change from one category to the next. The big difference between male and female may be due to boys and adults not considering "indecent exposure" an offense and of not reporting sexual exploration between two boys of similar age.

In comparison to neglect and physical abuse, sexual abuse (1,975 cases) is statistically minor. Physical abuse for the same states and year totalled 26,438 cases and for neglect 58,055 cases. Why then this national attention to such a *statistically* minor kind of behavior? One has to understand Western society's history in dealing with children on one hand and sexuality on the other (the first and last chapters of this book) for a disheartening example of mismanaged benevolence. Children and sexuality have no place together; the conventional wisdom infers that sex is too complex for children and adolescents to fully comprehend, it is potentially violent and dirty, and it is one area that invites exploitation between parties holding different amounts of power. Part of today's discovery of sexual abuse of children stems from the national attention being focused on rape or violence in general, including physical abuse of children. Since most reported victims are females, the re-emergence of the feminist movement also accounts for the emphasis today. In addition, the social science of victimology is gaining acceptance among universities and research centers. Whatever the cause, our shared interest should present opportunity to provide research and resources to address the issue. There are crimes against children of omission and commission on all sides. We think we know what is right for children, but we know little about children's rights.

Table I

AGE, SEX, AND TYPE OF SEXUAL ABUSE
(AMERICAN HUMANE ASSOCIATION 1978)
N=1975

TYPE	0-2yrs	3-5yrs	6-8yrs	9-11yrs	12-14yrs	15-17yrs	TOTALS
Rape	M - 0	M - 1	M - 2	M - 4	M - 0	M - 3	10 Cases
	F - 4	F - 19	F - 24	F - 32	F - 58	F - 37	174 Cases
Sexual Molestation	M - 6	M - 16	M - 12	M - 13	M - 18	M - 7	72 Cases
	F - 17	F - 72	F - 83	F - 83	F - 126	F - 107	493 Cases
Deviant Sex Act	M - 2	M - 12	M - 18	M - 30	M - 23	M - 7	92 Cases
	F - 5	F - 19	F - 26	F - 33	F - 19	F - 18	120 Cases
Sex Abuse Unspecified	M - 12	M - 15	M - 22	M - 13	M - 27	M - 10	99 Cases
	F - 19	F - 43	F - 75	F - 86	F - 165	F - 98	486 Cases
Incest	M - 2	M - 2	M - 4	M - 7	M - 13	M - 7	35 Cases
	F - 4	F - 12	F - 25	F - 60	F - 145	F - 128	374 Cases

1. American Humane Association: *Protecting the Child Victim of Sex Crimes.* Denver, 1966, p. 2.
2. American Humane Association: *Child Victims of Incest.* Denver, 1968, p. 5.
3. H. Gagnon: Female child victims of sex offenses, *Social Problems, 13;* 191, 1965.
4. A. Kinsey: *Sexual Behavior in the Human Female.* New York: Pocket Books, 1953, p. 117.
5. C. Hayman et al.: Rape in the District of Columbia, *American Journal of Obstetrics and Gynecology, 113(1);* 92, 1973.

6. J. Peters: The Philadelphia rape study. In I. Drapkin and E. Viano: *Victimology*, Vol 3. Lexington, Mass.: D.C. Health, 1975, p. 193.
7. P. Bart: Rape doesn't end in a kiss. *Viva, 2(9):* 39, 1975.
8. A. Jaffe et al.: Sexual abuse of children: An epidemological study. *American Journal of Diseases of Children, 129(6):* 689, 1975.
9. American Humane Association: *National Analysis of Official Child Neglect and Abuse Reporting*. Denver, 1978.

CONTENTS

THE LEGAL CONTROL OF THE SEXUAL ABUSE OF CHILDREN

"History is a drunk in the snow with his feet sticking out."

John Baskin, 1976

THE SEXUAL ABUSE OF CHILDREN AND MINORS: A SHORT HISTORY OF LEGAL CONTROL EFFORTS

LeRoy G. Schultz

The history of childhood in Western society makes for disheartening reading, but when combined with sexuality over time the picture becomes one of unadultered ugliness. The evolution of childhood and sexuality is characterized by superstition, unreasonable fears, folklore, religious fanaticism, medical sadism, and fundamental ignorance. The discovery of "childhood" and "adolescence" came late, and the "century of the child" later yet. The combination of 2000 years of Christianity and premature excursions into the lofts of misunderstood human behavior science have shaped our present values regarding children and sexuality and legal control efforts. The history of sex and children is an unpleasant walk through a house of horrors, a disgusting heritage that, even so, can not be disowned. The past is not dumb, and no one desires to repeat the errors of yesteryear. Its flawed condition should not hide the fact that it is all we have to build upon.[1] In our present efforts to protect children from sexual abuse and, at the same time, to avoid sexually neglecting them, we need not reinvent the wheel or the rack. "Our history suggests that we would do well to be wary of the presumption that we can get . . . outside our history itself in our effort to do abstract justice in the creation or recovery of rights for children."[2]

This short history is divided into two arbitrary time phases: the first up to the year 1800 and the second from 1800 to the present. Since so little has been recorded on both children and sexuality over time, what follows is necessarily broad and is slender on historical documentation. The first phase, up to 1800, is characterized as a dark time period in which children and minors were

3

indiscriminately used as sexual objects as the norm by various adults in the child's social space. The second phase, after 1800, marked society's efforts to kill off the child's natural sexual development "for his own good." During these two phases, the basic legal structure was built with the passage of criminal law designed to sexually protect children and minors from adults and from themselves.

At Risk as Norm

The taboo against using children as sex objects is only a few hundred years old. Little effort was made to determine, or concern shown for, the ages of children by parents or the children themselves.[3] Life was short and the age demarcations of child, adolescent, and adult were not discovered until the seventeenth and eighteenth centuries. As early as 100 A.D., young male children were circumcised to help reduce their potential sexual arousal[4] while others were castrated in infancy to enhance their sexual appeal as boy prostitutes. The early cities of Europe, particularly those of Rome and Greece, permitted marriages between boys and adult men, boy houses of prostitution, and rent-a-boy sexual services.[4] The sexual abuse of boys, by today's standards, may have been nearly universal for slave boys. In early Rome, upper-class boys were instructed to wear distinctive necklaces lest their fathers engage in sexual behavior with their own sons by mistake in public bathhouses. Nor was the boy the only sex object. Petronias (455 A.D.) described his rape of a seven-year-old girl with the aid of older women, who stood and watched, applauding the rapist. In general, the major sexual interest was in boys not girls.

Masturbation of children was thought to hasten growth and strength and to help children fall asleep. The life span for all was short by today's standard, menstruation signaled marriagability for girls, marriage to children was common, as was routinely having intercourse in front of, or involving, children. Sleeping arrangements were necessarily crude and simple, with all sleeping in one room. Bedrooms separate from other rooms were a late architectural development for all except the wealthy. In the late

1600s, moralists recommended separate beds for children[5] but separate bedrooms for children did not follow for some 200 years.[6] The clergy were the first to speak to the issue. Dominic in 1405 warned parents to avoid nudity in front of children because of its sexual temptations.[4] The sexual interest in children persisted, particularly among the wealthy. Cellini, the renowned sculptor, pupil of Michelangelo, was a child-molester. In 1440 Baron de Rais, the Protector of Joan of Arc, was put to death for the rape-murder of 800 children.[7,8]

The need for some form of child protection law was felt in the early 1500s in England. A law was passed in 1548 protecting boys from sodomy and in 1576 protecting girls under ten from forcible rape, with both offenses carrying the death penalty.[9] While Christianity may have recognized childhood innocence and the need to protect and preserve it in earlier times, secular law did not reflect this as a state interest until the 1500 to 1600 period. Since many girls were married by age thirteen, the age of consent was set low by today's standards. Boys were protected also. Hans Boesch, in his classic *Child Life in Germany* (1900), reported laws punishing boys of ages twelve to fourteen years arrested as customers in brothels.

The books of Gerson in 1706 indicated that children should be responsible for protecting themselves from sexual abuse, and parents should induce guilt when discovering children masturbating.[4] In this same period, the prominent educator Pascal offered parents advice for controlling sexual molestation.[4] He warned parents to supervise children at all times, to never pamper them, to avoid nudity near adults, to never let them be alone with servants, and to enforce sexual modesty in the home. These simple rules may be the first concrete help parents received from any source in controlling sexual abuse. The concept of childhood innocence gained further ground when the censorship of children's literature commenced.[10] Children's innocence was to be enforced not just where adults were involved but where the child himself showed any sexual precocity. For example, parents were instructed to keep candles burning in children's sleeping areas at night so that they could be checked for masturbation or self-stimulation.[10] Servants, house staff, and the clergy were told to refrain from developing close or friendly relationships with children for fear of the potential for sexual arousal. Teachers and tutors could no longer beat the naked buttocks of children as a disciplinary measure. Children could experience up to 1,000 enemas during their early years to assist the removal of "evil" from their bodies.[4] Children were now to be considered sexually dangerous, with innocence and asexuality to be enforced, which foretold of the coming attack on children's sexual integrity by a "well-meaning" society.

Sex Law Reform

Following the French Revolution, sexual conduct was somewhat liberalized under the Napoleonic Code. The Code removed the death penalty for sex crimes against children and decriminalized voluntary sexual acts between adults. This required various countries to set the age of consent, or to define adulthood. Most European countries followed the French experience in decriminalizing some sexual behaviors and softening penalties. However, both England and United States were to insist on retaining the old sex laws, with harsh punishments and little enlightenment in sexual attitudes. The English legal scholar and statesman Blackstone (1723-1780), while quite rational regarding other types of law reform, was virtually retarded when it came to applying this same rationality to sexual conduct. He refused to clearly define the sexual acts to be criminalized for fear such descriptions would sexually arouse the public.[6] Blackstone apparently had little choice but to legally operationalize the sexual superstitions and ignorance of his time. For example, in sex crimes against children, both victim and offender were equally guilty and both were to be punished, a condition not likely to result in complaints to the police. Sex offense charges could not be sustained unless a third party witnessed the offense, a condition unlikely in view of the privacy of the sexual act. Blackstone's semantic prudery confused everyone since "crime against nature" and "gross indeceny" proved vague and legally difficult to make uniform. The efforts of Blackstone, despite criticism from hindsight, represent the first budding effort at protecting both child sex victim and offender.

Further efforts at child protection occurréd under the English Tory, Robert Peel, Home Secretary from 1823 to 1830. He insisted on the death penalty for sexual assaults on girls under the age of consent. Under English law, the age of consent moved from age ten to age twelve in 1861, to age thirteen in 1875, and to age sixteen in 1885[11] although a girl could legally marry at age twelve. English law exempted child-beating or abuse from the definition of sexual assault. In 1861, a law was passed protecting children from homosexual attack, and in 1869, protecting children from exhibitionism. Pornographic books dealing with childhood seduction and rape gained popularity, along with photographs of children and adults in sexual activities, from 1780 to 1800.[12,13] Increasing the age of consent to sixteen years in 1885 (England) marked society's most intruding intervention "on behalf" of the sexual welfare of minors. The "age of consent" issue emerged from exposure of the so-called "white slave trade"[6] in England. Girls, ages fourteen to sixteen, were for the most part voluntarily entering prostitution in large numbers to escape poverty and rural unemployment. Pimps openly advertized, promising good wages and travel. The English social worker Josephine Butler[14,16] became interested in the plight of young prostitutes and was incensed by the lack of legal protection of minors. She formed powerful alliances with feminist groups, the Y.W.C.A., and the W.C.T.U. with the goal of rescuing the minor prostitutes. It seems the minors could not or would not be rescued from prostitution, the wages being unmatchable by current legal employment structure. Butler and her supporters seized upon the idea of raising the age of consent to sixteen years, thus authorizing police to arrest prostitutes under age. After a bitter struggle, the age of consent was raised to age sixteen years in 1885.

The American Experience

Since the ecclesiastical courts of England were not transferred to the new America, the Colonies insisted on strict enforcement of Puritan ethics and scriptural law. The sparse sanctions of common law were not enough, and special laws were enacted punishing all nonmarital sexual activities.[17]

Much like England, America was noting a sharp rise in prostitution among minors, and America was to follow the English example in raising the age of consent, using the same protest tactics.

Between 1877 and 1885, a powerful coalition was formed calling itself the Social Purity Alliance, made up of feminists, social workers, the Y.W.C.A., The Salvation Army, and the W.C.T.U.[22] The group's mission was to structurally preserve childhood innocence as long as possible, rescuing "sexual drunkards," improving child-rearing habits, rescuing "fallen women," all by raising the age of sexual consent as high as possible. The group rejected the older theological view that prostitutes were "fallen from grace," but explained "sexual incontinence" as a crime, or in the case of minors, sexual delinquency. The Alliance focused its attention on the "white slave traffic" and its violation of the civil liberties of minors, and it quickly lost any concern for volunteer rescuing effort and went after outright governmental control of the problem.

In 1883, another group formed calling itself the White Cross Society.[18] Its aim was to teach young men sexual self-control through church education and the denial of sex as a commitment to the feminist movement. It joined forces with the Social Purity Alliance and took as their first major goal the criminalization of the brothel. It was by working on the brothel problem that child prostitution was discovered, and changing the age of consent become the corrective strategy. Between 1886 and 1895, the Alliance and its supporters were successful in raising the age of consent in most states after a bitter struggle. (See Chapter Appendix).

Not all of the members of the feminist movement were in support of raising the age of consent. Other social forces were at work. Janet E. R. Reese, M.D., contended that premarital sexual expression should not be labeled as sex crime in women; Elizabeth Blackwell, M.D., spoke of all women's sexual needs; and Victoria Woodhull supported the "free love" concept—all three were ignored by their feminist sisters. Mrs. Francis Willard raised the question in 1891: "Are our girls to be as free to please themselves in the lawless gratification of every instinct. . .and passion as our boys?"[18] The answer was an overwhelming sexist "no." The girl's body now belonged to the state, and her protection became a state function, but the age of consent was to be uniformized with disregard for individual preferences and with disregard for social class and ethnic differences in sexualization, creating a new crime called statutory rape.

The sexual protection of children and minors was to take a grim turn in another direction.

Society as a Child Molestor

Parents in the eighteenth and nineteenth centuries seeking advice from "experts," whether physicians, teachers, or the clergy, were not aware that the experts were afflicted with the sexual ignorance of the time and they could only echo it. Once sexuality and morality in children were given over to the physician specifically, the sexual abuse of children was to take an incredible turn.[19,20]

Sexual feelings in children and "sexual precocity" led to self-abuse, and "self-pollution" and were etiologically responsible for almost every known pediatric ailment of the time. The child and minor were viewed as a simple undisciplined animal who needed protection from its own sexual instincts. "The spirit of children must at all costs be broken—not out of spite, but for their own good."[19] Added to medical intimidation and fear-mongering was parental loss of sexual control of minors during the long period from puberty to marriage (the only approved sex outlet) and from the increasingly earlier age of menstruation in girls, the former due to the necessity of employment and career before marriage for the male, the latter due to increased nutrition and health.[21] What innocence there was in children must be preserved to the last minute, the family was to be "God's reformatory," and a frenzy of antimasturbation efforts commenced. The fear was that masturbation in boys caused insanity and early death, and (sexism of the times) girls would become nymphomaniacs or prostitutes. The "unnatural" acts of children were to be suppressed. The emergence of the idea of childhood as based on weakness and need for protection demanded that parents deny that children had sexual feelings, drives, and gratification-means.[21]

This form of sexual abuse of children "for their own good" occurred in two time phases. Phase one, 1850-1879, marked the period of forced sexual underdevelopment via surgery and phase two, 1875-1925, via physical and/or psychological constraints.

Surgical procedures practiced only upon children consisted of partial or complete removal of the clitoris in young girls (sometimes without anesthesia), slitting or infibulating the penis in young boys, cauterization of clitoris or penis, castration of extra-sexually active boys, and cutting out nerves of both male and female genitalia. [22,23] As late as 1936, an American medical textbook recommended that masturbation be controlled in children by circumcision.[24]

The use of constraints[19] for desexualizing children consisted of encasing the child in canvas and splints, encasing in plaster of paris, blistering the genitalia with red mercury, terror-therapy, and if all failed, committing the child to the then prevalent "masturbation sanitoria." Parents could purchase chastity belts or girdles made of leather, bone, and padlocks, to prevent "touching." An iron spike ring could be placed around the penis or child-proof iron gloves could be placed on the children's hands. Other methods consisted of immersing the child or his organs in ice water, dressing the child caught masturbating in uniforms that told the community about it, placing bells on the hands, strapping hands to bedsides, handcuffs, over-exercising the child, child-battery, a wide range of guilt or trauma induction methods, and carrying a picture of one's mother. Mercifully, by 1925, raping children's sex organs came to a slow end as a cure for sexual development. In more modern times, the adult urge to control sexual development was to take the form of denying children a sex education for fear of early sexual autonomy.

In 1871, both sexual and physical abuse gained sufficient recognition as a problem for the formation of the First Society for the Prevention of Cruelty to Children (New York). The idea of some community responsibility to protect children slowly gained acceptance. This responsibility took two forms. The community's criminal law was to sexually protect children from adults, and the juvenile code was to continue the trend of sexually protecting the child from himself. From 1890 to 1960 the "child saving movement" was to appoint itself as guardian of children's sexual morality.[25][27] The movement aimed at imposing criminal-like sanctions on conduct "unbecoming youth" (sexual development among other things) and disqualifying youth from adult privileges.

In 1892 the first women's prison was established *for* sexual offenders, and life sentences for girls who were both sexually active and mentally retarded were recommended by feminist reformer Josephine Lowell.[28] A sexual interest manifested by females was a sign of sickness, since the current assumption was one of asexuality.[29] Later, a new vocabulary commenced with imprisoning phases such as the contradictory "statutory rape," "status offenses—Pens," "ungovernability," and a new social condemnation pushed by psychiatrists and social workers, under the guise of a diagnosis, "sexually acting out."[30,34]

The "best interests of the child" called for more restriction in the interests of morality or therapy, then protection from physical danger and a transfer from "God's reformatory" to the court and social services. Client or citizen participation in law-making and policy formulation were unheard of as the state moved in to regulate the pleasures of children and minors in an effort to protect them.

Current Protective Laws

The details of current law were worked out in the Middle Ages and transported to America. They were constructed as if they could withstand time and could hardly have anticipated the rapid changes in human sexual expression; that the laws have undergone virtually no further change as far as children and minors are concerned. One exception was the new offense of statutory rape.[35] The intent of this law was, as one court declared with biblical zeal, "to prohibit a girl, while passing through the years of adolescence from voluntarily becoming the author of her own shame and to set her apart from the lusts of men" and to "erect a barrier of years around a willful girlhood."[36] The state's moral duty to all girls was to offer resistence for them. The attached appendix lists the current age of consent in the fifty states. Most state age levels are unrealistic,[37, 39] and only recently has a proposal been made to lower the age to fourteen years in accordance with this reality.[31] Current "age of consent" levels reflect a romantic clinging to yesterday's concept of virtue and more importantly, ends up stigmatizing sexual experimentation by adolescents as criminal. In 1971, there were 13,099 young girls in America's delinquency institutions, of which two-thirds consisted of those with nondelinquent behavior, a large portion involving girls voluntarily making love with a male.[40]

The states very seldom offer boys sexual protection from females; exceptions are listed in the appendix, with one court ruling "under the law a girl may be older and more aggressive, the real seducer, a common prostitute who seduces a 15 year old boy (but) the boy will be guilty and the girl innocent."[41]

The sexual protection of girls and boys below age fourteen years is another matter, and it should not be confused with realistic sexual emancipation of those over fourteen years. All fifty states have well-established and well-accepted laws protecting the sexual integrity of young children. The laws of California can be cited as typical of most state laws in operation today.[44] These laws prohibit persons from loitering, delaying, lingering, or idling near areas where children gather; prohibit acts that sexually stimulate children under age fourteen; prohibit touching any parts of the child's body, even through clothing, or removal of a child's underclothing with sexual intent; and prohibits any person from willfully and lewdly committing any lascivious act upon or with the body, or any part thereof, with intent of arousing, appealing to, or gratifying the lust or passion or sexual desires of such persons or child (Cal. Penal Code 653 and 288). Further clarification of child molesting ruled that putting one's arm around a child's shoulder indoors at night could be a sexual offense,[45] and even accidentally allowing children to witness sexual intercourse by parents has been criminalized.[46]

In addition to the above laws addressing sexual molestation, other laws also sexually protect children; for example, rape, exhibitionism, sodomy, incest, prostitution, contributing to the delinquency of a minor, and more recently, protecting children from exploitation in films and magazines.[47] Added protection is also assured with civil penalties for various professions whose members do not report sexual abuse when encountering it in their practice.[48]

Conclusion

Society's sexual interest in children and minors has been historically chronic and may be more common today than is comfortable to admit.[49, 51] To be sexually vulnerable in a moral vacuum was replaced over time by a morality induced, socially sanctioned sexual abuse. The self-serving assumption that adolescents should have no sexuality and, if so, that it should be policed generated a status offense category for girls, making them the "little bitches" of *parens patriae*. In all historical periods children have served adult ends. Sex control laws, if carried too far, have an illusory quality and aim at prohibiting nonexistent harms. The future should include reasonable protection of children's sexual integrity, flexible enough to reflect a variety of life-styles and concepts of sexual expression, without the destruction of the human potential for sexual love by repression in childhood and adolescence.

APPENDIX
Age Of Consent To Sexual Intercourse*

State	1886 Female	1895 Female	1897 M	1897 F
ALABAMA	N.D.	--	--	--
ALASKA	N.D.	16	16	16
ARIZONA	N.D.	18	18	14
ARKANSAS	N.D.	16	17	16
CALIFORNIA	N.D.	14	18	14
COLORADO	10	18	14	18
CONNECTICUT	10	16	14	14
DELAWARE	7	7	18	18
DISTRICT OF COLUMBIA	N.D.	16	14	16
FLORIDA	10	10	14	17
GEORGIA	10	14	17	10
HAWAII	N.D.	N.D.	N.D.	N.D.

State	1886 Female	1895 Female	1897 M	F
IDAHO	N.D.	18	18	14
ILLINOIS	N.D.	14	17	14
INDIANA	N.D.	14	18	14
IOWA	N.D.	13	16	14
KANSAS	10	18	15	18
KENTUCKY	12	12	14	12
LOUISIANA	12	12	14	12
MAINE	10	14	14	14
MARYLAND	10	14	14	14
MASSACHUSETTS	10	16	14	16
MICHIGAN	N.D.	16	18	14
MINNESOTA	10	16	18	14
MISSISSIPPI	12	10	14	16
MISSOURI	N.D.	18	15	14
MONTANA	10	16	18	15
NEBRASKA	N.D.	18	18	16
NEVADA	N.D.	12	18	14
NEW HAMPSHIRE	10	13	14	13
NEW JERSEY	10	16	14	16
NEW MEXICO	10	14	13	14
NEW YORK	10	18	18	18
NORTH CAROLINA	10	10	16	10
NORTH DAKOTA	10	16	18	14
OHIO	N.D.	14	18	14
OKLAHOMA	N.D.	N.D.	18	15
OREGON	N.D.	16	18	14
PENNSYLVANIA	10	16	14	16
RHODE ISLAND	10	16	14	16
SOUTH CAROLINA	10	10	14	10
SOUTH DAKOTA	10	16	18	16
TENNESSEE	10	12	14	16
TEXAS	10	14	16	12
UTAH	N.D.	13	14	13
VERMONT	N.D.	14	14	14
VIRGINIA	N.D.	12	14	12
WASHINGTON	N.D.	16	21	16
WEST VIRGINIA	12	12	14	14
WISCONSIN	10	14	18	12
WYOMING	10	18	18	18

*Data from W. Bliss, *The Encyclopedia of Social Reform*, New York: Funk and Wagnell, 1897, p. 10-11.

D. Pivar, *Purity Crusade*, West Port, Connecticut: Greenwood Press, 1973, pp. 141-143.

REFERENCES

1. M. Yudof: The dilemma of children's autonomy. *Policy Analysis,* 2:387-407, 1976.
2. M. Zuckerman: Children's rights: The failure of reform: *Policy Analysis,* 2:384,1976.
3. E. Haeberle: Historical roots of sexual oppression. In H. and J. Gochros: *The Sexually Oppressed:* New York, Association Press, 1977, p. 15.
4. L. deMause: *The History of Childhood.* New York, Psychohistory Press, 1974, pp. 39-73.
5. D. Hunt: *Parents and Children in History.* New York, Basic Books, 1970, p. 165.
6. V. Bullough: *Sexual Variance in Society and History.* New York, John Wiley and Sons, 1976, p. 540.
7. D. Lipton: *The Faces of Crime and Genius.* New York, Barnes, 1970, p. 18.
8. C. Ruggiero: Sexual criminality in early Renaissance. *Journal of Social History,* 8:18-37, 1975.
9. L. Radzinowicz: *History of English Criminal Law,* Vol. 1. New York, Macmillan, 1948, pp. 631-632.
10. P. Aries: *Centuries of Childhood.* New York, Vantage, 1962, p. 109.
11. D. West: Thoughts on sex law reforms. In R. Hood: *Crime, Criminology and Public Policy.* New York, Free Press, 1974, p. 469-488.
12. M. Rugoff: *Prudery and Passion.* New York, Putnam, 1971, pp. 300-320.
13. A. Moll: *The Sexual Life of the Child.* New York, Macmillan, 1913, p. 224.
14. A. Butler: *Portrait of Josephine Butler.* London, Faber and Faber, 1954, pp. 137-141.
15. M. Mawby: Social action and crime theory: Josephine Butler. *Howard Journal of Penology,* 14:30-42, 1975.
16. M. Pearson: *The 5 Pound Virgins.* New York, Saturday Review Press, 1972.
17. A. Gigeroff: *Sexual Deviation in the Criminal Law.* Toronto, University of Toronto Press, 1968, pp. 52-82.
18. D. Pivar:*Purity Crusade, Sexual Morality and Social Control, 1868-1900* Westport, Cn, Greenwood, 1973.
19. A. Comfort: *The Anxiety Makers.* London, Nelson, 1967, pp. 69-113.
20. J. and R. Haller: *The Physician and Sexuality in Victorian America.* Urbana, University of Illinois Press, 1974.
21. R. Newman: Masturbation, madness and the modern concept of childhood and adolescence. *Journal of Social History,* 8:6-7, 1975.
22. R. Spitz: Authority and masturbation. *Yearbook of Psychoanalysis,* 9:110-125, 1953.
23. H. Engelhardt: The disease of masturbation: values and concepts. *Bulletin of the History of Medicine,* 48:234-248, 1974
24. A. Holt: *Diseases of Infancy and Childhood.* New York, 1936.
25. A. Platt: *The Child Saviors.* Chicago, University of Chicago Press, 1969.
26. J. Gillis: *Youth and History.* New York, Academic Press, 1974. pp. 133-184.

27. J. Kett: Adolescence and youth in 19th century America. *Journal of Interdisciplinary History, 2*:283-298, 1971.

28. R. Mennel: *Thorns and Thistles: Juvenile Delinquency in the U.S., 1825-1940*. Hanover, N.H., University Press of New England, 1973, p. 71 and 99.

29. G. Barker-Benfield: Sexual Surgery. In *The Horrors of the Half Known Life*. New York, Harper and Row, 1976, pp. 120-134.

30. L. Kanowitz: Law and the single girl. *St. Louis University Law Journal, 11*:672-686, 1967.

31. Sexual Law Reform Society: *Law in Relation to Sexual Behavior*. London, SLRS, 1974.

32. Policy Statement: Jurisdiction over status offenses should be removed from the juvenile court. *Crime and Delinquency, 21*:97-99, 1975.

33. Note: Ungovernability: The unjustified jurisdiction. *Yale Law Journal, 83*:1382-1409, 1974.

34. A. Friedman et al.: *Therapy with Families of Sexually Acting Out Girls*. New York, Springer, 1971, pp. 1-20.

35. People v. Ratz, 115 Cal. 132, 46 Pac., 915 (1896).

36. G. Mueller: *Legal Regulation of Sexual Conduct*, New York, Oceana, 1961, p. 16.

37. F. Furstenberg: *Unplanned Parenthood*. New York, Free Press, 1976. He reports 50 percent of a large sample of girls were sexually active by 15th or 16th birthday (p. 40-42)

38. R. Sorenson:*Adolescent Sexuality in Contemporary America*. New York, World, 1973. Sorenson reports 13 percent of all sexually active teenagers started at age twelve or younger (p. 214)

39. M. Zelnick and J. Kanter: Sexuality and contraceptive experiences of young unmarried women in U.S., 1976 and 1971. *Family Planning Perspectives, 9*:55-73, 1977.

40. K. Wooden: *Weeping in the Playtime of Others*. New York, McGraw-Hill, 1976, p. 119.

41. 138 Cal. 467, 71 Pac. 564 (1903).

42. People v. Curiale, 137 Cal. 534, 538 70 Pac. 468, 470 (1902)

43. The present law in Denmark, Belgium, Norway, and Sweden allows for punishment of female seducers of boys; see, *English studies in Criminal Science*, Vol. 9. London, Macmillan, 1957, Part 6.

44. S. Benefield et. al.: *The Sex Code of California*. Sansalito, Ca, Graphic Arts, 1973.

45. People v. Webb, 158 Cal. 2v. 537 (1958).

46. 145 Cal. App. 2d. 473, 302 P.2d. 603 (1966).

47. L. Schultz: *Kiddie Porn: A Social Policy Analysis*. Morgantown, West Virginia University, School of Social Work, 1977.

48. B. Fraser: A pragmatic alternative to current legislative approaches to child abuse. *American Criminal Law Review, 12*:103-144, 1974.

49. R. Lloyd: *For Love or Money*. New York, Vanguard, 1976.
50. K. Freund et al.: The female child as surrogate object. *Archives of Sexual Behavior*, 2:119-132, 1972.
51. C.B.S. T.V.: "Kiddie Porn." *60 Minutes*, 1977.

Chapter 2

SEXUAL VICTIMIZATION OF CHILDREN: AN URBAN MENTAL HEALTH CENTER SURVEY*

CAROLYN SWIFT

Children have been sexually exploited from ancient times through the present century (DeMause, 1974). The phenomenon has not been systematically studied, however. Scientific literature on the subject is extremely limited. The scant data available—mostly surveys and anecdotal accounts—are open to the criticisms of memory deficit and subjective distortion inherent in retrospective studies. Disagreement over the definition of sexual abuse, methodological problems involved in observing and measuring private events, and societal taboos complicate scientific attempts to explore the subject. Authorities differ as to whether sexual abuse of children should be regarded as child abuse. Walters disagrees with the classification of sexual abuse as physical abuse on the reporting form of the Children's Division of the American Humane Association. According to him sexual abuse is not physical abuse, "and to view it as such only confuses our understanding of both phenomena" (Walters, 1975). Gil defines child abuse as "nonaccidental physical attack or physical injury, including minimal as well as fatal injury, inflicted upon children by persons caring for them . . . 'Sexual attack', however, has been excluded from the definition provided it does not involve other physical attack, because perpetrators of sexual attacks are assumed to have motivations different from perpetrators of non-sexual physical abuse" (Gil, 1968). Even if one accepts the position that sexual abuse of children does not constitute child abuse, it is clear that the two types of behavior are

*Reprinted by permission from *Victimology: An International Journal*, Vol. 2 (1977) No. 2, Pp. 322-326 © 1977 Visage Press Inc. All rights reserved.

correlated. DeFrancis (1971) found that emotional neglect existed in 79 percent of families in which the children suffered sexual abuse, with physical abuse in 11 percent of these cases. The high rate of emotional neglect may account in part for the predominance in the literature of the theme of cooperation and/or seduction on the part of the child, and the related finding that few children defined as sexually victimized appear to suffer damaging or long-lasting effects from the experience (Bender and Grugett, 1952; Gagnon, 1970; Burton, 1968; Walters, 1975). Burton (1968) demonstrated in an empirical study using a control group that sexually victimized children show significantly more affection-seeking behavior, supporting the hypothesis that affectional needs make these children more vulnerable to victimization.

No national statistics documenting the sexual abuse of children exist. Not all states track sexual child abuse and those that do often include categories of sexual victimization not comparable to those of other states (such as "exposed to immoral, unstable behavior"). Available data are usually based on samples of female children—or are not retrievable by sex. Female children indisputedly constitute a major population at risk for sexual exploitation. The fact that young males are also at substantial risk for sexual exploitation is generally ignored by social scientists as well as the public. Prevention and treatment programs continue to be targeted to female children. Gagnon (1970) estimates that 500,000 female children from four to thirteen are sexually victimized annually—20-25 percent of middle class children and 33-40 percent of children raised in lower class environments. A five-month study in California in 1965-66 showed sexual abuse cases constituted 14 percent of reports of child abuse during that period (Helfer and Kempe, 1968). DeFrancis (1965) estimated between 3,000 and 4,000 cases of sexual abuse per year in New York City. While estimates of sexual abuse of female children are scattered and incomplete, those for male children are even less well documented. Lloyd (1976) estimates there are a minimum of 300,000 boy prostitutes in the United States. Differences in samples and definitions of sexual abuse, as well as the disparity of unknown proportion between reported and actual incidence, make generalizations hazardous.

Several studies provide evidence that the incidence of sexual victimization of male children may approach—perhaps equal or surpass—that of female children when differential reporting and society's double standard toward nudity are taken into account. A classic study conducted in 1937 by Bender and Blau used as subjects 16 "unselected successive admissions of prepuberty children who were admitted for observation and recommendation to the children's ward of the psychiatric division of Bellevue Hospital, following sexual relations with adults" (p. 50). Of the 16 admissions, five or approximately one-third were boys. There appears to have been little attempt to follow with appropriate research the possibility suggested by this early study that a substantial proportion of sexual victims are young males. Landis (1956), in a survey of 1,800 college students, found that roughly one-third—30 percent of the males and 35 percent of the females—reported at least one childhood experience with a sexual deviate. Of these victims, 40 percent of the males and 35.5 percent of the females reported three or more such experiences. Over 80 percent of the experiences reported by males involved homosexual advances (compared with 1.5 percent for females). The most frequent experiences reported by females were exposure to exhibitionism (54.8 percent) and sexual fondling (26.9 percent). Males reported these two categories at much lower rates (4.7 percent and .4 percent, respectively). The discrepancy between the frequency of victimization of males and females by exhibitionists appears to be an artifact resulting from society's double standard toward male and female nudity. Males are not assumed to be harmed by exposure to nudity. If exhibitionism were removed from the list of "deviate" experiences reported in Landis' survey, reports of sexual victimization of male children would equal or surpass those of female children. Walters (1975) found in a survey of the prepubertal sexual experience of 412 college students (both males and females) that 38 percent reported receiving sexual signals from adults—21 percent reported receiving verbal signals, and 17 percent reported physical contact. Problems of definition in both surveys limit the generalizability of the results—what appears to be a "sexual signal" or "homosexual approach" to one child may not be so interpreted by another. However, the fact that a third of the subjects in both surveys reported incidents of childhood sexual victimization provides a rough estimate for the general population.

In 1975 the author conducted a survey among 30 clinicians (psychologists, psychiatrists and social workers) at a midwestern mental health center to determine the incidence of child sexual abuse as reflected in caseloads over a twelve month period. For the purposes of the survey sexual abuse was defined as "rape, forced oral or anal intercourse; or penetration of the oral, vaginal or anal orifices with an object; molestation." Clinicians were instructed to "think back over your caseload for the last year to remember any case in which the client mentioned sexual abuse of a minor, whether or not the abuse was a central problem in the case." By definition, all of the acts reported involved physical sexual abuse. Although clinicians were also asked to note reports of acts of exhibitionism, none were reported. The 20 clinicians who returned the survey reported a total of 74 cases of child sexual abuse in four categories: children or adolescents in treatment reporting a history of sexual victimization; adults in treatment reporting sexual abuse (by other persons) of their children; adults in treatment reporting that they were themselves sexually abused as children; and adults in treatment reporting that they had committed acts of sexual abuse against children. Two of the 20 clinicians reported no cases of sexual abuse against children. Two of the 20 clinicians reported no cases in any of the categories. The respondents reported treating 21 minors (7 males, 14 females) with a history of sexual victimization. While most of these clients are currently in late adolescence, the abuse reportedly occurred earlier: in early childhood and early adolescence for the girls and in early adolescence (11-14) for the boys. (These data corroborate Landis' findings concerning the different ages at which male and female children are sexually abused—early childhood for girls, early adolescence for boys.) The abuser was the father, stepfather, or foster father in 52 percent of the cases. Father-son incest accounted for one case of the male abuse and mother-son incest was reported once. It is notable that a third of the cases reported involve male children as victims.

The survey showed five adults in treatment who reported

sexual abuse of their children by others. All five adults were female, and the sexual abuse reported involved their female children. In three cases the reported abuser was the father. The responding clinicians listed a total of 36 adult clients who reported having been sexually abused as children (7 males, 29 females). Most of these clients, now between 26 and 35 years of age, report the abuse occurred when they were in early adolescence. The abuser was the father or stepfather in 60 percent of the cases. Over half of the cases of male victimization involved incest—two between father and son and two between brothers. The other cases involved homosexual attacks by strangers—in jail, in a boy scout camp, and on the street. The clinicians reported a caseload of 12 males who admitted having committed acts of sexual abuse against children (two male and twelve female victims). One male child was reportedly victimized by his grandfather, the other by a neighbor. Of the twelve cases of female victimization, seven of the abusers were the fathers of the victim. The data from this survey confirm two consistent findings in the literature on sexual child abuse: the abusers are almost always male, and in over half of the cases they are related to the child, usually the father. The survey also supports a conclusion at odds with popular consensus: young males are at substantial risk for sexual victimization. The survey showed young males constituted 33 percent of the child caseload reporting sexual abuse, 19 percent of the adult caseload reporting sexual abuse as children, and 16 percent of the victims of self-confessed abusers seen in treatment at the mental health center. These figures are probably underestimates, given the pressures operating in our society to suppress revelations of behavior subjected to social censure, such as incest, homosexuality, and child abuse.

One of the cultural handicaps that contributes to the blind spots professionals share with the general public in this field is the taboo attached to the observation and reporting of sexual behavior. The more deviant the behavior the greater the taboo. The accepted norm of sexual behavior is heterosexual genital intercourse between married adults. Other heterosexual acts between consenting adults are proscribed in many states regardless of the marital status of the parties involved. Homosexual acts between consenting adults are likewise prohibited in many states. While the commission of sexual intercourse with a child is regarded as a deviant act, there appears to be degrees of deviance, with concomitant degrees of taboo, within the area of sexual abuse of children as well as adults. Homosexual attacks of children carry a double stigma since they violate the heterosexual norm as well as the prohibition of the use of a child as a sexual partner. There is evidence that boys report their sexual experiences with deviates less frequently than girls. In Landis' survey only 16.5 percent of the victimized boys reported the incident to their parents compared with 43 percent of the victimized girls. Differential preparation of sons and daughters around the issue of sexual victimization may account in part for the discrepancy in reporting: only 26.8 percent of the boys in Landis' survey reported parental attempts to prepare them to deal with such an experience, compared with 44.1 percent of the girls.

The taboos surrounding sexual behavior, particularly deviant behavior, discourage children from reporting sexual victimization out of fear of punishment, shame, or because they pick up the implicit message that such things are not to be talked about. Parents and helping professionals are frequently uncomfortable in dealing with descriptions of explicit sexual behavior from children (Chaneles, 1967). In their uncertainty as to how to advise the child their horror may lead them to discount the child's veracity or suppress discussion or reference to the event. The silence of 84 percent of the victimized boys in Landis' study testifies to the efficacy of the taboo attached to the doubly stigmatized act of homosexual attack of a child. The importance of establishing empirically the incidence of sexual abuse of young males and the reporting of these events lies in the possibility that it is this group that constitutes a high risk for committing sexual offenses later in life. The phenomenon of the repetitive cycle of child abuse is a familiar theme in the literature. If further research corroborates the hypothesis that sexually victimized boys grow up to be sexual abusers, programs directed to the early identification and treatment of victimized boys would, hopefully, result in the prevention of sexual offenses by this population in later life.

REFERENCES

Bender, Lauretta and Blau, Abraham. 1937. "The Reaction of Children to Sexual Relations with Adults." *American Journal of Orthopsychiatry*, Vol. 7 (October), pp. 500-518.

Bender, Lauretta and Grugett, A. 1952. "A Follow up Report on Children Having Atypical Sexual Experience." *American Journal of Orthopsychiatry*, Vol 22.

Burton, Lindy. 1968. *Vulnerable Children*. New York: Schocken Books.

Chaneles, Sol. 1967. "Family Structure of Child Sex Victims." American Humane Association Publication: Implications for Casework.

DeFrancis, Vincent. 1971. "Protecting the Child Victim of Sex Crime Committed by Adults." Federal Probation, September, pp. 15-20.

DeMause, Lloyd, ed. 1974. *The History of Childhood*. New York: The Psychohistory Press.

Gagnon, John H. 1970. "Female Child Victims of Sex Offenses." In *Studies in Human Sexual Behavior: The American Scene*, Ailon Shiloh, ed. Springfield, Illinois: Chas. C Thomas, pp. 398-419.

Gil, David G. 1968. "California Pilot Study." In *The Battered Child*, Helfer, Ray E. and Kempe, Henry C., eds., University of Chicago Press, pp. 216-225.

Helfer, Ray E. and Kempe, Henry C., eds., 1968. *The Battered Child*, University of Chicago Press.

Landis, Judson T. 1956. "Experiences of 500 Children with Adult Sexual Deviation." *Psychiatric Quarterly Supplement*, Vol. 30, pp. 91-109.

Lloyd, Robin. 1976. *For Money or Love: Boy Prostitution in America*. New York: Vanguard Press, Inc.

Walters, David R. 1975. *Physical and Sexual Abuse of Children Causes and Treatment*. Indiana University Press.

Chapter 3

SEXUAL MOLESTATION OF CHILDREN: THE LAST FRONTIER IN CHILD ABUSE*

Suzanne M. Sgroi

CASE NO. 1: A Florida newspaper tersely reported to its readers early in 1975 that the city's youngest rape victim to date was only two months old at the time of the sexual assault. No other comment was offered.

CASE NO. 2: Two and one-half-year-old Jerry was admitted to the hospital because he cried when he passed urine and his mother noticed a discharge of pus from his penis. When his problem proved to be an acute gonorrhea infection, public health authorities investigated his home and found that Jerry's mother, father and an older sibling were all infected. His doctor was persuaded that a non-sexual mode of transmission had occurred because the family members were reported to share the same bed frequently. All of the family members were treated for infection simultaneously. Jerry's parents were counseled to avoid allowing their children to sleep in "contaminated sheets," and the case was closed.

An epilogue, however, was written several months later when an alert nursery school teacher noted that Judy, Jerry's 4-year-old sister, consistently refused to take her turn riding a rocking horse during playtime. When asked why, she replied "It hurts." A careful examination by the school's pediatrician that same day revealed the presence of sperm in Judy's vagina. An immediate joint police-Protective Services investigation of the family revealed that Jerry's and Judy's father had a long history of previous incidents of child-molesting although none had ever been proved. Their mother admitted she was aware that both

*From *Children Today*, 18-21, 44, May-June 1975.

25

children had been sexually assaulted by their father on numerous occasions.

CASE NO. 3: Stephanie, at age 17 months, was brought to a hospital emergency room by her mother who had noticed blood in the baby's diaper after she returned home from work. On examination, the child was found to have a small anal fissure that bled freely when touched. There was no previous history of abnormality or trauma and the mother was reassured that the fissure could be easily corrected surgically if it did not heal by itself. Several weeks later, Stephanie was found dead in her crib— a victim of asphyxiation. An autopsy revealed the presence of semen in her mouth and throat. When apprehended, the baby-sitter, a 19-year-old boy, freely admitted to sexual abuse of the child but protested "I didn't mean to kill her!"

Any member of the "helping professions" who is searching for an effective method to make himself unpopular with his peer group can probably achieve that goal by frequent involvement in cases such as those described above. The professional who becomes sufficiently concerned and knowledgeable about sexual abuse of children to be consistently alert to the possibility that sexual molestation *may* have occurred will often face a spectrum of reactions from his colleagues that range from incredulity to frank hostility. For although the pioneering efforts of many distinguished professionals and dedicated lay people over the past decade have made child abuse a national issue, the problem of sexual molestation of children remains a taboo topic in many areas.

This is not to argue that the problem of child abuse has been "solved" anywhere in the United States. It is, however, fair to assert that sexual abuse of children is the last remaining component of the maltreatment syndrome in children that has yet to be faced head-on. In medical parlance, child molestation is the least popular diagnosis. In the vernacular, it is not nearly so "in" a topic as child battering or neglect. Combatting these forms of maltreatment is publicly applauded and encouraged. But somehow, protecting children against sex crimes has received far less community sanction. It seems to be "too dirty," "too Freudian" or perhaps "too close to home." Thus one who becomes concerned with this particular aspect of child protection must be prepared to cope with a very high degree of resistance, innuendo and even harassment from some, as well as indifference from others. The pressure from one's peer group as well as the community to ignore, minimize or cover up the situation may be extreme.

Incidence of Molestation

No one knows the true incidence of child molestation in the United States today. Vincent DeFrancis, director of the Children's Division of the American Humane Association, conducted a comprehensive 3-year study of child molestation in New York City that was reported in 1969.[1] His estimate of approximately 3,000 cases each year in New York City alone is probably conservative. Considering the widespread reluctance to recognize and report this condition, it must be assumed that the reported incidents represent a small fraction of the cases.

Nevertheless, the reporting of suspected sexual abuse of children is encompassed in the child abuse reporting statutes of many states. Recent strengthening of these statutes and the establishment of child abuse hotlines has markedly increased the reporting of all forms of child maltreatment. In Connecticut, for example, passage of an expanded child abuse reporting law (P.A. 73-205, effective October 1, 1973), which involves a $500 fine for mandated reporters who fail to report suspected child abuse, resulted in 1,957 reported cases in fiscal year 1974—an increase of *nearly 200 percent* over the preceding fiscal year. A breakdown of the total by reporting source is shown in Table 3-I.

The opening of the Care-Line, a 24-hour statewide toll-free child abuse prevention and information line, probably had a significant impact since it facilitated the reporting process for many professionals and private citizens who called to express concern about children. The Connecticut Child Welfare Association (CCWA), a private statewide citizens' organization which operates the Care-Line, has also conducted a continuing education effort aimed at both the general public and the professional groups who have been required to report cases of suspected child abuse since 1971. Connecticut's Municipal Police Training Council has cooperated by incorporating lectures on child abuse detection and reporting into their mandatory training program for all newly-hired police officers in 166 of the state's 169 towns. These child abuse training sessions were initiated in 1972 as part of the CCWA Child Advocacy Project and have been conducted by Association staff at 6-week intervals ever since. In October 1973 the two groups jointly sponsored and taught three one-day seminars on child abuse which were attended by higher ranking police officers from all over the state. It is therefore not surprising that the percentage of reports of suspected child abuse by police officers increased markedly in F.Y. 1974, while reports by hospitals decreased proportionately and those by private physicians remained at the same low level—five percent.

Table 3-I
TOTAL NUMBER OF CHILDREN REPORTED AS SUSPECTED ABUSED IN CONNECTICUT*

	Physicians	Hospitals	Police	Schools	Social Workers	CCWA Care-Line	Others	Total
F.Y. 1973 number	37	205	107	122	65	†	133	669
percent	5.5%	30.2%	16%	18.2%	9.8%	†	19.9%	100%
F.Y. 1974 number	98	396	456	401	327	104	175	1957
percent	5%	20.3%	23.3%	20.5%	16.7%	5.3%	8.9%	100%

*Connecticut State Welfare Department statistics.
†A statewide toll-free child abuse hotline has been operated by the Connecticut Child Welfare Association, a private citizen's organization, since October 1, 1973.

It is noteworthy that during this same reporting period, the total number of reports of suspected sexual abuse of children in Connecticut increased, while the proportion of such reports to total child abuse reporting statistics declined slightly. Table 3-II shows a breakdown of sexual abuse by type of report.

Table 3-II
REPORTS OF SUSPECTED SEXUAL ABUSE OF CHILDREN IN CONNECTICUT*

	Incest & Rape	Sexual Moles- tation	Venereal Disease	Total Sexual Abuse	Total Cases of Suspected Child Abuse	% Sexual Abuse
F.Y. 1973	19	57	†	76	669	11.4%
F.Y. 1974	47	108	17	172	1957	8.8%

*Connecticut State Welfare Department statistics
†Acquired venereal disease in children under age 13 years did not become reportable as suspected child abuse until fiscal year 1974 (October 1, 1973).

In fiscal years 1973 and 1974 in Connecticut, the relationship of the perpetrator to the child in all cases of suspected abuse was that of a parent or a parent-substitute in 80 percent of the cases. This complements DeFrancis' finding that parents were involved in the sexual molestation of children in 72 percent of the cases studied—either by perpetration of the offense (25 percent) or else by acts of omission or commission.[2] The most frequently named perpetrator in cases of sexual abuse is the father or a male relative or boyfriend—virtually always someone who has ready access to the child in his or her home. Ages of victims may range from early infancy (one to two months) all the way to 17 or 18 years.

Recognizing Sexual Abuse

Why is sexual molestation of children the last frontier in child abuse? And what are the major obstacles to identifying the sexually abused child?

In practical terms, the answers are lack of recognition of the phenomenon, failure to obtain adequate medical corroboration of the event, and reluctance to report. If one accepts the premise that it is impossible to protect the child victim of sexual molestation unless we know that he exists, these obstacles take on major importance. Each is rooted in ignorance and taboo and must be considered accordingly.

Recognition of sexual molestation in a child is entirely dependent on the individual's inherent willingness to entertain the possibility that the condition may exist. Unfortunately, willingness to consider the diagnosis of suspected child sexual molestation frequently seems to vary in inverse proportion to the individual's level of training. That is, the more advanced the training of some, the less willing they are to suspect molestation.

The lack of preparation and willingness of many physicians to assist patients with sexual problems in general has often been noted. When the patient is a child, these deficiencies are extremely serious.

If the victim of alleged sexual assault is a child, a complete physical examination with careful attention to any other signs of physical abuse or neglect must accompany the routinized perineal examination and laboratory tests. The examination is not complete unless the child is carefully scrutinized for evidence of oral and/or anal penetration as well as genital sexual contact. This includes inspection for trauma as well as laboratory tests for the presence of semen and venereal disease.

Unfortunately, all too few health professionals are trained to look for or to recognize the signs of rectal and urogenital gonorrhea infections in young children. This not only requires a high index of suspicion but again an inherent willingness to entertain the diagnosis of acquired venereal disease in a child. With the exception of congenital syphilis and gonococcal eye infection in newborns, the presence of a gonorrhea or syphilis infection in a child makes it imperative that sexual molestation be suspected unless or until it is ruled out by a careful joint medical and protective services investigation. The U.S. Public Health Service, which operates the National Communicable Disease Center in Atlanta, Georgia, has recently cautioned that "with gonococcal infection in children, the possibility of child abuse must be considered!"[3]

Medical Corroboration of Abuse

The next major obstacle to identifying and helping the child victim of sexual abuse is failure to obtain immediate medical corroboration of the assault. This occurs most frequently on the grounds that physical examination of the child will aggravate and intensify the psychological trauma that may already have been experienced. However, this attitude has little basis in fact and may be detrimental in the extreme to the future protection of the child. A gentle and thorough examination, as outlined above, conducted by a knowledgeable examiner, will be well tolerated by most children. The experience not only can be non-threatening but it may also be reassuring and welcomed by a child victim who is old enough to worry that he or she may have been harmed by the assault. For example, the examiner may find numerous opportunities to assure the child that all is well, that no harm has occurred or else that any injury incurred can be alleviated.

It is well to avoid repeated questioning of the child about circumstances relating to the incident of sexual abuse at any time. Such questioning is particularly to be avoided during the physical examination. Since repeated examinations may indeed be traumatic, the first should be comprehensive enough to preclude the necessity for further examinations if the child's condition does not require them.

Preventing a recurrence of sexual abuse should be a twin therapeutic goal along with preventing and alleviating any psychological damage incurred by the sexually molested child. Each of these goals should have equal priority. The therapist who counsels against a comprehensive and compassionate examination of the child in a case of suspected sexual assault (including, of course, a physical examination) effectively circumvents an adequate Protective Services investigation of the case. It is a known fact that judicial proceedings against child molesters virtually require that medical evidence of sexual assault be presented. Without such evidence, it is practically impossible to protect the child against repeated sexual assault by preventing or monitoring access of the child-molesting adult to the victim, especially in the intra-family situation.

The frequently recommended alternative of removing the child temporarily or permanently from the "at risk" situation by transferring custody from his or her parents to the state has the disadvantage of risking serious damage to the child by the act of premature separation from the "psychological parent." Thus the totality of risks must be carefully weighed in selecting what the authors of *Beyond the Best Interest of the Child* term "the least detrimental alternative."[4]

Regardless of the consequences, it would be unusual in any state for a child to be removed permanently from his parents to protect him from sexual abuse if corroborating medical evidence were not presented to verify that sexual molestation of that child had already occurred within the family. To put it another way, the future protection of a child victim of sexual assault is virtually impossible without a carefully recorded examination by a knowledgeable physician.

Reporting Sexual Abuse

Failure to report to the statutory authority is the last major obstacle to identifying the sexually abused child. Sexual abuse of a minor is a reportable condition in every state in the United States. Such a report is the triggering mechanism for a Protective Services investigation of the child and his family—thereby providing a conduit for professional help and community resources to strengthen and improve the home situation or, occasionally, to remove a child from an untenably dangerous environment. Nevertheless, sexual abuse of children is grossly underreported.

It is unconscionable that any member of the "helping professions" would violate the law as well as withhold potential help from the child victim by failure to report suspected sexual abuse. In most areas it is particularly inappropriate to withhold reports to the statutory authority on the grounds that more effective therapy for delicate internal family matters can be provided surreptitiously by a private agency or private practitioner. Since the success of the private agency's efforts to monitor the home situation for indications of recurrent abuse is directly dependent upon the family's voluntary compliance (which may cease at any time), such reasoning is fallacious. A far more appropriate course for the private help source who discovers the abuse is to report immediately and request to "service" the case in cooperation with the statutory authority. In most cases, cooperation with the frequently superior resources of the private source of help will be eagerly welcomed by the public agency. The result: a higher level of service available to the family as well as increased protection for the child.

For too long health professionals have skirted the issue of reporting suspected sexual molestation when an unmistakable diagnosis of acquired venereal disease has been made in a child. We have been content to do contact investigation within the family circle and to treat other family members—parents, aunts and uncles, older siblings, etc.—for venereal disease without asking why or how a 6-year-old boy acquired a gonorrheal urethritis or a 3-year-old girl contracted pelvic infection with gonococci. Because of reluctance to entertain the possibility of sexual molestation of a child by an adult, we have often postulated modes of transmission of venereal disease to children within the family circle that were long ago discarded in relation to adults, such as the possibility of transmission via clothing, towels and bedsheets. In view of what we know about the epidemiology of gonorrhea and syphilis in adults, it is absurd to cling to an erroneous double standard when we deal with acquired venereal disease in children. We must assume that these children have had some type of sexual contact, most probably with an adult, and investigate accordingly.

In the past, there has been some concern by public health authorities about violation of confidentiality by sharing a report of venereal disease in a child with the statutory agency mandated to investigate suspected child abuse. Connecticut is the first state in the United States to clarify this issue in its child abuse reporting statute. According to the Connecticut law, all reports of acquired venereal disease in children under 13 years of age must be reported to Protective Services as well as to the State Health Department. In this way a simultaneous Protective Services investigation of the family may, if necessary, initiate steps to protect the child from further sexual molestation while public health authorities do contact investigation and treatment to prevent further transmission of the disease.

Identifying Abused Children

Since we cannot help the sexually abused child and his family unless we know they exist, how then can the major obstacles to identification detailed in this article be overcome? The key role of the physician in obtaining adequate medical corroboration of sexual abuse has not been minimized. Nevertheless, any concerned individual, especially when professionally involved with some aspect of child care, can do much to enhance recognition and reporting of this phenomenon.

First, since this is a phenomenon that thrives and proliferates in darkness, we need to open windows and doors and promote open public discussion of the topic. Increased public awareness is best stimulated by people who care enough to snatch every opportunity to arouse society's consciousness of the child victim of sexual abuse. Only then will the public sanction so vital to identifying and assisting these children be forthcoming.

Instead of wasting time during a crisis situation in helpless frustration with medical personnel who are uncooperative or unknowledgeable in this area, those who are concerned should identify and establish a relationship with reliable sources of medical help in advance. Knowledgeable and receptive physicians and health professionals in the community should be sought out so that ways to improve medical services to child victims of sexual assault can be jointly explored. Emergency rooms or private practitioners who do the most effective and sensitive job should be identified, encouraged and patronized. The services of new demonstration programs in this area should also be identified and sought.

Connecticut has recently received funding from the Children's Bureau, OCD to establish a Child Abuse and Neglect Demonstration Center that will enable a multidisciplinary consortium of agencies to work cooperatively toward diagnosis and treatment of families where child abuse, neglect or sexual molestation is a danger. One of the center's charges will be to delineate a workable range of effective services for child protection. As a last resort, it may be necessary to utilize legal and judicial means to identify and enforce the basic minimum standard of medical services that the sexually abused child is entitled to receive.

Lastly, it behooves every professional who deals with children to be aware that sexual molestation exists, to recognize danger signals—especially in high-risk children—and to be knowledgeable about his or her state's reporting laws and sources of help. Sexual abuse of children is certainly not the problem of any single profession or segment of society. A strong united effort is required to push back the last frontier in child abuse and assist the sexually molested child.

References

[1]*DeFrancis, Vincent.* "Protecting the Child Victim of Sex Crimes Committed by Adults," *Children's Division, American Humane Association, Denver, 1969.*

[2]*Ibid.*

[3]*"Gonorrhea: The Latest Word,"* Emergency Medicine, *Vol 7, No. 2, February 1975, pp. 132-138.*

[4]*Goldstein, Joseph et al.* Beyond the Best Interest of the Child, *Macmillan Publishing Co., Inc., New York, 1973.*

DIAGNOSIS AND TREATMENT

"Sexual abuse, alone with other forms of child abuse, is a reportable condition in most states. However, it presents special problems to. . .professionals because of the difficulties in substantiating the suspected diagnosis. . . Reporting entails the risk of being subpoenaed by the court without the tangible evidence that helps to substantiate a diagnosis in other forms of child abuse."

Dr. B. Herjanic and Dr. R. Wilbois: Journal of the American Medical Association, January 23, 1978.

Chapter 4

DIAGNOSIS AND TREATMENT—
INTRODUCTION

LeRoy G. Schultz

The literature on diagnosis does not indicate that professionals agree on any of the effects of sexual abuse on minors.
Whatever the effect on the minor, it is presumed to be related to
four factors: the amount of physical violence employed in the
sexual encounter, the age difference between the partners or
victim and offender, the type and depth of relationship established between partners or victim and offender, and the number
of sexual acts over time. The sparse literature does not substantiate these four generalizations. We seem to flounder when
elements such as ingratiation, promise, or entreaty, rather than
physical force, are used to gain compliance from the minor, or
when some child victims report enjoying and prolonging the
sexual relationship with adults.

As Germaine Greer put it, "From the child's point of view and
from the commonsense point of view, there is an enormous
difference between intercourse with a willing little girl and the
forcible penetration of the small vagina of a terrified child. One
woman I know enjoyed sex with an uncle all through her
childhood, and never realized that anything was unusual until
she went away to school. What disturbed her then was not what
her uncle had done but the attitude of her teachers and the school
psychiatrist. They assumed that she must have been traumatized
and disgusted and therefore in need of very special help. In order
to capitulate to their expectations, she began to fake symptoms
that she did not feel, until at length she began to feel truly guilty
about not having been guilty. She ended up judging herself very
harshly for this innate lechery."[1]

We simply do not have any criteria to determine how each
minor will react to the sexual event, but it seems clear that some

victim's personality may be plastic and highly adaptive, without indication of trauma.

The effects of sexual victimization as reported in the earlier literature appear a reflection of the historical *zeitgeist* of the time. They have been exaggerated, in part, due to a naivete and misunderstanding of the role of sexuality in the development of minors, an underestimate of the normal child's adoptive capacity, and the use of the medical profession to support morality. Since no more than 5 to 10 percent of sexual abuse involves physical injury, the presumed trauma has to be psychological or social. It may be useful for professionals to assume trauma is absent unless clear evidence contraindicates. Much of the literature is couched in acceptable access, where well-meaning emotional noise masks statistical reality. We seem to artificially create "norms" for minors and then justify departures from them as traumatic. Such fabrication is professionally unethical and possibly damaging to minors involved in sexual behaviors with others. What inappropriate trauma ideology does is to pit the professional (true believer) against the child or his parents who may feel otherwise. The risk is that a type of self-fulfilling prophecy emerges that manages to produce the problem it claims to abhor, but which it, in fact, must have in order to sustain the ideology it is based upon. The problem resists a neat fit to any theory. While data are scanty, the conception of all child victims being sacrificed to adult lust would seem unfounded. Sexual behavior between adult and child or between two minors is neither harmful or harmless always.

Another weakness in trauma theory is its inability to define its limits. The earlier literature dealt with a generation of minors not exposed to television sexuality, sexual books for children, so-called "men's" magazines, the sexual revolution in free verbalization of sexuality among peers and within some families. Some children watch their mother deliver a sibling, an act that earlier would be defined as traumatic for many children (*Newsweek*, May 30, 1977, p. 90). *Trauma* is a word that moved from physical medicine to mental health through the work of Freud.[2] The word *trauma* was originally meant to describe any experience that called up distressing effects and later changed to describe a state of psychic helplessness.[3] Today the word is used loosely, to describe all kinds of events with adjectives like "upsetting" or "shattering." The difficulty for some child victims centers on forcing them to take a short-lived distasteful act (in the child's mind), with few permanent consequences, and to blow it all out of proportion, forcing the child to reorient his ideas to the confused adult interpretation of the event. Compounding the difficulty further, the child is given the heavy responsibility of convicting the offender in a confusing law enforcement process. Since we all are expected to react severely to child-adult sexual encounters, such a reaction is bound to insure the *unlikelihood* of victims escaping the difficulties produced by the definition and interpretation. There is a remarkable void in professional literature on the topic of iatrogenesis, where the helping process is damaging or useless.[4] Needed are professional criteria to determine when the best interests of the child mandate intervention, and when to do nothing. Early learning, unless repeated over time, is no more than a link in the child's developmental chain. It is the "here and now" that has the powerful effect on behavior. It is no longer defensible, if it ever was, to apply diagnostic and treatment models appropriate to those minor victims who are truly traumatized, physically or mentally, to the large majority who are not, thus placing some control on possible iatrogenesis. This is not to be construed as condoning child-adult sexuality, but to put the child's welfare first. No professional wants to create sex dysfunction in children. Another hidden muted finding in the literature is one possibly positive or healthy result of child-adult sexual interactions. Kinsey found in his research on females who experienced child-adult sexuality that such children on reaching adulthood were more responsive sexually than the rest of the population.[5] A similar finding resulted from a study of German sex victims.[6] The fact of positive result is not condoning of such behavior, but highlights the need for open-minded research. To the extent that we put a utilitarian gloss on our disapproval of child-adult sexual encounter, we risk remaining professionally deaf to contradictory psychological evidence.

The following four chapters reflect these realistic aspects, and many more. Helpful guidelines for many aspects of the post-victimization process are provided; they have utility for all practitioners.

REFERENCES

1. G. Greer: Seduction is a four-letter word. New York, John Cushman Associates, Inc., 1975.
2. *The Standard Edition of the Complete Psychological Works of Sigmund Freud*, Vol. 2. London, Hogarth, 1955.
3. *The Standard Edition of the Complete Psychological Works of Sigmund Freud*, Vol. 20. London, Hogarth, 1955.
4. C. Torry: Iatrogenic anguish caused by child psychiatry. *Psychology Today*, :24, March 1977.
5. P. Arnow: An interview with Dr. Wardell Pomeroy. *Multi-Media Resource Guide*, *2(1)*:53, Fall 1977.
6. G. Kirchhoff and C. Thelen: Hidden victimization by sex offenders in Germany. In E. Viano (Ed.): *Victims and Society*. Washington, D.C., Visage, 1976.

———————————— Chapter 5 ————————————

THE SEXUALLY MISUSED CHILD*
RENEE S. T. BRANT, M.D., AND VERONICA B, TISZA, M.D.

This paper, based on a study of pediatric emergency room records and on clinical experience, suggests that sexual misuse of children often goes unrecognized, and that this diagnosis must be considered in all children seen for genital injury, irritation, and infection. It is concluded that sexual misuse is most often a symptom of family dysfunction; preliminary guidelines for case management are offered.

Sexual abuse is a subject laden with strong taboos, which have contributed to the failure of professionals to identify the sexually abused child and have made treatment of the child and family more difficult. While the psychiatric literature contains several important retrospective studies of individuals who experienced sexual trauma as children and subsequently came to psychiatric attention, [2,6] there are few papers about early identification and management of these cases.

In recent years, however, as more cases have come to the attention of professionals, the sexually abused child has been the object of increasing concern. In part, this is due to the inclusion of sexual abuse as a reportable condition in the child abuse reporting statutes of many states.[4] Sensitization of professionals to the problem of child abuse, a social climate that allows for freer communication about sexuality, and the recent focus on the sexually assaulted female have contributed to increasing public and professional awareness of this group of vulnerable children.

Our interest in the sexual abuse of children grew out of our

*From *American Journal of Orthopsychiatry*, 47 (1):80-90, Jan 1977. Copyright © 1977, the American Orthpsychiatric Association, Inc. Reproduced by permission.

work as child psychiatrists in consultation to the emergency room and pediatric gynecology clinic at The Children's Hospital Medical Center in Boston. We were interested in learning about the nature of the cases that were presented to a pediatric hospital, and the mode of presentation. We began with a retrospective study of the emergency room log covering a one-year period from March 1, 1973 to March 1, 1974. We searched for chief complaints or diagnoses that might lead one to suspect that a child had been sexually abused. We reviewed the records of patients presenting chief complaints of molestation, rape, incest, sexual abuse, dysuria, and genital irritation, trauma or infection, as well as cases of adolescent pregnancy. Out of approximately 56,000 emergency room visits during that year, 52 cases of possible sexual abuse were found. Fewer than five had been reported to the child abuse team in the hospital. According to the records, in at least 25 percent of the cases, professionals had not considered the diagnosis of sexual abuse, although retrospectively we considered this diagnosis possible. Emergency examination often failed to include relevant social, family, and behavioral data that would be important in making a diagnosis. These preliminary findings convinced us of the need to better understand the mode of presentation of these cases and to sensitize and educate hospital personnel in order to facilitate case recognition and management.

In pursuing our study, we became aware of limitations inherent in the use of the term "sexual abuse" to describe the phenomenon we were studying. The term derives from a legal rather than a mental health perspective, and tends to make one view cases in terms of adult "abusers" and child victims. In the course of our work we discovered that children are not always the passive victims of adults. Rather, sexual abuse is usually a manifestation of family pathology, and several family members as well as the child as usually active in perpetuating the "abuse." From a mental health perspective, we feel the term "sexual misuse" is preferable; it is less pejorative and does not compel one to think only in terms of victims and abusers. We see sexual misuse of a child as a manifestation of family dysfunction in which all to some extent suffer. In this paper "sexual misuse" means exposure of a child to sexual stimulation inappropriate for the child's age, level of psychosexual development, and role in the family. We use the appearance of physical or behavioral symptoms in the child and evidence of family dysfunction as criteria for determining the inappropriateness of the stimulation, and recognize that that which is "inappropriate" may vary according to the family and ethnic or sociocultural context.

The case material that follows is drawn from emergency room and gynecology clinic cases in which we have acted as consultants. Through this material we hope to illustrate various modes of presentation of cases of sexual misuse and to give some idea of the spectrum of cases appearing in a pediatric setting. We will also discuss high risk situations in which children appear to be especially vulnerable to sexual misuse.

Family Aspects

Our work with sexually misused children, as well as the work of others, indicates that sexual misuse in most cases is a reflection of family pathology. Studies of sexual abuse universally indicate that the person responsible for misusing the child is frequently known to the child. DeFrancis's New York study[4] found that the parent or parent-substitute was involved in 72 percent of the cases studied, either by perpetration of the misuse (25 percent) or by acts of omission.[4] Most studies point to the father, a male relative, or a boyfriend of the mother as the most frequent perpetrator of the abuse. Mothers are often unconsciously, if not consciously, aware of the misuse and contribute to its perpetuation through denial, passivity, and failure to provide adequate protection for the child. While most attention is directed toward the male "abuser" and the female child victim, there are instances in which the mother overstimulates a male child, especially when the father is absent from the family. Cases in which children are misused by adults of the same sex are also not uncommon. Finally, sexual misuse may be a consequence of mutual genital masturbation or sexual play among deprived children in disorganized and poorly supervised home settings. Even when children are separated from their family of origin and are placed in foster care, the family dynamics may be recreated and may continue to play an important role.

The importance of the family dynamics is obvious in most of the following case material. A family-oriented approach to case recognition is mandatory. In addition to examining the child, the examiner must be cognizant of parental anxiety and behavior, as well as parent-child interaction. These observations are important in assessing whether a child is being misused within the family.

Modes of Presentation

The first step in the recognition of cases of sexual misuse is willingness to entertain the possibility that the situation may exist. Social and cultural taboos and values, personal anxiety, and ignorance may contribute to failure to recognize these cases in emergency settings. It is often particularly difficult for a mental health or medical worker to acknowledge that sexual misuse may occur in middle-class and upper-class families. Professionals must be aware of their anxieties, which may interfere with their ability to recognize such cases. They must also be aware of the various ways in which these cases may be presented to medical settings.

Sometimes parents or children will state "molestation" or "rape" as a chief complaint. At times the chief complaint appears appropriate and is borne out by examination. At other times the complaint may be more a reflection of fantasy and anxiety than of reality. Even in such cases one must be concerned, for it is possible that preventive work may keep the fantasy from becoming a reality. There are some cases in which the examiner may never be certain about what in reality did happen; these require active outreach and close follow-up.

Case 1

The psychiatrist was asked to see a four-year-old girl who was brought to the emergency room by her anxious parents. The child was apparently playing with a friend when a strange man walked up to them and asked directions to a nearby apartment. The four-year-old was left alone with the man for a minute or two by her friend, who returned subsequently. The four-year-old ran home to her parents. Upon hearing of the incident, they immediately brought her to the emergency room, fearful that she had been molested. Medical and psychiatric examination of the child gave no evidence of sexual misuse. She was functioning well at school and at home. In follow-up visits with the parents, the psychiatrist discovered that both the father's sister and the mother of the child had been subjected to sexual misuse as children.

Chief complaints cannot always be taken at face value. Sometimes a parent will project onto the child anxieties that actually reflect unresolved conflicts from the parent's past. The examiner must be sensitive to the emotional concerns of parent and child and must search for the source of the anxiety that gives rise to the chief complaint.

The age of a child may be important in determining how a case is presented. Infants may be subjected to innappropriate stimulation. At times this may take the form of excessive attention to and manipulation of the baby's genitals. Reddened or traumatized genitalia in infants should lead the examiner to consider whether the child is being inappropriately stimulated. Infants may respond to overstimulation with more generalized symptoms, including eating and sleeping disturbances and altered activity level.

Toddlers and school-age children have difficulty verbalizing fears and concerns. They are likely, however, to present physical and behavioral signs and symptoms. Physical complaints may range from stomachache to dysuria, and symptoms of increased fearfulness, insomnia, and attentional problems. The presence of genital irritation, laceration, abrasion, bleeding, discharge, or infection should lead the examiner to include sexual misuse in the differential diagnosis. Frequently the history accompanying a case of genital injury indicated that the child fell in the bathtub or suffered some accidental trauma; in cases of vulvar irritation it is not unusual for the examiner to assume, sometimes too readily, that bubble bath is the cause. While such histories and explanations may be true, it is important to entertain the possibilty that the child has been misused. History-taking must be tactful, with some focus on the child's general behavior and adaptation within the family and at school. As stated previously, observing parental behavior and noting the quality of parent-child interaction are equally important. Follow-up study in a nonthreatening setting is especially significant in cases that leave the experienced examiner with an uneasy feeling regarding the etiology of physical signs and symptoms.

Venereal disease in children is being reported with increasing frequency and must be considered in any child presenting genital irritation, discharge, or infection. In Maryland, a family-centered approach was used to screen for new cases of gonorrhea. Family members of index cases were screened. Sixteen percent of the family members investigated were identified as new cases of gonorrhea. Among the children found to have gonorrhea, one-third were male. The average age of the male child patients was seven to ten years. The average age of the female child patients was three to five years.[9] With the recognition that venereal disease is often family centered comes the question of how children within a family contract the infection. Although some studies indicate that children may contract venereal infection as a consequence of poor hygiene and by means other than direct genital contact, most studies of the transmission of venereal disease indicate direct contact.[1,8] Sexual misuse must be considered in the case of any child with venereal disease.

Case 2

> Three siblings, one boy and two girls, all under the age of eight, were diagnosed and treated in the emergency room for genital gonoccus infection. The source of infection was not ascertained but the sexual misuse of the oldest child by an adult in the family seemed likely. The children's general hygiene was extremely poor. The family was a disorganized and chaotic one. It was reliably learned that the children engaged in mutual genital play.

Other less specific symptoms in children may include enuresis, hyperactivity, altered sleeping patterns, fears, phobias, overly compulsive behavior, learning problems, compulsive masturbation, precocious "sexual" play, excessive curiosity about sexual matters, and separation anxiety.

Case 3

The mother of a seven-year-old girl, the second of three children, called the emergency psychiatrist after she learned that the child had been engaging in mutual masturbation with her maternal granduncle. He had lost his wife several months earlier, and the child had been sent to spend weekends with him to relieve his loneliness. During this period the child became enuretic. The mother had noticed increased activity level, sleeping problems, night fears, and a surge of sexual curiosity. The child's pre-existing preoccupation with cleanliness also assumed compulsive proportions. The mother learned about the child's experiences from a young aunt in whom the child had confided.

The mother had chronic somatic complaints. Because of her illness and preoccupations, she was unable to meet her family's dependency needs. The patient turned to the father, who accepted a special relationship with his capable and precocious daughter, and she in turn assumed the role of "little mother" to the rest of the family. She was assigned the caretaking role in relation to the old uncle, who because of his need and impaired judgment misused her. She carried her secret, with all its pleasure and guilt, for several months, developing a host of anxiety symptoms before she revealed it to the young aunt. The family dynamics of this case are similar to those found in cases of incest.

Adolescents are sometimes able to verbalize concerns about sexual misuse but it is rare for them to come to a medical setting with a direct complaint. They may act out their distress by running away from home and engaging in delinquent behavior, including prostitution. Often adolescents who have been sexually misused come to a medical setting after becoming pregnant.

Case 4

A child protective agency worker brought a pregnant 15-year-old to the gynecology clinic to seek an abortion. The adolescent appeared very childlike and immature. It was considered likely an older male in the foster home had impregnated the girl. She had a history of alleged sexual misuse two years previously by her mother's boyfriend and was repeatedly exposed to physical abuse. In the foster home she seemed to invite sexual activity in a childlike, naive manner, admittedly seeing it as a way to get close to people. She expressed the fantasy that having a child might be a way for her to return to her own mother, who had abandoned her.

One should always inquire into the circumstances under which an adolescent became pregnant. Often pregnancy is a consequence of sexual misuse in the family or rape. Anxiety, denial, and guilt often prevent adolescents from seeking medical attention sooner.

Spectrum of Cases

Our emergency room and clinical experiences indicate that cases of sexual misuse cover a broad spectrum. At one end are cases involving sometimes subtle interactions within families, in which the boundaries defining relationships are blurred and it is often difficult to separate family members' actions from their underlying fantasies. Frequently, it is not possible to view the child as a passive victim in such cases; the child may in fact be an active participant. Father and daughter, for example, may be involved in physical games, such as the daughter's playing at riding a horse while being bounced upon her father's leg. At times such physical games generate more excitement and stimulation than a child is able to manage. Lonely mothers may engage in covert sexual misuse of their sons. Undue amounts of physical contact between mother and son, prolonged physical care, and lack of permission to "grow up" and gradually separate from the mother may result in a host of neurotic and psychosomatic symptoms, with the boy's anger turned toward himself or, more frequently, discharged toward the mother as adolescence approaches.

Case 5

> A mother brought her seven-year-old son to the clinic, complaining of his refusal to attend school and his clinging behavior. The father had left the home two years previously, leaving mother and son alone. Mother and son slept together, and the mother showed undue preoccupation in tending to the physical needs of the boy, bathing and dressing him, and supervising the minute details of his everyday functioning.

Under usual circumstances the loving caresses of a parent or close relative serve to increase a child's sense of self-esteem and feelings of being pleasing and lovable. There are instances, however, when the physical contact may turn into frank genital stimulation because of the adult's feelings of loneliness and need, possibly combined with weakened impulse control and poor judgment. Tender fondling by the parent may transgress strict boundaries; in the twilight state of mutual affection, unconscious wishes and vivid fantasies may merge, and incest may become an emotional experience for a child even without direct genital contact.

The sometimes subtle transition between the loving caress and genital stimulation places Freud's[5] initial theory concerning incestuous relationships in his hysterical patient's childhood in a somewhat different perspective.[5] It is hard to define the point at which pleasurable stimulation is experienced as overstimulation, and the child, flooded with excitement, feels overwhelmed and helpless, fears loss of control, and becomes symptomatic. It is also difficult to ascertain at what point an experience engenders an individual child's reaction of anxiety and guilt. The examiner must consider the child's presenting symptoms and general functioning and adaptation in trying to ascertain whether family interactions are overly stimulating for the child. In observing family interactions, it is helpful to keep in mind the notion of boundaries within families, those implicit and explicit rules that govern relationships between family members.[7] When roles and boundaries between parent and child remain clear, there is less chance that a child will be inappropriately stimulated.

At the other end of the spectrum of cases of sexual misuse are the gross transgressions, including incest within the family and violent assault of a child by a stranger in the form of molestation or rape.

Long-term cases of incest do not come to the medical setting very frequently. Occasionally the family equilibrium will be drastically disrupted, and an angry and upset parent will bring the child to the emergency room. Often the parent brings the child because of anger toward the spouse and guilt, rather than because of real concern about the child. The child may not show acute symptoms.

Case 6

A mother came to the emergency room at 3 A.M. with her two adolescent daughters, aged twelve and fourteen. She claimed to have just discovered that her husband had been having intercourse with both girls for one or two years at times when she was not at home. The mother appeared very angry. Apparently, she had just fought with her husband about another matter and feared he would leave her. In her anger she had gone to the police to initiate criminal action against her husband and had then brought the girls to the emergency room. The girls appeared shy and confused and were reluctant to speak to medical and psychiatric personnel. They were hospitalized to assure their immediate protection and the case was brought to the state child abuse unit. The mother became very distressed about the possible consequences of her legal action. Her distress was communicated to the children. The children refused to testify at a court hearing. Shortly thereafter the parents left the state with their two children.

In a minority of the cases in which we were consulted, children were the victims of assault by a stranger. In some of the cases, lack of adequate protection of the child by the parent appeared to contribute to the child's being placed in a vulnerable position. In other cases, family pathology did not appear contributory.

Case 7

An eleven-year-old girl was walking home from a skating rink along a familiar route in the daytime. A man in a parked car forced her into his vehicle and, under threat of violence, forced her to perform fellatio. Intercourse was attempted, but there was no penetration. The man released the child at the same place he picked her up. She went home to her parents and tearfully told them what happened. They immediately brought her to the emergency room. Initially, the parents and child appeared composed and controlled in their response. Subsequently, the child developed some anxiety and mild phobic symptoms which soon abated. The mother and the parental relationship proved to be the vulnerable points in the family system. One week after the incident the father reported that his wife had become acutely anxious and guilty. He feared that she was "falling apart" and that the stability of the marriage was threatened. A short-term crisis intervention program, which included individual work with mother and child, as well as some couples meetings and family meetings, helped the family work through its reaction.

A family approach to diagnosis and treatment is advised even in cases in which the child is attacked by a stranger. It is not unusual for the reaction to an assault upon a child to permeate the entire family system.

Male children may also be the objects of sexual misuse both within the family and outside the family. Far fewer males than females come to the attention of personnel in medical settings. It is not known whether males are in fact misused less often than females or whether other factors contribute to males' seeking medical attention less often.

Case 8

The emergency psychiatrist was asked to see a ten-year-old boy whose mother and younger brother were in psychotherapy in the child psychiatry clinic. The boy had been playing with friends when an adolescent male approached the group. He assaulted the ten-year-old, and forced him to engage in fellatio and mutual masturbation, while the other children managed to run away. The boy then ran home and told his mother what happened. She took him to the psychiatrist on emergency call.

High Risk Situations

In working with sexually misused children and their families, we became aware of circumstances in which children appeared to be at increased risk for sexual misuse. Awareness of these circumstances may assist medical personnel in recognizing cases, and hopefully may facilitate preventive work.

In many cases, a parent of a sexually misused child had been misused as a child. It is possible that children of parents who were misused are at risk for sexual misuse. Parents may unconsciously or consciously participate in creating the circumstances that foster the repetition.

Case 9

A 16-year-old girl came to the emergency room after being raped by a man she did not know, who entered her family's apartment. Her mother had been drinking in a bar that evening, and became intoxicated. By means that were never clear, her keys came into the possession of a man in the bar, who then left the bar, entered her apartment, and raped her daughter. Subsequently, the mother revealed that she had been raped when she was sixteen.

Children who have been physically or sexually misused are at high risk for repeated misuse. Often, through the repetition compulsion, they provoke further misuse in an attempt to master the traumatic event. These children may receive gratification and pleasure as a consequence of the misuse; and unable to satisfy needs in other ways, they may continue to seek pleasure, need satisfaction, or a masochistic experience by provoking continued misuse.

Case 10

A five-year-old with vaginal bleeding and vulvovaginal irritation was brought to the emergency room by her mother. Included in the child's background were episodes of physical abuse in early infancy and a foster placement in which she was sexually misused by an adolescent. The child had been returned to her natural mother. She had been visiting the home of her estranged father and was sleeping in the bedroom with the seven- and-eight-year-old sons of the father's girlfriend. The five-year-old claimed that during the night the boys stuck her genitals with pins. She told her father the next morning but he did nothing. She repeated the story to her mother, who initially did not respond. The next day when the mother noticed bloody spots on the child's underwear, she took her to the emergency room. The child was a bright, precocious, seductive five-year-old who sat with her legs spread apart. She spoke of boyfriends in school whom she hugged and played with in the bathroom. She spoke with sadness of her father's absence from the family and of her anger at her mother, who would not let her see the father more often.

It appears that this child responded to the many hurts in her life by turning her anger toward her mother and by directing her longing for closeness toward her father and other males. Neither parent was able to protect this bright, precocious, deprived child, and she continued her quest for closeness through provoking age-inappropriate "sexual" contact, thus making herself vulnerable for repeated sexual misuse.

Many of the cases of sexual misuse cited above involve children in foster placement. Many of the children placed in foster care have either experienced or witnessed physical and sexual assault.

If not adequately cared for, supervised, and protected, they are at high risk not only to invite assault, but also to become the sadistic attacker, through identification with the aggressor. For example, mutual masturbation is common among needy children in poorly supervised settings who sleep in close proximity. Feelings of deprivation drive them to provide one another with much needed closeness and pleasure. Masturbation may help them relieve tensions caused by the episodic overstimulation to which they are exposed. Among children who were victims or witnesses of aggression, mutual genital exploration may turn into aggressive genital attack.

Case 11

A five-year-old with injured genitals was brought to the emergency room. She was a member of a large foster family. Apparently she was engaged in sexual games with two slightly older boys who, in the process of mutual exploration, overpowered her and forced a pencil into her vagina.

Much care must be taken in the placement of such children to protect them from repeating past experiences. Much sensitivity and tactful help is needed to protect the foster parents from the awakening of intrafamilial conflict in which the foster child may play the role of unconscious fomenter and ultimate scapegoat.

Finally, single-parent families may constitute one more setting in which children are at greater risk for sexual misuse. Lonely, needy, isolated parents often turn to their children for warmth and closeness. Sometimes this results in inappropriate stimulation of the child.

Sexual Abuse and the Law

We have noted the continuum of sexual abuse-misuse, ranging from outright attack to those subtle instances in which it becomes difficult to separate fantasies and actions or to differentiate appropriate expressions of parent-child affection from misuse. We have been writing from a clinical vantage point, and our definitions are intended for use in clinical settings. One must, of necessity, differentiate between the clinical definition of sexual misuse and the legal definition of "sexual abuse." The legal definition differs in that its purpose is to identify those blatant cases in which the state feels obligated to interfere in the life of a family and child for the purpose of assuring protection of the child. The reporting of a case and activation of governmental involvement have vast implications for the life and privacy of the child and family as well as for their treatment. We would by no means advocate that all cases coming under our definition of sexual misuse be reported to governmental agencies. The decision as to where to draw the line in reporting cases is necessarily arbitrary and may differ from state to state.

Every state in the United States has enacted a statute requiring reporting of cases of child abuse by certain groups of persons. In some states, sexual abuse is included in the definition of what is reportable. In Massachusetts, for example, the Regulations of the Department of Public Welfare include as reportable abuse "the commission of a sex offense against a child as defined in the criminal laws of Massachusetts." The child abuse reporting statute states that a reportable condition is one that results in "serious physical or emotional injury."[3] Professionals must therefore assess which of the cases of sexual abuse lead to injury that is "serious" enough to merit reporting. We have also found it necessary to use the court or protective agencies in those cases in which we doubt that parents can adequately protect their children from further harm, even if therapeutic support is offered. One can often identify such parents by their lack of guilt and anxiety in the medical setting.

Cases of sexual abuse may also come under the jurisdiction of criminal courts. It is not unusual for parents to turn to criminal courts in moments of anger and then subsequently to regret their actions. The criminal process is long and complicated and often creates stresses for children and their families beyond those resulting from the actual misuse. Children are often caught in the middle of these proceedings. Although there are trends toward closing courtrooms to the public and having the judge see the child in his chambers, the process is often traumatic for child and family; support throughout the trial process constitutes an important part of the treatment program.

Guidelines For Acute Case Management

In the course of working with cases of sexual misuse and abuse in emergency and clinic settings we have developed some preliminary guidelines for acute management of these cases.

1. Support System

An interdisciplinary support system is essential for professionals working with these children and their families. The high level of anxiety generated by these cases, problems in sorting out reality and fantasy, and the strong feelings that workers experience in response to these children and their parents necessitate back-up for the workers. A team approach is often helpful for purposes of providing mutual support and sharing the responsibility of decision-making. Ideally, the team might include physicians (pediatricians, child psychiatrists), a nurse, and a social worker, with access to other consultants, including gynecologists, attorneys, and specialists in child protection. Liaison with the courts, judges, and governmental child protective agencies is helpful for those cases in which the child is thought to be in serious jeopardy.

2. Child and Family Focus

One must attempt to understand the symptom of sexual abuse in terms of its impact on a given child's development and its meaning within the context of the family system. Whether or not misuse actually occurs within the family, a family focus must be maintained to ascertain whether family factors contributed to placing the child in a vulnerable position and to gauge the family's reaction to the event. One should determine the clarity of role definitions within the family and the boundaries between generations. Often in families that misuse children, roles, rules, and boundaries are indistinct.

3. Safety and Controls

Early in working with a family one must assess the capacity of the family to provide safety and protection for all of its members and must determine the minimum steps necessary to assure protection. Assessment of a parent's capacity for impulse control and reality testing, and of the nature of the parent's superego, is important in this determination. Certainly, no therapeutic work can proceed unless people feel safe. Decisions regarding safety should be shared by members of the therapeutic team, and the family should be involved when possible. Sometimes the presence of a therapeutic person is sufficient to make family members feel safe. In situations where safety is less certain, the child protective agencies should be consulted, and, if necessary, the courts involved early in the process. To increase the impact of super-vision upon a family, the measures may include monitoring of the intact family by a child protective caseworker or the court, temporary foster placement of a child, removal of a parent from the home, and, in extreme cases, the permanent placement of the child away from the home. When sexual misuse occurs within families in which there is a serious lack of protection, our preference as therapists has been to work in coordination with the civil courts rather than the criminal courts, when this is possible. Using the court as monitor and protector, one can proceed with therapeutic work directed toward the entire family and decide whether the long-range goal of keeping the family intact is tenable. A split between the protective function provided by the courts and the therapeutic function of the team can be very important in more serious cases. The distressed families often direct anger and mistrust toward the "protectors" and are better able to form treatment alliances with "therapists" when they perceive the protectors as being separate from the therapists. Of course, in situations where the two functions are split, it is esstential that the "therapists" and "protectors" maintain contact and cooperation.

4. The Solution as a Problem

We must make sure that the "solutions" we impose on children and their families do not become part of the problem. For example, temporary placement of a child may provide a short-term solution by removing the child from a dangerous situation. However, there are dangers inherent in separating the child from the family and it is not unusual to hear of cases in which children experience repeated sexual misuse within foster homes.Placement of a child necessitates education and support for the foster parents as well as continued work with the child and the family of origin. Court proceedings are often part of the solutions we impose. Especially in criminal cases, these proceedings can be traumatic for children and other family members. We are obliged to find means to provide support and minimize repeated trauma. Even in hospital settings, where these cases appear in emergency rooms or clinics, the manner in which the cases are approached by hospital personnel may have a significant impact on the child and family, for better or worse.

REFERENCES

1. ASNES, R. ET AL. 1972. Gonococcal infection in children. J. Pediat. 81: 192-193.
2. BENDER, L. AND BLAU, A. 1937. Reaction of children to sexual relations with adults. Amer. J. Orthopsychiat. 7:500-51.
3. DeFRANCIS, V. 1974. Child Abuse Legislation in the 1970's. The American Humane Association, Denver.
4. DeFRANCIS, V. 1969. Protecting the Child Victim of Sex Crimes Committed by Adults. The American Humane Association, Denver.
5. FREUD, S. AND BREVER, J. 1955. Studies on Hysteria. *In* The Standard Edition of the Complete Psychological Works of Freud, Vol. II, J. Strachey, ed. The Hogarth Press, London.
6. KATÁN, A. 1973. The children who were raped. Psychoanalytic Study of the Child 28:208-224.
7. MINUCHIN, S. 1975. Families and Family Therapy. Harvard University Press, Cambridge, Mass.
8. SHORE, W. AND WINKELSTEIN, G. 1971. Nonvenereal transmission of gonococcal infections to children. J. Pediatrics 79:661-663.
9. SINGER, R. 1975. Presentation at workshop on sexual abuse of children. 52nd Annual Meeting of the American Orthopsychiatric Association, Washington, D.C. (unpublished)

Chapter 6

OBSERVATIONS AFTER SEXUAL TRAUMATA SUFFERED IN CHILDHOOD*

HEINZ BRUNOLD

Public opinion judges sexual offenders with especial severity and emotionalism. Why this is so will not be considered here. But an investigation of the question would certainly be rewarding: an astonishing number of repressed guilt feelings would surely come to light.

For sexual crimes against children there is exceptionally rigorous condemnation, normally accompanied in newspaper reports and court judgments by the statement that such experiences inflict lasting psychological damage on the child. Assertions of this general kind are, however, in no way proved.

Doctors come to know a number of psychologically damaged patients whose disturbances can be traced back to sexual affronts in childhood. There is a tendency to generalize from these and to give practically no thought to the possibility that there may be children who are able partially or entirely to assimilate such experiences, at least sufficiently for their later life to be unaffected.

In the present study I set myself the task of finding a substantial number of persons, now grown up, who as children were the victims of sexual delinquents, and trying to discover damage which could be traced back to the sexual experience in childhood.

The subjects of the investigation were found through court records. There were originally a little over 100 children who had been victims of sexual assaults. Naturally not all could be traced; very few did not agree to help in the investigation. To achieve a

*From *Excerpta Criminologica*, Jan/Feb 1964. Courtesy of Swets & Zeitlinger B.V., Lisse, The Netherlands.

moderately clear picture, some selection was made. For example, only those children were chosen who had suffered relatively serious assaults, i.e. had undergone an intensive physical contact (once or repeatedly) such as intensive onanistic acts, mutual onanism, cunnilingus, fellatio, acts resembling coitus, normal coitus. Exhibitionistic acts, showing of pornographic pictures and so on were not considered, although of course it is quite conceivable that visual impressions of a sexual kind can lead to difficulties in later development. A further selection was made by including only children who were aged 5 years or more at the time of the offence, on the assumption that from this age onwards an assault of a sexual nature would be experienced on a largely conscious level. Children over 15 years old were also excluded, since today children of this age may be regarded as sufficiently developed to be able to accept and assimilate sexual experiences as adults. Further, the period of time between the offence and the follow-up was arbitrarily fixed at a minimum of 15 years (the average for all cases studied was 23 years). After imposing these various limitations 62 cases were left (50 girls and 12 boys) who could be followed up. This is, of course, not a large number, but even so, the findings may not be without interest.

Almost exactly half the 62 children came from urban areas, the other half from rural or small-town environments.

The follow-up consisted in each case of one or more interviews of at least one hour, and additional enquiries from family doctors, guardianship, authorities etc., as necessary. There was in general a surprising willingness to give information, once the purpose of the investigation had been explained.

Although the victims of sexual crimes could be studied and assessed from the most varied points of view, the investigator was forced by other circumstances to restrict himself to relatively few. The factors mainly considered were background, especially family conditions, schooling, later occupation and marital relationships. Personality was not in general considered.

The first conclusion is that apparently children from urban and from rural/small-town environments are exposed to approximately equal risks from sexual delinquents. It is remarkable that the majority of the children came from the lower social strata, such as labourers' families, and especially from families where both parents go out to work and the children are largely left to themselves or lack the security of an orderly family life.

It is striking that well over half the children came from clearly unfavourable family backgrounds (parents' broken marriage, etc.). About one third were children of divorced parents, or had a parent who had been divorced previously. This may be relevant to the fact that in 15 cases the step-father was the offender. Lack of pocket money clearly favoured susceptibility, and in fact the majority of the children were lured by small amounts of money, sweets or other small presents. Less than half a dozen of the children had previously received a scanty explanation of sexual matters.

Boys of about 12 were the most exposed to risk; for girls the age was about ½ to 1 year less, which may be connected with their earlier maturation.

It has already been mentioned that poor marital relationships of the parents and neglected up-bringing markedly increased the susceptibility. Intelligence alone, on the other hand—as measured by performance at school—played a comparatively small part (but three of the girls were definitely mentally deficient).

There was a decided desire to attract attention and act importantly, especially among the girls; also pride at receiving notice and respect from an adult. Ten girls were led to the offender by their own friends, which happened in the case of only one of the boys. No child was aware of suffering from any serious psychic abnormality before the commission of the offence. Understandably, the occurrence of a sexual offence was clearly favoured by the existence of a subordinate relationship towards the offender.

In more than a third of the cases the offenders were fathers, step- or foster-fathers, teachers, clergymen or close acquaintances of the family. One teacher was the culprit in several of the cases considered. Large families, on the other hand, did not favour these occurrences in the observed cases; nor did extra-marital or pre-marital birth of the child.

. It seems rather surprising that two-thirds of the children apparently offered no resistance, or at least very little, to the offender's intentions, and that in more than half tne cases the offence was repeated with the same person: in several cases there were even intimate relationships over a number of years, of which one or two lasted after the child was grown up and had married someone else.

In the following figures concerning the nature of the offences against the 50 girls and 12 boys it should be remembered that the figures will add up to more than the total number of cases, as frequent unlawful acts took place with the same child.

With the girls there was always a more or less intensive handling of the body and genitals. Cunnilinction occurred in 11 cases, fellatio by the girl in at least 6, actions akin to coitus in 24 and actual coitus in vaginam in 19 cases.

With all the boys there were active or passive onanistic acts, and in 11 cases mutual onanism. Active and passive fellatio took place in 4, coitus inter femora in 2 and coitus in anum in 3 cases.

The great majority of the offences took place in the home of the offender.

As far as can be seen from the records no child actively offered itself to the offender, but as has been mentioned, several children voluntarily allowed themselves to be taken to the offender by others, who were also involved; this may have been from curiosity or more often in the expectation of a small reward.

Since it is generally not possible, in investigations such as this, to adduce, without lengthy analytical procedures, positive proof of deeper psychic damage, the questions were aimed primarily at discovering the earlier and present attitude of the victims to the acts they were subjected to, and the consequences; in addition their subsequent social development was considered.

It is remarkable that the authorities seldom took any special action to care for the children after the offences had become known. Of the 50 girls and 12 boys, 45 and 9 respectively were left in their own families, even when conditions were hardly favourable. Three girls were, however, placed in another family, and 2 girls and 3 boys in institutions. The environment in which the 62 children grew up after the offences could be considered good in about half the cases, dubious in about a third, and poor in the remainder.

At the time of the study, 35 of the female former victims and 10 of the male were married, of which however 8 women and 2 men appeared to be living in unsatisfactory marital circumstances; in 5 of these cases an earlier marriage had already been dissolved (without any certain indication that the causes could be traced back to the earlier sexual experiences).

As regards occupation, 12 of the female subjects are today working in factories, 8 are shop assistants, another 8 are housewives only, 4 each are tailoresses, domestic servants, and clerks, and one each are book-shop assistant, children's nurse, deaconess, manageress, and marriage consultant. Of the 12 men, 7 are labourers, 2 each are skilled craftsmen and salesmen, and the last is a dance musician.

In general the persons studied are living in the same or similar social circumstances as those from which they originated. Only in a very few cases is there a certain improvement in social status. There was virtually no sign of any descent on the social ladder.

As objective (documented) injury resulting from the offences suffered, it must be mentioned that 3 girls were infected with gonorrhea and pregnancy occurred in 4 cases (with 2 illegal terminations). In one further case a 5-year-old girl suffered serious bodily injuries.

With the exception of one woman, who declared that her whole life had been 'ruined' and who suffers from massive feelings of inferiority, all the subjects denied that there was any lasting damage as a result of the sexual assaults. Some (about 8) did however admit that they had suffered, for some time after the offences, from feelings of shame and revulsion. Several women asserted that the investigations by the police or in court had made a considerably worse impact on them than the offence.

About 10 of the women mentioned that their sexuality had been prematurely awakened by their experiences, but did not feel this to be harmful. It is indeed questionable whether the heightened sexual sensibility mentioned in a few cases can be interpreted as injurious, provided that this does not lead to promiscuous sexual behaviour—which did however happen in two or three of the cases studied.

In about 3 of the female victims, sexual frigidity exists to a more or less marked extent. The principal cause of this neurotic reaction must presumably be the sexual trauma suffered in childhood, even though other factors may play a part. One of the boys has become an active homosexual, almost certainly as a result of the offences, and has himself been punished for paedophilic homosexual misconduct.

Altogether it may be said that probably about a tenth of the children suffered injury of a lasting kind; a serious number, although in view of commonly held opinions one would have expected it to be higher.

The following points, emerging from the follow-up investigations, seem worth noting:

1. Children from good environment and family conditions suffered less injury as a result of the offences, especially when the environment continued to be good afterwards.
2. Children of the lower social classes are in greater danger of sexual assault, especially in families where both parents are out at work so that the children are largely left to themselves without supervision.
3. Sexual offenses of whatever kind, repeated over a long period of time, more often cause lasting injury than single occurrences.
4. The age at which the offence occurs was not, in the present sample, a significant factor in the causation of lasting injury.

The constantly expressed fears that sexual traumata suffered in childhood lead to lasting psychic injury are not, in the present follow-up survey at least, to be accepted without qualification. It is true that this follow-up is based on relatively simple criteria and may contain erroneous information, especially since it was necessary to rely largely on facts provided by the persons concerned. But if their statements can to some extent be believed, of which most cases there is hardly any doubt, it may be said in general that lasting psychological injury as a result of sexual assaults suffered in infancy is not very common.

Very often, associated circumstances such as judicial hearings had a much greater impact than the actual offences.

Feelings of shame and revulsion did, however, appear in many victims for some time afterwards, but in general they were assimilated relatively quickly, so that lasting injury cannot be said to have occurred.

Psychological injury of a permanent nature must be expected in about a tenth of the children concerned—a number which is still far too high and can apparently be diminished only by a reduction in the number of sexual offenders. There remain the children themselves.

If it is found that in the cases considered the children were never, or seldom, or inadequately instructed or warned, it could be concluded that suitable sexual instruction and explanation, in good time, of the dangers should reduce the number of offences. Such a task naturally falls first and foremost to the parents. The tendency of parents, however, to want to withdraw more and more from educational tasks and duties has unfortunately become general, so that the hopes in general do not seem very encouraging.

The question then arises whether the school (teachers and school doctors) and also the family doctor should give more attention to this problem than they appear to have done until now.

Special instruction and warning are certainly called for when both parents are out at work and the necessary supervision and control of the home are lacking.

It should be apparent that the danger is particularly great for children in an unloving family environment, who are consequently in need of love and hence particularly susceptible to the approaches of paedophiliacs.

The effects are disastrous when the family itself sets an example of fecklessness and lack of control, especially in sexual respects, so that the child cannot experience the moral authority and exemplary behaviour which it always seeks.

—————— **Chapter 7** ——————

SEXUAL TRAUMA OF CHILDREN AND ADOLESCENTS: PRESSURE, SEX, AND SECRECY*

ANN WOLBERT BURGESS, D.N.SC.
AND LYNDA LYTLE HOLMSTROM, PH.D.

I think the reason why a lot of kids don't do anything, don't tell anybody, is because an adult is an authority figure and somehow they have been forced to do something wrong by an authority, and therefore it must have been right.

An accessory-to-sex victim, now age 23

This paper describes our work with a group of sexual trauma victims—primarily children and adolescents—whom we call accessory-to-sex victims. In this type of sexual situation, victims are pressured into sexual activity by a person who stands in a power position over them as through age, authority, or some other way. The victim in unable to consent because of either personality or cognitive development. The emotional reactions of victims result from their being pressured into sexual activity and from the added tension of keeping the act secret. This accessory-to-sex situation is in contrast to our prior work with rape victims, described in an earlier paper,[1] in which the sexual assault of rape was clearly against the victim's will as well as generating a life-threatening situation.

The Victim Counseling Program was established at Boston City Hospital in July, 1972, as a voluntary service project staffed by a psychiatric nurse (AWB) and a sociologist (LLH). There were two objectives of the project: (1) to provide counseling services to victims of forcible rape, attempted rape, sexual assault, and child molesting; and (2) to study the problems victims encountered as they proceeded through the institutions designed

*From *Nursing Clinics of North America*, 10(3):551-563, Sept 1975. Courtesy of W. B. Saunders Company, Philadelphia.

to help them—that is, the hospital, the police, the court. In the first year, 146 victims were seen, of whom 109 were adult women, 34 were pre-adult females, and 3 were pre-adult males. The second year of the project was designed to train and supervise emergency department personnel (primarily nurses) to implement victim counseling into their repertoire of services.

The third year of the project has expanded to include consultation by staff for other hospitals and institutions as they begin to develop programs for victims. We believe nurses are an important professional group to provide diagnostic and intervention services to sexual assault victims because of their bio-psycho-social skills and their presence in facilities where victims seek services. And we especially believe that nurses could play a key role in counseling children and adolescents in issues regarding human sexuality.

The Victims and the Activity

Over a two-year period, we looked at all cases admitted through the emergency services of the Boston City Hospital with the chief complaint of "I've been raped" and devised three diagnostic categories: rape trauma, accessory-to-sex, and sex-stress situations. We identified a sub-sample of 33 accessory-to-sex victims from the total sample; this sub-sample included 29 females and 4 males. We have also included 9 referral cases which provide the data on the silent reaction to accessory-to-sex incidents. Of the 42 total subjects, 36 were female, 6 were male, and 27 were white and 15 black victims.

The accessory cases were categorized according to whether the incident occurred once, several times within a short period of time, or over an extended period of months or years. Cases were categorized as attempted rather than completed if there was only mention of semisexual activity or extremely minimal sexual contact such as the offender briefly touching the victim. Silent reactions to accessory-to-sex incidents are those in which the victim remained silent for a long amount of time—years. The majority of victims—27 of the total 42—were under age 9 and almost half of these 27 victims were traumatized over a period of years.

Relationship of Offender to Victim

Almost half of the offenders were family members. Of these 20 men, 10 were assuming the role of father in the home; 6 of the offenders were uncle of the victim; 3 situations involved a grandfather and one situation involved a cousin. Four of the offenders were involved with 10 of the victims, which emphasizes the frequency with which one family member is able to gain access to more than one female or male child in the family. One reason that these people have repeated access to the child is because they are family members and their presence is not questioned by the family.

Pressuring the Victim into Sexual Activity

The offender stands in a relationship of dominance to the victim. Ambivalence as a component of the decision-making process is a characteristic of the child's or young person's emotional life, and the offender trades on this. Georg Simmel, in discussing domination as a form of interaction, states that the desire for domination is aimed at breaking the internal resistance of the subordinate.[2]

In accessory-to-sex incidents, the offender pressures the victim into being an accessory to the sexual activity, that is, to go along with it at least once. The victim may be totally unaware that sexual activity is part of the offer. One victim described her happy visits to her grandparent's farm and how she enjoyed being thrown into the haystack. One day the grandfather said he would throw her into the haystack and give her a silver dollar if she did something with him. The child went along with him assuming it would be as she had previously experienced the fun, but it turned out very differently.

As in this example, some method of pressure or offer is made to the person—i.e., being thrown into the haystack. Three main types of pressure were noted in the victim sample as shown in the following chart.

Method of Pressure

Material goods	19
Misrepresenting moral standards	13
Need for human contact	3
No data	7

MATERIAL GOODS. Children are most likely to be offered some type of material good such as candy or money. In one case involving a 6-year-old girl and 6-year-old male cousin, the girl said:

> Big Bobby asked me and Joey to come see his puppies. Then he said he'd give us some money to take down our pants.

The situation advanced to where the girl was further pressured into sexual activity and penetration was attempted by the offender.

MISREPRESENTING MORAL STANDARDS. Family members can pressure the child by telling the child it is "okay to do". As one victim said, "If an adult tells you to do something you do it." In the case of a 5-year-old, a neighbor-offender pressured the child into "playing house" with him. The matter came to the attention of the mother when she discovered blood in her child's pants.

Young people often do not have the ability to consent when confronted with pressure by material goods or when an adult misrepresents moral standards. Children under age 6 and latency age children may know that sexual situations between themselves and adults are wrong, but a concept of sexuality has not been incorporated into their life style and they go along with the pressure from the adult in the situation. The following example illustrates this inability to make a decision until it was too late.

> He had me lay down . . . and then he showed me his penis and I remember his talking to me and telling me he was going to put that inside of me and he showed me where he was going to put it and he made me touch my vagina and he made me touch his penis. That's when I decided that there was no way—I looked at this thing and I looked at me and thought "no way." And I got upset and I tried to get away from him but he said, "Oh, I'm going to throw you in the haystack; everything will be all right,

everything will be okay." And he kept telling me that. Then he started to enter me and I can just remember the pain.

NEED FOR HUMAN CONTACT. The majority of accessory-to-sex victims are children and adolescents. However, our sample did include some adult women who did not have the cognitive or emotional development to be able to consent or not to consent. These women were extremely isolated and impoverished socially and emotionally and they were enticed by men by their needs for warmth and contact.

Types of Sexual Activity and Victims' Reactions

The type of sexual activity of the offender varies. Each case in the victim sample was counted once for the type of sexual activity and if multiple activities were used—which was frequent—penetration or the one closest to penetration was cited. Penetration had the highest incidence in this victim sample—15 of the 42 victims—with hand-genital contact next with 10 victims, followed by fairly equal numbers of victims reporting mouth-genital contact, attempted penetration, and approach and pressure only with no sexual contact.

Physical Reaction to Sexual Activity

Children usually described the experience in terms of whether it hurt, a negative reaction, or was pleasurable, a positive reaction. Those who indicated neither reaction were categorized as neutral.

Over half the victims experienced a negative reaction to the sexual activity. Sometimes the negative reaction serves to disrupt the offender's intent and he leaves the situation as in the following case.

A 6 year old girl stated that a man followed her into her building and offered her a bag of candy. She said "He took me inside the hall and put his hands in my pants and pinched me and I cried." The man left the scene at that point and the child ran to tell her mother. The mother noted blood on the child's pants, notified the police and brought the child to the hospital.

There were some victims—7 out of 12—who found the sexual activity pleasurable. These tend to be cases in which hand-genital contact was used rather than penetration. One 19-year-old woman recounting her childhood experience with her grand-father said:

> He would sit me in his lap with my legs slightly spread apart and stroke my inner thighs, labia and genital area. . . . I found it very pleasurable. I would have my back against his torso, my head on his chest and sometimes fall asleep. He was always so warm and gentle and he would tell me stories.

Pressuring the Victim into Secrecy

If the offender is successful with his victim, he must try now to conceal the deviate behavior from others. More likely than not, he will try to pledge the victim to secrecy in several ways. The child may not necessarily be aware of the existence of the secret, as in situations in which the act is gentle and pleasurable and the child does not believe it is wrong. The offender may say this is something secret between them or, in some cases, he may threaten harm to the child if she does tell.

In most situations, the burden of the pressure to keep the secret is psychologically experienced as fear. Victims have spontaneously described the following fears which they said bound them to the secret.

FEAR OF PUNISHMENT. The victim often fears punishment if she tells. As one victim said:

> I don't remember anything wrong with it till Dad began to threaten me if I told. . . . There was pressure to go along with him . . .he said he would punish me if I told mother.

FEAR OF REPERCUSSIONS FROM TELLING. Some victims do not think they would be believed. As one 23-year-old victim said in reflecting back on why she did not tell her parents, "You know, to this day, I don't think they [parents] would have believed me."

Some victims never tell because they fear the reaction the outside person will have to the disclosure. One victim said she just knew her parents "never would have acted right." Or the child may fear being blamed for the activity. One victim said:

> I think I never told because father [offender] might have said I was lying or I was a bad child and no one would like me again.

In two separate situations, the children were blamed after the disclosure. One 19-year-old male victim said, "Mother made us feel we were the cause of her brother being bad and wouldn't let us talk to our cousins."

FEAR OF ABANDONMENT OR REJECTION. Children may fear that revealing the secret will cause catastrophic results. As one victim said:

> I thought it would be terrible to be separated from the family. I thought something terrible would happen if I told. . . . The fear of rejection was really great as a child.

COMMUNICATION BARRIER. Children do have difficulty sometimes putting a description of the activity into words, and oftentimes the child tells another companion who, in turn, tells an outside person. Children may not know the adult words. One victim describes this:

> . . . that's extremely rare where a kid would really be able to waltz up to Mom and say, "Guess what? Guess what your father did to me? Is it wrong for Grandpa to stick his thing into me?" I mean, can you imagine?

Disclosure of the Secret

In many situations, the secret is broken and this is a crucial point. A secret disclosed without both parties' consent may be termed betrayal. Thus, there is the ever-present tension that the

secret may be betrayed. Simmel describes a secret being sur-
rounded by temptation and possibility of betrayal; and the
external danger of being discovered is interwoven with the
internal danger of giving oneself away.[3]

Disclosure of Sexual Activity

The disclosure of the activity becomes a key clinical factor. The
emotional reaction of the victim is greatly influenced by how and
when the secret is disclosed and the resulting behavior on the part
of the outside person. There are several ways in which the secret
may by disclosed.

DIRECT CONFRONTATION. There are times when the act will
be observed by others and direct confrontation will occur. In the
case of a 12-year-old mentally retarded girl who was seen being
led into a neighbor's house, the police were notified and, upon
entering the room of the man, found the offender in the act of
intercourse with the girl. Or there are situations in which the
child is confronted with the fact that someone has found out
about the sexual activity. One 19-year-old woman recounts her
childhood experience in which her mother confronted her as
follows:

> One time when I came back from a weekend with my grandparents my
> mother wouldn't talk to me . . . she finally said she was disgusted with me
> and that she knew what my grandfather and I were doing and that I
> would have to tell a priest in confession . . . I knew what she meant
> because no one else did what he did . . . she wouldn't talk to me for days
> and I was upset and mad at her. It was her father and he told me to and I
> was supposed to obey elders and I didn't think it was wrong. So why was
> she mad at me? Why wasn't she mad at him?

VICTIM TELLS SOMEONE. Some victims are able to directly tell
a parent or outside person about the sexual activity. For example,
one 9-year-old was able to tell her mother that her stepfather had
been "fooling" with her.

THE CLUE. Visible clues were provided by many victims who
were unable to tell someone directly. These clues included
walking home without any clothes, children staying out all

night, and a pregnancy. The more subtle clues were the mother
noticing an accumulation of nickels and dimes or new clothes.
Another mother asked why the children were eating lollipops all
the time and was told, "Uncle Jimmy gave it to me and told me
not to tell you." Or the child may draw a picture or write a note.
One mother told how she discovered the situation.

> My daughter half hinted at it and I had a funny feeling something was
> wrong so I pumped her. We were sitting at the table having coffee and my
> husband asked her to do something and she said no. I asked her to do
> something and she did it. Later she asked me if I knew why she did things
> for me and not for my husband. I said no. And she said she would tell me
> some other time—it was grown-up stuff. Well, I got this awful feeling
> and I knew I had to find out so I asked her. She said she couldn't tell me
> but would draw it . . . I took one look at what she drew on the paper and I
> went kookey.

SIGNS AND SYMPTOMS. If the sexual activity continues over
time, signs and symptoms often develop and these may be
brought to the attention of a professional.

Some parents observe the signs such as the child staying inside
more frequently, not wanting to go to school, crying with no
provocation, taking an excessive number of baths, or a sudden
onset of bedwetting, and they become suspicious and seek
professional help. The following illustrates this:

> The mother of a 15-year-old girl stated to the nurse, "Mary is taking baths
> constantly and keeps complaining of stomach aches. She gets very upset
> when one of our neighbors comes around. She used to like going riding
> with him and he took her for cokes and donuts. . . . I am suspicious of
> what might be going on."

It was learned that the 35-year-old neighbor had been pressuring
the girl into sexual activity and this was producing the somatic
and behavioral symptoms.

A variety of symptoms may be described by the child and the
parent or the professional decodes the message. The symptoms
may be gastrointestinal, where the child makes a complaint of a
stomach ache or a urinary tract infection develops, or the child
develops a medical condition such as pneumonia or mononu-

cleosis. The following case illustrates how a silent reaction was missed during the first hospitalization but picked up the next time by the mother and the physician and nurse.

> 11-year-old girl admitted with two-day history of right lower quadrant pain which is absent now; sharp and intermittent without exacerbation or worsening over a two-day period; no vomiting or diarrhea. Sore throat for one day. No other remarkable findings except that one year ago was admitted to another hospital and was hospitalized 5 days and diagnosed to have pelvic inflammation.
>
> A careful history obtained from the patient and her mother separately revealed the following:
>
> Patient told mother last evening that she was sexually assaulted by her father four times. Parents are now separated, divorce proceedings in progress. The child states that six months ago she and her four siblings were staying alone with their father (mother had left house for 4 weeks following parental argument). Father would either put the other children to bed early or send them on errands and then tell the patient to go to his bed. She would do so. He would then ask her to pull down her pants and he would do likewise. He would put "Vaseline on his pickle" and would "put it into her." She did not look, turned her head and screamed. She thought it went "into her bum." She was lying on her back each time. This scene happened two times previously approximately one year ago when her mother was absent from the home. The patient told her two siblings that her father told her that if she ever told anyone he would kill her so she never told anyone till last evening. The mother was questioning her about ordinary games played when she stayed with her father and the patient then related the "dirty game" story. Mother became disturbed and brought the child to the clinic and wants to press charges against her husband.

Clinical Implications

Management of the Victim

Nurses are key professionals to diagnose and intervene with the child or adolescent victim of sexual trauma. Very often the child is brought into a clinic or emergency room where the nurse is the first person to assess the situation. We have found several techniques useful in our work with victims which we recommend that all nurses become familiar with.

ENCOURAGING THE CHILD TO TALK. Many of the children spontaneously talked about the incident although the family found it difficult to discuss. The parents need to talk about how they are encouraging or discouraging the child to talk about it. One mother said, "She talks about it. I tell her to forget it. She gets nervous when his name is mentioned." Another mother said:

> She has brought it up three times today. I try to ignore it so she won't think about it but she keeps talking about it.

In this situation, the mother was encouraged to talk about her feelings and told it was a normal sign for the girl to talk about it and that when she had talked enough about it she would probably stop. And she did.

DRAW-A-PICTURE. Some children will return for clinic visits as part of the treatment regimen. The method of drawing pictures of what happened as a method to insure the child was settling the experience was discovered early in our work with two sisters, ages 9 and 10, who had been molested by their stepfather. The sisters had seen the hospital child psychiatrist and later said to a victim counselor:

> I was afraid he was going to ask me to draw a picture of what happened but he didn't.

Further in the conversation one sister said, "I know what he was trying to get me to say. He was a psychiatrist and wanted to know my reaction." The sisters were quite amenable to using crayons to draw the scene, which included two stick figures lying side by side in bed. This prompted further discussion of the actual details of the activity and the children were quite intent to talk about the details they had drawn on the paper. It is our belief that encouraging the children to talk about their experiences is an open and healthy way to deal with the tensions that have built up over the secrecy process.

OBSERVING SYMPTOMS OVER TIME. Parents need to be instructed about the possible physical and behavioral symptoms that can develop in the child from the pressure of the situation, and that are considered within the normal range for this reaction to a stress situation.

Minor phobic symptoms may be reported when the victim sees or hears the offender's name or sees him. One 12-year-old mentally retarded girl who was unable to verbalize her concerns would run into the house whenever she would see the offender in the neighborhood. Another victim described her change in behavior:

> . . . afterwards I just wanted to get away from him. I was afraid to go where he was after that. Didn't like visiting there any more in the summer. I stayed in the house a lot . . . used the chamber pot under the bed rather than using the bathroom.

Changes in sleep patterns may be noted as well as the occurrence of dreams and nightmares. One victim described a recurrent dream that she had around the age of 7 and 8 which reveals her feeling of being trapped in the situation.

> Round disk figures were making me do things. Like in one instance I was in a safety pin race with elephants and I was walking so slowly; I couldn't walk fast and the elephants would beat me. I remember feeling this terror that something terrible would happen if they beat me and each time I would wake up before the end of the race . . . I couldn't do what I wanted to do . . . I couldn't move fast enough.

Management of Silent Reaction to Accessory-to-Sex Syndrome

We have defined a silent reaction to accessory-to-sex activity when the child has kept the burden of the secret of the activity within herself. This creates considerable tension, and victims have several reactions to having to keep the secret.

CO-CONSPIRACY DYAD. Two victims of the same offender agreed that they did not feel guilty about the sexual experience, but rather about the fact that they had kept it hidden from a parent. In this situation, when the secret was dissolved, a split occurred in the family and this was equally upsetting to the victims.

In another silent reaction the victim said:

> It's the lying and the hiding and the not talking about it that is bad. It has
> to be put into perspective—need to talk about it rather than make it such
> a hideous thing.

RESISTANCE TECHNIQUES. There are techniques that children
will use that aid in their avoiding the sexual activity. However,
they do not betray the secret and they do not disobey the pledge to
secrecy, but they do play a game. One victim said:

> He said I would get another silver dollar if I did it. And I said I did not
> want to do it right then but that I would do it some other time. And for
> the next several years I played that little game: "Well, I can't do it now, I
> have to do this for my mother." I was never so diligent for my mother
> except when we were visiting.

In a situation involving a father and two daughters, the one
victim described how her sister managed to avoid the father:

> My sister said my father was doing the same thing . . . but she wasn't
> afraid to talk back—be aggressive about it and he left her alone. . . . She
> would get emotionally sick now that I think back. She would throw up
> her food when she was upset. She cried a lot and had nightmares—that
> would be when he was after her and this kept him away from her.

SYMPTOM FORMATION. Symptoms will develop as the person
is pressured to keep the secret over time; these are related to the
tension inherent in the fear of disclosure. Fears become exaggerated as in the following case.

> I felt anxiety, frustration and constant fear—a real paranoia that
> someone would find out. It affected my relationships with my peers. I
> lived in a shell and escaped by reading . . . I was always afraid of people
> and thought something terrible would happen if people found out.

The fear may be exaggerated to the degree that the woman feels
that her sexual partners will know she has had such an experience
and she may even fear blackmail. One victim said, "I was afraid if
I ever told a man or anyone that I might be blackmailed."

The fear may be expressed through recurrent dreams as in the
following:

> I am riding on my father's shoulders down the main street of the town where we lived. I am naked from the waist down. As we walk my father has oral sex with me and everyone sees us.

The symptom of flashback during subsequent sexual experiences may be reported. One victim describes this:

> . . . sometimes when I'm not quite ready to have sex and [he] starts to enter me, I just black into that. I just think of that, the pain; it is a similar pain . . .I can't deal with it at all.

REPORTING A SILENT REACTION. What triggers the person to reveal the incident to another person is clinically important. It may be a timely question, it may be an association to a conversation, or it may be the concern of the interviewer. One victim said the first person she told was a close friend over the telephone when they were both drunk. Another victim could not tell until the significant parties involved were dead.

One notable feature when the silence is broken is the characteristic of the unresolved issue phenomenon. The incident has been encapsulated within the psychic structure for so long that when the person finally discloses the secret, the emotional affect can be quite strong, as in the following case.

> . . . I am going to get hysterical in a minute and that's really terrible. I always giggle when I get very upset. I'm sorry. . . . You know, he was wearing green work pants with a metal zipper. I never thought of that before either, I never really sat down and discussed it in detail. He unbuttoned his shirt, god . . . all of a sudden I just have this feeling of this hairy chest on my chest . . . like remembering him rubbing my chest . . . with his chest.

When the nurse diagnoses a silent reaction to a sexual trauma situation, the details of the incident should be discussed fully in order to start the process of resolving the incident into motion.

Discussion

In the limited number of research articles on the subject of the psychological components of the reaction of child victims to sexual offenses, the issues of victim participation and the child's personality structure are stressed. Abraham[4] discusses sexual trauma as a form of infantile sexual activity which is often desired by the child unconsciously. Bender and Blau[5] in their report on 16 cases in children between ages 5 and 12 state there is evidence that the child derived some emotional satisfaction from the experience and that the child in some cases was the initiator or seducer. In the follow-up of this group, Bender and Grugett[6] describe how children use charm in their role of seducer. Weiss et al.[7] report on the child's personality which favored the occurrence of the sexual activity. In contrast to these positions, Melanie Klein has stated that the experience of a seduction or rape by an adult may have serious effects on the child.[8]

In reviewing our data on child and adolescent victims, we have tried to avoid traditional ways of viewing the problem and instead to describe, from the victim's point of view, the dynamics involved between offender and victim regarding the issues of inability to consent, adaptive behavior, secrecy, and disclosure of the secret.

Our data matches that of Gagnon and Simon,[9] who discuss social network reactions and state that these may further complicate the child's reaction to disclosing the sexual activity. Our data clearly indicates that a syndrome of symptom reaction is the result of the pressure to keep the activity secret as well as the result of the disclosure. However, our data also shows that the child does react, in some way, to being involved in the sexual activity itself.

It may be speculated that there are many children with silent reaction to sexual trauma. The child who responds to the pressure to go along with the sexual activity with an adult may be viewed as showing adaptive response for survival in the environment. Case finding for this type of sexual child abuse will not be easy.

The study raises many questions. If the child goes along with the sexual activity and thus adapts to the situation, are there trauma effects? If so, is it the sexual component that is traumatizing to the developing personality or is it the threat of adult aggression and fear of disclosure and punishment?

What are the psychodynamic consequences when the sexual incident is not dealt with? Will the victim develop neurotic and personality defects? Will there be a lack of social controls or lack of adult identification? What does happen if the child is deprived of childhood experiences and overstimulated with fears, sexual activity, and aggression? What implications are there for the development of a concept of sexuality?

Only long-term study can begin to look at some of these areas. It is our hope that this data may encourage further in-depth exploration of the effects of the repetition of sexual trauma on the developing personalityg of the child, and the rights of children to their own sexual development.

REFERENCES

1. Burgess, A. W., and Holmstrom, L. L.: Rape trauma syndrome. *Am. J. Psychiatry*, 131:981-986, Sept., 1974.
2. Simmel, Georg: Soziologie, 1908. *The Sociology of George Simmel*, ed. and trans. by K. H. Wolff. New York, Free Press of Glencoe, 1950, p. 181.
3. Ibid, p. 334.
4. Abraham, Karl: *The Experiencing of Sexual Trauma as a Form of Sexual Activity*, 1907. Selected Papers, trans. by D. Bryon and A. Strachey. London, Hogarth Press, 1927, p. 47.
5. Bender, Lauretta and Blau, Abram: The reaction of children to sexual relations with adults. *Am J. Orthopsychiatry*, 7:500-518, Oct., 1937.
6. Bender, Lauretta and Grugett, A. E., Jr.: A follow-up report on children who had atypical sexual experience. *Am. J. Orthopsychiatry*, 22:825-837, 1952.
7. Weiss, Joseph, Rogers, Estelle, Darwin, Mirim and Dutton, Charles: A study of girl sex victims. *Psychiatric Quarterly*, 29:1-27, Jan., 1955.
8. Klein, Melanie: *The Psychoanalysis of Children*. London, Hogarth Press, 1932.
9. Gagnon, John, and Simon, William: The child molester: Surprising advice for worried parents. *Redbook*, February, 1969.

Chapter 8

SEXUAL ASSAULT CENTER EMERGENCY ROOM PROTOCOL: CHILD/ADOLESCENT PATIENTS

STAFF, SEXUAL ASSAULT CENTER
HARBORVIEW MEDICAL CENTER
SEATTLE, WASHINGTON

Information for All Involved With Patient

1. See immediately. Even though no physical trauma may be present, victims of sexual assault should receive high priority (immediately following acutely ill or injured patients).
2. Provide maximum support to parents as well as to the child/adolescent victim. Do not be judgmental nor allow emotional responses, e.g. anger or outrage, to interfere with providing optimal care.
3. Only those *directly* involved in care should talk with the patient; give the patient and parents your name and explain your role.
4. Do not discuss sexual assault cases with anyone without the consent of the parent or legal guardian and the patient, if an adolescent.
5. "Rape" and "sexual assault" are legal, not medical, terms. Do not use other than as "history of sexual assault."
6. The chart may be legal evidence. "Hearsay" statements from those who first see the child/adolescent may be admissible in court. All statements should be accurate, objective, and legible.

Emergency Room Personnel

1. Provide private facilities for the victim. Complete registration there.

2. Contact the emergency room physician immediately if there is evidence of moderate to severe physical trauma.
3. Obtain consent for care from the parents or legal guardian. If such consent cannot be obtained, contact the hospital administrator or the juvenile court for temporary consent. Examination of the adolescent should not be done without her/his consent unless a life-threatening emergency exists.
4. Contact social worker immediately.
5. If the assault occurred within the past 48 hours, contact the pediatric resident immediately. If the assault occurred more than 48 hours ago, the social worker will ascertain need for medical care.
6. The sexual assault tray and vaginal kit (containing Pedersen and pediatric specula) should be placed in examination room. (Check and replace items daily.)
7. Chaperone pelvic examination. A female chaperone (hospital employee) should be present for all pelvic examinations. Do not have the patient undress until just before the physical examination.

Social Worker

1. Assess immediate emotional needs of child and parents. Respond appropriately.
2. Confirm that the pediatric resident has been notified.
3. History: Obtain alone or in conjunction with the physician.

    (a) Ascertain as much of the history as possible from parents or accompanying persons first, away from patient.
    (b) See patient alone to obtain history (unless parent or other person is needed for support, i.e. in the very young child).
    (c) Determine and use the patient's terminology for parts of the body, sexual acts, etc. Use aids, i.e. toys and picture books, as needed. Questions should be appropriate for age and developmental level.
    (d) Obtain a directed history of the assault. Do not ask "why" questions, e.g. "Why did you go to his house?" Phrase the questions in terms of "who, what, where, when,"

e.g. "Did the offender use oral, finger, penile contact to mouth, vulva, vagina, rectum?" "How long ago did it happen?" "Did penetration or ejaculation occur?" "What kind of force, threat or enticement was used?" "From whom did the patient seek help?"

(e) When the physician arrives, present history and impressions (out of patient's hearing) and complete history-taking conjointly.

4. Explain to patient and parents the reasons for questions asked, types of medical/legal tests needed, and possible treatment.

5. Obtain special consents, i.e. for photographs, release of clothing, and release of information (specify to whom).

6. Assist with the physical examination, if indicated.

7. Discuss reporting to police and/or children's protective service. Police may be contacted to come to the emergency room for an initial report.

8. Assessment and counseling:
   (a) Assess behavior and affect. Ascertain support systems of patient and family. Do not return child home unless the environment is safe. Document changes in housing.
   (b) Explain anticipated emotional problems. Give patient and parents (Sexual Assault Center) SAC handout.
   (c) Encourage consulting with the Sexual Assault Center.

9. Record on Sexual Assault Report form services offered to patient:
   (a) Medical appointment for follow-up care.
   (b) Ongoing counseling or advocacy by SAC.
   (c) Children's protective service referral, when indicated. (Referral to CPS is legally mandated when the offender is a family member or when the home environment does not protect the child from further sexual abuse.)
   (d) Referrals made to other agencies.
   (e) Victim's compensation brochure, form, and brief explanation.

Physician

1. Medical History: Ascertain history from social worker and parents. Corroborate with patient. Do not needlessly repeat questions. Use "History of Sexual Assault" form.

   (a) Use vocabulary appropriate for age and developmental level. Use patient's words to describe and explain meaning if needed, i.e. "He put his 'thing' (penis) in me." Use picture books or toys as aids as needed.

   (b) Ascertain activity post-assault: changes of clothing; bathing; douching; urinating; defecating; drinking.

   (c) Obtain menstrual, contraceptive, VD history as needed.

   (d) Obtain pertinent medical history: chronic illnesses; allergies; etc.

   (e) Discuss VD prophylaxis, hormonal pregnancy prevention, and abortion. Ascertain patient's feelings in these areas.

2. Approach to Examination:

   (a) Be gentle and empathetic. Explain what you are doing in a calm manner and voice. Take time to relax the apprehensive patient.

   (b) If supportive, have parent stay with child during the examination. Allow the adolescent the option of having whom s/he wishes to be present.

   (c) Allow the patient to feel as much in control of his/her body during the examination as possible. Verbalize an understanding of his/her anxiety.

   (d) Use appropriate gowns and drapes to ensure modesty and decrease feelings of vulnerability.

   (e) Unless there is physical trauma that is apparent or must be ruled out, the complete examination does not need to be done, i.e. use of stirrups and speculum. All tests can be done with a glass pipette and cotton swabs.

   (1) A small child may lie across the mother's lap in a "frog-leg" position.

   (2) An older child may lie on the examination table in the same position.

(3) An adolescent may lie on the table in the same position or in stirrups.

(f) Use a *reasonable* approach. Use only those parts of the protocol appropriate for age of child and type of assault.

3. Physical Examination: Perform with hospital employee as chaperone.
   (a) General: Document emotional status, general appearance of patient and clothing.
   (b) Document areas of trauma on a diagram and•describe in detail.
   (c) Examine areas involved in sexual assault, i.e. oral, vaginal, rectal, or penile. Very carefully document even minor trauma to these areas. Photograph areas of trauma as indicated (per evidence collection checklist).
   (d) Ask patient to point with finger to exact area involved. Ask how much further offender penetrated.
   (e) Describe developmental level (Tanner Stage), external genitalia, type and condition of hymen, and diameter of introitus.
   (f) Do examination as indicated by age of patient, type of assault, and degree of injury. If injuries are extensive or cannot be determined due to lack of cooperation, consider examination and treatment under general anesthesia.

4. Medical Tests:
   (a) Culture body orifices involved for gonorrhea. If history is uncertain, culture all orifices.
   (b) Obtain gravindex to rule out pregnancy as indicated.
   (c) Obtain VDRL baseline. May be deferred in the young child or apprehensive adolescent.

5. Legal Tests:
   (a) UV light—semen fluoresces. Examine areas of body and clothing involved (in dark after visual adaptation).
       (1) Save clothing fluorescing for police (as per evidence collection checklist).
       (2) Swab body areas fluorescing with saline moistened swabs. Place swabs in red top tubes. (Follow evidence collection checklist.)

(b) Wet mount preparation:
  (1) Aspirate or swab areas of body involved (pharynx, rectum, vaginal pool). Saline moistened swabs may be used; however, aspiration with a glass pipette after flushing area with 2 cc of saline is preferred.
  (2) Place drop of secretions on glass slide, plus drop of saline; examine immediately.
  (3) Physician should examine several fields under high power with light source turned down. Document presence or absence of sperm and number of motile/nonmotile seen per high power field.
(c) Permanent smears:
  (1) Physician will make two preparations. One slide will be a routine PAP from the endocervix and vaginal wall areas (may be deferred in child). The second slide will be a smear from the posterior vaginal pool, rectum, pharynx as indicated. Obtain in the same manner as the wet mount.
  (2) Put both slides promptly into the PAP bottle, back to back.
    Do not allow to air dry. (Follow evidence collection checklist.)
  (3) Physician will complete and sign PAP form noting "History of Sexual Assault; please do routine PAP and document presence or absence of sperm."
(d) Acid Phosphatase:
  (1) Collect in same manner as for wet mount preparation.
  (2) Place saline moistened swabs or secretions from pipette in red top tube. (Follow evidence collection checklist.)
(e) Other tests—as indicated or as police request (mainly to identify assailant), i.e. ABO antigens (collect as for acid phosphatase); fingernail scrapings; pubic hair combings.
6. Treatment:
  (a) Injuries—treat and/or consult with other specialities as indicated. Give tetanus prophylaxis as indicated by history; follow CDC-Public Health recommendations

(available in ER).

(b) Pregnancy prophylaxis—may be given *if* a vaginal assault occurred at mid-cycle, without contraception, and patient understands risks and side effects of estrogens to be given and is willing to have an abortion should pregnancy occur despite medication. *Do not prescribe* if there has been other unprotected intercourse during this cycle or any possibility of pre-existing pregnancy. Obtain a negative gravindex before instituting therapy.

　　(1) Hormonal therapy—Estinyl®: 2.5 mg b.i.d. for 5 days OR stilbesterol: 25 mgm b.i.d. for 5 days.

　　(2) Antinauseant therapy—Bendectin® (ii h.s. as needed for nausea and vomiting). Give routinely to use as needed.

(c) VD prophylaxis

　　(1) Not given routinely but as indicated, e.g. high patient anxiety, possibility patient will not return for follow-up care, known disease, or multiple rapists.

　　(2) Therapy (over 12 years of age):

　　　　(a) Probenecid® 1 gm orally + Ampillin® 3.5 gm orally stat; OR

　　　　(b) Probenecid 1 gm orally followed in 20 minutes by procaine penicillin G 4.8 million units im; or

　　　　(c) If penicillin allergy, spectinomycin 4 gm im or tetracycline 500 mgm q.i.d. × 4 days.

　　(3) Therapy (under 12 years of age): use age and weight appropriate dosages.

(d) Treatment for anxiety and/or difficulty sleeping—as indicated (rarely needed in children under 12 years; use age appropriate dosage when given). Adult therapy as follows:

　　(1) Mellaril® 10 mgm one-half hour before sleep (may repeat once, if necessary; do not exceed 20 mgm/day. Give a 3-day supply (60 mgm); OR

      (2) Valium® 5 mgm one-half hour before sleep (may repeat once p.r.n.). Do not exceed 10 mgm/day. Give 3-day supply (30 mgm).

7. Final Care
   (a) Verbally express concern and availability for help as needed.
   (b) Reinforce social worker information; reinforce that patient is physically intact and is not responsible for the assault/abuse.
   (c) Discuss medical problems that may arise and encourage family to call as needed.

8. Final Diagnosis
   (a) History of Sexual Assault.
   (b) Presence or absence of sperm.
   (c) Specific diagnosis of injuries, contusions, lacerations, etc.
   (d) Other pertinent medical diagnoses.

9. Follow-up
   (a) Pediatric clinic appointment in one week.
   (b) Repeat gonorrhea cultures at follow-up visit; VDRL in 8 weeks; other as indicated.
   (c) Consultation from other specialties as indicated.

INCEST

". . . in the U.S. today, there are a great many cultural factors, especially illegality and censure by society, which work to make such child-adult sex relationships damaging even though there may be nothing essentially damaging in them. That we are presently paying a higher price than need be for protecting children from sexual exploitation is probable: If we ever care enough to give the matter thorough study, we probably can give as much or more protection while reducing emotional penalties which may fall as heavily on the child as on adult participant in these cases."

R. Masters: *Sex Driven People*. Los Angeles, Sherbourne, 1966, p. 118

Chapter 9

INCEST—INTRODUCTION

LeRoy G. Schultz

Incest represents the most time honored problem in Western civilization. No generation has successfully come to grips with it. However, it has fallen on new times. Giving it a new perspective are several social forces: the re-emergence of the feminist movement, the new childrens/adolescent rights movement, and national attention and focus on child abuse in general. Next to child rape, incest incites the most outrage, hysteria, and counter-aggression in adults. Part of this springs from the lack of knowledge about incest, or research-produced knowledge, and an abundance of folklore, superstitition, and simple ignorance. Paradoxically, "getting even" with the incest perpetrator or convicting him draws into motion a series of actors' behaviors from the victim's social space that can transform a benign sexual event, in the victim's perception, into a traumatic situation. Professionals have little to guide them in deciding on what cases to leave alone. In some instances they have no choice but to report it to some authority under the child abuse law. Such a criteria is presently needed. Universal condemnation of incest with older adolescents (ages 14 and up) can no longer be counted upon from families or professionals. Some researchers, social workers, psychiatrists, and incest participants are challenging the conventional wisdom that has characterized society's attitude and reaction to incest. Social scientists' and various moralists' views on incest are as numerous as there are viewers; the common man is beset by baffling problems in distinction and choice. He may only have a weakly supported taboo from yesteryear to guide him. There are numerous theories given by "authorities" of both religion and science as to what causes incest. Among them are individual character defect in incest perpetrator, mental retar-

93

dation in participants, general immaturity, poor judgment, sexism, sexual dysfunction in wives, natural evilness, changing economics, a fanatically family-centered society, and a sensate focused society, to name a few. Participants are not so esoteric in motivation: whether knowing causes can shape solutions has not been raised as a question to date. Only recently have various "authorities" raised the prospect that some types of incest may be either a positive-healthy experience or at worse, neutral and dull, with perhaps one-third of sample cases indicating some post-incest adjustment problems. Extensive research on this aspect is required and is in progress. Whether such research findings (supporting positive or neutral reactions) will influence family's and children's policy in this country is in doubt, since entrenched values are not easily reached by research findings of a contrary nature. Another problemsome area is the question of post-offense "trauma"; does it occur in all victims, despite age, type of relationship to offender, length of relationship, etc.? The professional choice of the word *trauma* may be a misleading one. Actually, *trauma* is a word that evolved from physical medicine and later in history was transferred to the mental functions of human beings. It was used by earlier psychiatrists and social workers only as a metaphor, but more recently has been projected into the social and psychological, as if it were a physical, life-threatening injury, without more than hearsay justification. Another semantic problem centers on the word *victim*, a form of verbal overkill. It is used to describe all manner and degree of traditional pain and suffering. Today, professionals speak of victims of loneliness, divorce, old age, childhood, acne, left-handedness, a first sexual experience, and masturbation, just to name a recent few. In short, if we define every kind of experience as being victimogenic, then we artificially create a new generation of victims in a self-fulfilling charade. Iatrogenesis has not been seriously examined by any of the helping professions. To what extent are current approaches to the incest victim themselves traumatogenic? Depending upon one's choice of evidence or indicators, one's political leaning, the professional degree the holder has, and the period of history during which one graduated, the size and severity of the incest trauma can be seen as

producing guilt-induced incapacities, creating neurosis or psychosis, creating drug addicts and prostitutes, inducing sexual
precocity, supporting lesbianism, and turning out child porno
stars, or whatever the current professional "hype" will support.
The "research" upon which such suppositions regarding cause
and effect are based are nonexistent or very weak at best. Some
reflect a gross violation of simple research principles. What may
be likely is that the professions use their resources to "cloak with
science" the current moral or political position. What is so
outrageous is that being made aware of professionals' interpretation of incest experiences creates, for participants, a concern
to work out whether these imputations may in fact be true. In the
absence of someone to invalidate these possibilities, such versions
may be incorporated into the process of becoming a victim, with
subsequent self-doubt and insecurity.

Most of the "research" regarding incest ends up being rhetori-
cally manipulative, abounding in cliches and myths. So power-
fully have these myths been propagated and received that to
question them is to invite abuse and disbelief. It is as if these
incest "findings" were beyond dispute and that the ultimate test
had been conducted. Many of the studies confuse moral damage
with psychological damage. Such finality is indefensible to the
open-minded. The literature does not support a causal relationship between incest and any single piece of pre- or post-incest
behavior, yet policy and practice assume such a relationship.

Part of the solution to the incest problem centers on two issues
society steadfastly refuses to address but which must be faced. Our
obsession with the sanctity and privacy of the family, while
having some justification, if carried too far is a major barrier to
adequate incest-controlling policy. Until families stop treating
children like property or objects, some governmental intrusion
into family life is essential for some children and adolescents.
Second, we refuse to readdress in each generation the changing
"age of consent" question. While we are able on the one hand to
admit to children's need for sexual response, with the other hand
we slap the emerging child down for asserting his sexual freedom.
While pro-genital one way, we are anti-sexual in others. At what
age is a person capable of making his own sexual decisions and

with whom? We seldom ask the children or adolescents. We try to prevent persons from making mistakes, or becoming victims of their own mistakes, but seldom do we protect them from the mistaken intentions of others. The "for your own good" argument weakens in direct proportion to age increments. Ageism is like racism and sexism. As the age of majority creeps downward (the iron age of twenty-one years was split in the early 1970s), each children's age group must prove its capabilities to a doubting adult group of powerholders, even though children cannot vote. The determination of the capabilities of different age groups is a job for researchers first, and the legislation should follow. Much of our opposition relates not so much to ageism as it does to our lack of integrating normal sexual expression in our lives throughout the age spectrum.

The four chapters in this section attempt to address some of these issues. The Herman-Hirschman contribution introduces the new feminist perspective on incest, and reports findings on fifteen cases of incest "after the fact." They end their chapter with sensible recommendations.

Yorukoglu and Kemph report on two cases of incest in which damages could not be found. This is a courageous piece of research, and despite twitterings of professional hostility was published. It is rare kind of research in that it flies directly into professional sacred cows and the conventional wisdom, in its need to individualize each case. If the chapter does nothing else, it gets us off the dead center of evaluating all incest victims homogenously.

Giarretto has developed a prototype or effective mode of treatment of one type of incest, that of father-daughter. It offers the beginning for therapists to model or from which to branch out into different approaches to meet different types of victim situations. With so many modes of therapy abounding, it may be just a matter of time before such modes are adapted to the incest situation.

The final chapter deals with policy problems and prospects for addressing the incest problem and raises many uncomfortable and costly issues facing those in the fight for children's rights.

Chapter 10

FATHER-DAUGHTER INCEST

Judith Herman and Lisa Hirschman

A Feminist Theoretical Perspective

The incest taboo is universal in human culture. Though it varies from one culture to another, it is generally considered by anthropologists to be the foundation of all kinship structures. Lévi-Strauss describes it as the basic social contract; Mead says its purpose is the preservation of the human social order.[1] All cultures, including our own, regard violations of the taboo with horror and dread. Death has not been considered too extreme a punishment in many societies. In our laws, some states punish incest by up to twenty years' imprisonment.[2]

In spite of the strength of the prohibition on incest, sexual relations between family members do occur. Because of the extreme secrecy which surrounds the violation of our most basic sexual taboo, we have little clinical literature and no accurate statistics on the prevalence of incest. This chapter attempts to review what is known about the occurrence of incest between parents and children, to discuss common social attitudes which pervade the existing clinical literature, and to offer a theoretical perspective which locates the incest taboo and its violations within the structure of patriarchy.

*From *Journal of Women in Culture and Society* 1977, vol. 2, no. 4: 735-756. © 1977 by The University of Chicago. All rights reserved.

The authors gratefully acknowledge the contributions of the incest victims themselves and of the therapists who shared their experience with us. For reasons of confidentiality, we cannot thank them by name.

1. Claude Lévi-Strauss, *The Elementary Structures of Kinship* (Boston: Beacon Press, 1969), p. 481; Margaret Mead, "Incest," in *International Encyclopedia of the Social Sciences*, ed. David L. Sills (New York: Crowell, Collier & Macmillan, 1968).

2. Herbert Maisch, *Incest* (London: Andre Deutsch, 1973), p. 69.

The Occurrence of Incest

The Children's Division of the American Humane Association estimates that a minimum of 80,000-100,000 children are sexually molested each year.[3] In the majority of these cases, the offender is well known to the child, and in about 25 percent of them, a relative. These estimates are based on New York City police records and the experience of social workers in a child protection agency. They are, therefore, projections based on observing poor and disorganized families who lack the resources to preserve secrecy. There is reason to believe, however, that most incest in fact occurs in intact families and entirely escapes the attention of social agencies. One in sixteen of the 8,000 white, middle-class women surveyed by Kinsey et al. reported sexual contact with an adult relative during childhood.[4] In the vast majority of these cases, the incident remained a secret.

A constant finding in all existing surveys is the overwhelming predominance of father-daughter incest. Weinberg, in a study of 200 court cases in the Chicago area, found 164 cases of father-daughter incest, compared with two cases of mother-son incest.[5] Maisch, in a study of court cases in the Federal Republic of Germany, reported that 90 percent of the cases involved fathers and daughters, step-fathers and step-daughters, or (infrequently) grandfathers and granddaughters.[6] Fathers and sons accounted for another 5 percent. Incest between mothers and sons occurred in only 4 percent of the cases. Incest appears to follow the general pattern of sexual abuse of children, in which 92 percent of the victims are female, and 97 percent of the offenders are male.[7]

It may be objected that these data are all based on court records and perhaps reflect only a difference in complaints rather than a difference in incidence. The Kinsey reports, however, confirm the impression of a major discrepancy between the childhood sexual

3. Vincent De Francis, ed., *Sexual Abuse of Children* (Denver: Children's Division of the American Humane Association, 1967).

4. Alfred Kinsey, W. B. Pomeroy, C. E. Martin, and P. Gebhard, *Sexual Behavior in the Human Female* (Philadelphia: Saunders & Co., 1953), pp. 116-22.

5. S. Kirson Weinberg, *Incest Behavior* (New York: Citadel Press, 1955).

6. See n. 2 above.

7. De Francis.

contacts of boys and girls. If, as noted above, more than 6 percent of the female sample reported sexual approaches by adult relatives, only a small number of the 12,000 men surveyed reported sexual contact with any adult, relative or stranger. (Exact figures were not reported.) Among these few, contact with adult males seemed to be more common than with adult females. As for mother-son incest, the authors concluded that "hetero-sexual incest occurs more frequently in the thinking of clinicians and social workers than it does in actual performance."[8] None of the existing literature, to our knowledge, makes any attempt to account for this striking discrepancy between the occurrence of father-daughter and mother-son incest.

Common Attitudes toward Incest in the Professional Literature

Because the subject of incest inspires such strong emotional responses, few authors have even attempted a dispassionate examination of its actual occurrence and effects. Those who have approached the subject have often been unable to avoid defensive reactions such as denial, distancing, or blaming. We undertake this discussion with the full recognition that we ourselves are not immune to these reactions, which may be far more apparent to our readers than to ourselves.

Undoubtedly the most famous and consequential instance of denial of the reality of incest occurs in Freud's 1897 letter to Fliess. In it, Freud reveals the process by which he came to disbelieve the reports of his female patients and develop his concepts of infantile sexuality and the infantile neurosis: "Then there was the astonishing thing that in every case blame was laid on perverse acts by the father, and realization of the unexpected frequency of hysteria, in every case of which the same thing applied, though it was hardly credible that perverted acts against children were so general."[9]

---

8. Alfred C. Kinsey, W. B. Pomeroy, and Clyde Martin, *Sexual Behavior in the Human Male* (Philadelphia: Saunder & Co., 1948), pp. 167, 558.

9. Freud, *The Origins of Psychoanalysis: Letters to Wilhelm Fliess, Drafts and Notes: 1887-1902* (New York: Basic Books, 1954), p. 215.

Freud's conclusion that the sexual approaches did not occur in fact was based simply on his unwillingness to believe that incest was such a common event in respectable families. To experience a sexual approach by a parent probably *was* unlikely for a boy: Freud concluded incorrectly that the same was true for girls. Rather than investigate further into the question of fact, Freud's followers chose to continue the presumption of fantasy and made the child's desire and fantasy the focus of psychological inquiry. The adult's desire (and capacity for action) were forgotten. Psychoanalytic investigation, then, while it placed the incest taboo at the center of the child's psychological development, did little to dispel the secrecy surrounding the actual occurrence of incest. As one child psychiatrist commented:

> Helene Deutsch and other followers of Freud have, in my opinion, gone too far in the direction of conceptualizing patients' reports of childhood sexual abuse in terms of fantasy. My own experience, both in private practice and with several hundred child victims brought to us . . . [at the Center for Rape Concern] . . . in Philadelphia, has convinced me that analysts too often dismissed as fantasy what was the real sexual molestation of a child. . . . As a result, the victim was isolated and her trauma compounded.[10]

Even those investigators who have paid attention to cases of actual incest have often shown a tendency to comment or make judgments concerning the guilt or innocence of the participants. An example:

> These children undoubtedly do not deserve completely the cloak of innocence with which they have been endowed by moralists, social reformers, and legislators. The history of the relationship in our cases usually suggests at least some cooperation of the child in the activity, and in some cases the child assumed an active role in initiating the relationship. . . . It is true that the child often rationalized with excuses of fear of physical harm or the enticement of gifts, but there were obviously secondary reasons. Even in the cases where physical force may have been

---

10.   Joseph Peters, "Letter to the Editor," *New York Times Book Review* (November 16, 1975).

applied by the adult, this did not wholly account for the frequent repetition of the practice.

Finally, a most striking feature was that these children were distinguished as unusually charming and attractive in their outward personalities. Thus, it was not remarkable that frequently we considered the possibility that the child might have been the actual seducer, rather than the one innocently seduced.[11]

In addition to denial and blame, much of the existing literature on incest shows evidence of social and emotional distancing between the investigators and their subjects. This sometimes takes the form of an assertion that incestuous behavior is accepted or condoned in some culture other than the investigator's own. Thus, a British study of Irish working-class people reports that father-daughter incest, which occurred in 4 percent of an unselected outpatient clinic population, was a "cultural phenomenon" precipitated by social isolation or crowding, and had "no pathological effects."[12] The several investigators who have also reported instances where children, in their judgment, were not harmed by the incest experience do not usually state the criteria on which this judgment is based.[13] Still other investigators seem fearful to commit themselves to an opinion on the question of harm. Thus, for example, although 70 percent of the victims in Maisch's survey showed evidence of disturbed personality development, the author is uncertain about ascribing this to the effects of incest per se.

A few investigators, however, have testified to the destructive effects of the incest experience on the development of the child. Sloane and Karpinski, who studied five incestuous families in rural Pennsylvania, conclude: "Indulgence in incest in the postadolescent period leads to serious repercussions in the girl, even in an environment where the moral standards are relaxed."[14]

---

11. L. Bender and A. Blau, "The Reaction of Children to Sexual Relations with Adults," *American Journal of Orthopsychiatry* 7 (1937): 500-518.

12. N. Lukianowitz, "Incest," *British Journal of Psychiatry* 120 (1972): 301-13.

13. Yokoguchi, "Children Not Severely Damaged by Incest with a Parent," *Journal of the American Academy of Child Psychiatry* 5 (1966): 111-24; J. B. Weiner, "Father-Daughter Incest," *Psychiatric Quarterly* 36 (1962): 1132-38.

14. P. Sloane and E. Karpinski, "Effects of Incest on the Participants," *American Journal of Orthopsychiatry* 12 (1942): 666-73.

Kaufman, Peck, and Tagiuri, in a thorough study of eleven victims and their families who were seen at a Boston clinic, report: "Depression and guilt were universal as clinical findings. ... The underlying craving for an adequate parent...dominated the lives of these girls."[15]

Several retrospective studies, including a recent report by Benward and Densen-Gerber, document a strong association between reported incest history and the later development of pomiscuity or prostitution.[16] In fact, failure to marry or promiscuity seems to be the only criterion generally accepted in the literature as conclusive evidence that the victim has been harmed.[17] We believe that this finding in itself testifies to the traditional bias which pervades the incest literature.

Our survey of what has been written about incest, then, raises several questions. Why does incest between fathers and daughers occur so much more frequently than incest between mothers and sons? Why, though this finding has been consistently documented in all available sources, has no previous attempt been made to explain it? Why does the incest victim find so little attention or compassion in the literature, while she finds so many authorities who are willing to assert either that the incest did not happen, that it did not harm her, or that she was to blame for it? We believe that a feminist perspective must be invoked in order to address these questions.

Incest and Patriarchy

In a patriarchal culture, such as our own, the incest taboo must have a different meaning for the two sexes and may be observed by men and women for different reasons.

Major theorists in the disciplines of both psychology and anthropology explain the importance of the incest taboo by

---

15. I. Kaufman, A. Peck, and L. Tagiuri, "The Family Constellation and Overt Incestuous Relations between Father and Daughter," *American Journal of Orthopsychiatry* 24 (1954): 266-79.

16. J. Benward and J. Densen-Gerber, *Incest as a Causative Factor in Anti-social Behavior: An Exploratory Study* (New York: Odyssey Institute, 1975).

17. Weinberg.

placing it at the center of an agreement to control warfare among men. It represents the first and most basic peace treaty. An essential element of the agreement is the concept that women are the possessions of men; the incest taboo represents an agreement as to how women shall be shared. Since virtually all known societies are dominated by men, all versions of the incest taboo are agreements among men regarding sexual access to women. As Mitchell points out, men create rules governing the exchange of women; women do not create rules governing the exchange of men.[18] Because the taboo is created and enforced by men, we argue that it may also be more easily and frequently violated by men.

The point at which the child learns the meaning of the incest taboo is the point of initiation into the social order. Boys and girls, however, learn different versions of the taboo. To paraphrase Freud once again, the boy learns that he may not consummate his sexual desires for his mother because his mother belongs to his father, and his father has the power to inflict the most terrible of punishments on him: to deprive him of his maleness.[19] In compensation, however, the boy learns that when he is a man he will one day possess women of his own.

When this little boy grows up, he will probably marry and may have a daughter. Although custom will eventually oblige him to give away his daughter in marriage to another man (note that mothers do not give away either daughters or sons), the taboo against sexual contact with his daughter will never carry the same force, either psychologically or socially, as the taboo which prohibited incest with his mother. *There is no punishing father to avenge father-daughter incest.*

What the little girl learns is not at all parallel. Her initiation into the patriarchal order begins with the realization that she is not only comparatively powerless as a child, but that she will remain so as a woman. She may acquire power only indirectly, as the favorite of a powerful man. As a child she may not possess her mother *or* her father; when she is an adult, her best hope is to *be* possessed by someone like her father. Thus, according to Freud

---

18. Juliet Mitchell, *Psychoanalysis and Feminism* (New York: Pantheon Books, 1974).
19. Freud, *Three Essays on the Theory of Sexuality* (New York: Avon Books, 1962).

she has less incentive than the boy to come to a full resolution of the Oedipus complex.[20] Since she has no hope of acquiring the privileges of an adult male, she can neither be rewarded for giving up her incestuous attachments, nor punished for refusing to do so. Chesler states the same conclusion more bluntly: "Women are encouraged to commit incest as a way of life. . . . As opposed to marrying our fathers, we marry men like our fathers . . . men who are older than us, have more money than us, more power than us, are taller than us, are stronger than us . . . our fathers."[21]

A patriarchal society, then, most abhors the idea of incest between mother and son, because this is an affront to the father's prerogatives. Though incest between father and daughter is also forbidden, the prohibition carries considerably less weight and is, therefore, more frequently violated. We believe this understanding of the asymmetrical nature of the incest taboo under patriarchy offers an explanation for the observed difference in the occurrence of mother-son and father-daughter incest.

If, as we propose, the taboo on father-daughter incest is relatively weak in a patriarchal family system, we might expect violations of the taboo to occur most frequently in families characterized by extreme paternal dominance. This is in fact the case. Incest offenders are frequently described as "family tyrants":

> These fathers, who are often quite incapable of relating their despotic claim to leadership to their social efforts for the family, tend toward abuses of authority of every conceivable kind, and they not infrequently endeavor to secure their dominant position by socially isolating the members of the family from the world outside. Swedish, American, and French surveys have pointed time and again to the patriarchal position of such fathers, who set up a "primitive family order."[22]

Thus the seduction of daughters is an abuse which is inherent in a father-dominated family system; we believe that the greater the

20. Freud, "Some Psychical Consequences of the Anatomical Distinction between the Sexes" (1925), "Female Sexuality" (1931), and "Femininity" (1933), all reprinted in *Women and Analysis*, ed. Jean Strouse (New York: Viking Press, 1974).
21. Phyllis Chesler, "Rape and Psychotherapy," in *Rape: The First Sourcebook for Women*, ed. Noreen Connell and Cassandra Wilson (New York: New American Library, 1974), p. 76.
22. Maisch, p. 140. See n. 2 above.

degree of male supremacy in any culture, the greater the likelihood of father-daughter incest.

A final speculative point: since, according to this formulation, women neither make nor enforce the incest taboo, why is it that women apparently observe the taboo so scrupulously? We do not know. We suspect that the answer may lie in the historic experience of women both as sexual property and as the primary caretakers of children. Having been frequently obliged to exchange sexual services for protection and care, women are in a position to understand the harmful effects of introducing sex into a relationship where there is a vast inequality of power. And, having throughout history been assigned the primary responsibility for the care of children, women may be in a position to understand more fully the needs of children, the difference between affectionate and erotic contact, and the appropriate limits of parental love.

A Clinical Report

The following is a clinical case study of fifteen victims of father-daughter incest. All the women were clients in psychotherapy who reported their incest experiences to their therapists after the fact. Seven were women whom the authors had personally evaluated or seen in psychotherapy. The remaining eight were clients in treatment with other therapists. No systematic case-finding effort was made; the authors simply questioned those practitioners who were best known to us through an informal network of female professionals. Four out of the first ten therapists we questioned reported that at least one of her clients had an incest history. We concluded from this admittedly small sample that a history of incest is frequently encountered in clinical practice.

Our combined group of six therapists (the authors and our four informants) had interviewed close to 1,000 clients in the past five years. In this population, the incidence of reported father-daughter incest was 2-3 percent. We believe this to be a minimum estimate, since in most cases no particular effort was made to elicit the history. Our estimate accords with the data of the Kinsey report,[23] in which 1.5 percent of the women surveyed stated that they had been molested by their fathers.

For the purposes of this study, we defined incest as overt sexual contact such as fondling, petting, masturbation, or intercourse between parent and child. We included only those cases in which there was no doubt in the daughter's mind that explicit and intentionally sexual contact occurred and that secrecy was required. Thus we did not include in our study the many women who reported seductive behaviors such as verbal sharing of sexual secrets, flirting, extreme possessiveness or jealousy, or intense interest in their bodies or their sexual activities on the part of their fathers. We recognize that these cases represent the extreme of a continuum of father-daughter relationships which range from the affectionate through the seductive to the overtly sexual. Information about the incest history was initially gathered from the therapists. Those clients who were willing to discuss their experiences with us in person were then interviewed directly.

The fifteen women who reported that they had been molested during childhood were in other respects quite ordinary women. Nothing obvious distinguished them from the general population of women entering psychotherapy (see Table 10-I). They ranged in age from fifteen to fifty-five. Most were in their early twenties at the time they first requested psychotherapy. They were all white. Four were single, seven married, and four separated or divorced. Half had children. The majority had at least some college education. They worked at common women's jobs: housewife, waitress, factory worker, office worker, prostitute, teacher, nurse. They complained mostly of depression and social isolation. Those who were married or recently separated complained of marital problems. The severity of their complaints seemed to be related to the degree of family disorganization and deprivation in their histories rather than to the incest history per se. Five of the women had been hospitalized at some point in their lives; three were or had been actively suicidal, and two were addicted to drugs or alcohol. Seven women brought up the incest history among their initial complaints; the rest revealed it only

---

23. Kinsey et al. (n. 4 above), p. 121.

after having established a relationship with the therapist. In some cases, the history was not disclosed for one, two, or even three years after therapy had begun.

TABLE 10-I

CHARACTERISTICS OF INCEST VICTIMS ENTERING THERAPY

Characteristic	Victims (N)
Age (years):	
15-20	3
21-25	7
26-30	2
30+	3
Marital Status:	
Single	4
Married	7
Separated or divorced	4
Occupation:	
Blue collar	4
White collar	4
Professional	3
Houseworker	1
Student	3
Education:	
High school not completed	4
High school completed	2
1-2 years college	3
College completed	5
Advanced degree	1
Presenting complaints:	
Marital problems	5
Depression	3
Anxiety	3
Social isolation	4
Drug or alcohol abuse	4
Suicide attempt	2

The incest histories were remarkably similar (see Table 10-II). The majority of the victims were oldest or only daughters and were between the ages of six and nine when they were first approached sexually by their fathers or male guardians (nine fathers, three stepfathers, a grandfather, a brother-in-law, and an uncle). The youngest girl was four years old; the oldest fourteen. The sexual contact usually took place repeatedly. In most cases the incestuous relationship lasted three years or more. Physical force was not used, and intercourse was rarely attempted with girls who had not reached puberty; the sexual contact was limited to masturbation and fondling. In three cases, the relationship was terminated when the father attempted intercourse.

TABLE 10-II
CHARACTERISTICS OF THE INCEST HISTORY

Characteristic	Incidence
Daughter's place in sibship:	
Oldest daughter	9
Only daughter	3
Middle or youngest daughter	1
Unknown	2
Daughter's age at onset of incestuous relationship (years):	
4	1
5	0
6	2
7	3
8	4
9	2
10	0
11	1
12	0
13	0
14	1
Unknown	1
Duration of incestuous relationship (years):	
Single incident	1
1-2	1
3-4	3
5-6	5
7-10	2
Unknown	3

LENORE: I had already started to develop breasts at age nine and had my period when I was eleven. All this time he's still calling me into bed for "little chats" with him. I basically trusted him although I felt funny about it. Then one time I was twelve or thirteen, he called me into bed and started undressing me. He gave this rationale about preparing me to be with boys. He kept saying I was safe as long as I didn't let them take my pants down. Meantime he was doing the same thing. I split. I knew what he was trying to do, and that it was wrong. That was the end of the overt sexual stuff. Not long after that he found an excuse to beat me.

In all but two of these fifteen cases the sexual relationship between father and daughter remained a secret, and there was no intervention in the family by the courts or child-protection authorities. Previous studies are based on court referrals and therefore give the erroneous impression that incest occurs predominantly in families at the lower end of the socioeconomic scale. This was not the case in the families of our victims. Of these, four fathers were blue-collar workers, two were white-collar workers, six were professionals, and the occupations of three were not known. The fathers' occupations cut across class lines. Several held jobs that required considerable personal competence and commanded social respect: college administrator, policeman, army officer, engineer. Others were skilled workers, foremen, or managers in factories or offices. All the mothers were houseworkers. Five of the fifteen families could certainly be considered disorganized, with histories of poverty, unemployment, frequent moves, alcoholism, violence, abandonment and foster care. Not surprisingly, the women who came from these families were those who complained of the most severe distress. The majority of the families, however, were apparently intact and maintained a facade of respectability.

The Incestuous Family Constellation

Both the apparently intact and the disorganized families shared certain common features in the pattern of family relationships. The most striking was the almost uniform estrangement of the mother and daughter, an estrangement that preceded the occurrence of overt incest. Over half the mothers were partially incapacitated by physical or mental illness or alcoholism and either assumed an invalid role within the home or were periodically absent because of hospitalization. Their oldest daughters were often obliged to take over the household duties. Anne-Marie remembered being hidden from the truant officer by her mother so that she could stay home and take care of the younger children. Her mother had tuberculosis. Claire's mother, who was not ill, went to work to support the family because her father, a severe alcoholic, brought home no money. In her absence, Claire did the housework and cooking and cared for her older brother.

At best, these mothers were seen by their daughters as helpless, frail, downtrodden victims, who were unable to take care of themselves, much less to protect their children.

> ANNE-MARIE: She used to say "give with one hand and you'll get with the other" but she gave with two hands and always went down. . . . She was nothing but a floor mat. She sold out herself and her self-respect. She was a love slave to my father.
> CLAIRE: I always felt sorry for her. She spent her life suffering, suffering, suffering.

Some of the mothers habitually confided in their oldest daughters and unburdened their troubles to them. Theresa felt her mother was "more like a sister." Joan's mother frequently clung to her and told her, "You're the only one who understands me." By contrast, the daughters felt unable to confide in their mothers. In particular, the daughters felt unable to go to their mothers for support or protection once their fathers had begun to make sexual advances to them. Some feared that their mothers would take action to expel the father from the house, but more commonly these daughters expected that their mothers would do nothing; in many cases the mothers tolerated a great deal of abuse themselves, and the daughters had learned not to expect any protection. Five of the women said they suspected that their mothers knew about the incest and tacitly condoned it. Two made attempts to bring up the subject but were put off by their mothers' denial or indifference.

Only two of the fifteen women actually told their mothers. Both had reason to regret it. Paula's mother reacted by committing her to an institution: "She was afraid I would become a lesbian or a whore." Sandra's mother initially took her husband to court. When she realized that a conviction would lead to his imprisonment, she reversed her testimony and publicly called her twelve-year-old daughter a "notorious liar and slut."

The message that these mothers transmitted over and over to their daughters was: your father first, you second. It is dangerous to fight back, for if I lose him I lose everything. For my own survival I must leave you to your own devices. I cannot defend you, and if necessary I will sacrifice you to your father.

At worst, the mother-daughter relations were marked by frank and open hostility. Some of the daughters stated they could remember no tenderness or caring in the relationship.

> MARTHA: She's always picking on me. She's so fuckin' cold.
> PAULA: She's an asshole. I really don't like my mom. I guess I am bitter. She's very selfish. She did a lousy job of bringing me up.

The most severe disruption in the mother-daughter relationship occurred in Rita's case. She remembers receiving severe beatings from her mother, and her father intervening to rescue her. Though the physical attacks were infrequent, Rita recalls her mother as implacably hostile and critical, and her father as by far the more nurturant parent.

Previous studies of incestuous families document the disturbance in the mother-daughter relationship as a constant finding.[24] In a study of eleven girls who were referred by courts to a child guidance center, Kaufman et al. reported that the girls uniformly saw their mothers as cruel, unjust and depriving, while the fathers were seen much more ambivalently: "These girls had long felt abandoned by the mother as a protective adult. This was their basic anxiety. . . . Though the original sexual experience with the father was at a genital level, the meaning of the sexual act was pregenital, and seemed to have the purpose of receiving some sort of parental interest."[25]

In contrast, almost all the victims expressed some warm feelings toward their fathers. Many described them in much more favorable terms than their mothers. Some examples:

> ANNE-MARIE: A handsome devil.
> THERESA: Good with kids. An honest, decent guy.

---

24. Maisch. See n. 2 above.
25. Kaufman et al., p. 270. See n. 15 above.

LENORE: He was my confidant.
RITA: My savior.

Although it may seem odd to have expressed such attitudes toward blatantly authoritarian fathers, there are explanations. These were men whose presentation to the outside world made them liked and often respected members of the community. The daughters responded to their fathers' social status and power and derived satisfaction from being their fathers' favorites. They were "daddy's special girls," and often they were special to no one else. Feelings of pity for the fathers were also common, especially where the fathers had lost social status. The daughters seemed much more willing to forgive their fathers' failings and weaknesses than to forgive their mothers, or themselves.

SANDRA: He was a sweet, decent man. My mother ruined him. I saw him lying in his bed in the hospital, and I kept thinking why don't they let him die. When he finally did, everyone cried at the funeral but me. I was glad he was dead. He had a miserable life. He had nothing. No one cared, not even me. I didn't help him much.

The daughters not only felt themselves abandoned by their mothers, but seemed to perceive their fathers as likewise deserted, and they felt the same pity for their fathers as they felt for themselves.

The victims rarely expressed anger toward their fathers, even about the incestuous act itself. Two of the three women who did express anger were women who had been repeatedly beaten as well as sexually abused by their fathers. Not surprisingly, they were angrier about the beatings than about the sexual act, which they viewed ambivalently. Most women expressed feelings of fear, disgust, and intense shame about the sexual contact and stated that they endured it because they felt they had no other choice. Several of the women stated that they learned to deal with the sexual approach by "tuning out" or pretending that it was not happening. Later, this response generalized to other relationships. Half of the women acknowledged, however, that they had felt some degree of pleasure in the sexual contact, a feeling which only increased their sense of guilt and confusion.

KITTY: I was in love with my father. He called me his special girlfriend.
LENORE: The whole issue is very complicated. I was very attracted to my father, and that just compounded the guilt.
PAULA: I was scared of him, but basically I liked him.

Though these women sometimes expressed a sense of disappointment and even contempt for their fathers, they did not feel as keenly the sense of betrayal as they felt toward their mothers. Having abandoned the hope of pleasing their mothers, they seemed relieved to have found some way of pleasing their fathers and gaining their attention.

Susan Brownmiller, in her study of rape as a paradigm of relations between men and women, refers briefly to father-daughter incest. Stressing the coercive aspect of the situation, she calls it "father-rape."[26] To label it thus is to understate the complexity of the relationship. The father's sexual approach is clearly an abuse of power and authority, and the daughter almost always understands it as such. But, unlike rape, it occurs in the context of a caring relationship. The victim feels overwhelmed by her father's superior power and unable to resist him; she may feel disgust, loathing, and shame. But at the same time she often feels that this is the only kind of love she can get, and prefers it to no love at all. The daughter is not raped, but seduced.

In fact, to describe what occurs as a rape is to minimize the harm to the child, for what is involved here is not simply an assault, it is a betrayal. A woman who has been raped can cope with the experience in the same way that she would react to any other intentionally cruel and harmful attack. She is not socially or psychologically dependent upon the rapist. She is free to hate him. But the daughter who has been molested is dependent on her father for protection and care. Her mother is not an ally. She has no recourse. She does not dare express, or even feel, the depths of her anger at being used. She must comply with her father's demands or risk losing the parental love that she needs. She is not

---

26. S. Brownmiller, *Against Our Will: Men, Women and Rape* (New York: Simon & Schuster, 1975), p. 281.

an adult. She cannot walk out of the situation (though she may try to run away). She must endure it, and find in it what compensations she can.

Although the victims reported that they felt helpless and powerless against their fathers, the incestuous relationship did give them some semblance of power within the family. Many of the daughters effectively replaced their mothers and became their fathers' surrogate wives. They were also deputy mothers to the younger children and were generally given some authority over them. While they resented being exploited and robbed of the freedom ordinarily granted to dependent children, they did gain some feeling of value and importance from the role they were given. Many girls felt an enormous sense of responsibility for holding the family together. They also knew that, as keepers of the incest secret, they had an extraordinary power which could be used to destroy the family. Their sexual contact with their fathers conferred on them a sense of possessing a dangerous, secret power over the lives of others, power which they derived from no other source. In this situation, keeping up appearances and doing whatever was necessary to maintain the integrity of the family became a necessary, expiating act at the same time that it increased the daughters' sense of isolation and shame.

> THERESA: I was mortified. My father and mother had fights so loud that you could hear them yelling all over the neighborhood. I used to think that my father was really yelling at my mother because she wouldn't give him sex. I felt I had to make it up to him.

What is most striking to us about this family constellation, in which the daughter replaces the mother in her traditional role, is the underlying assumption about that role shared apparently by all the family members. Customarily, a mother and wife in our society is one who nurtures and takes care of children and husband. If, for whatever reasons, the mother is unable to fulfill her ordinary functions, it is apparently assumed that some other female must be found to do it. The eldest daughter is a frequent choice. The father does not assume the wife's maternal role when she is incapacitated. He feels that his first right is to continue to receive the services which his wife formerly provided, sometimes including sexual services. He feels only secondarily responsible for giving care to his children. This view of the father's prerogative to be served not only is shared by the fathers and daughters in these families, but is often encouraged by societal attitudes. Fathers who feel abandoned by their wives are not generally expected or taught to assume primary parenting responsibilities. We should not find it surprising, then, that fathers occasionally turn to their daughters for services (domestic and sexual) that they had formerly expected of their wives.

The Victims

The fifteen women who reported their incest experiences were all clients in psychotherapy. That is to say, all had admitted to themselves and at least one other person that they were suffering and needed help. Although we do not know whether they speak for the vast majority of victims, some of their complaints are so similar that we believe that they represent a pattern common to most women who have endured prolonged sexual abuse in childhood at the hands of parents.

One of the most frequent complaints of the victims entering therapy was a sense of being different, and distant, from ordinary people. The sense of isolation and inability to make contact was expressed in many different ways:

> KITTY: I'm dead inside.
> LENORE: I have a problem getting close to people. I back off.
> LOIS: I can't communicate with anyone.

Their therapists described difficulty in forming relationships with them, confirming their assessment of themselves. Therapists frequently made comments like "I don't really know whether I'm in touch with her," or "she's one of the people that's been the hardest for me to figure out." These women complained that most of their relationships were superficial and empty, or else extremely conflictual. They expressed fear that they were unable to love. The sense of an absence of feeling was most marked in sexual relationships, although most women were sexually responsive in the narrow sense of the word; that is, capable of having orgasms.

In some cases, the suppression of feeling was clearly a defense which had been employed in the incestuous relationship in childhood. The distance or isolation of affect seemed originally to be a device set up as protection against the feelings aroused by the molesting father. One woman reported that when she "shut down," did not move or speak, her father would leave her alone. Another remembered that she would tell herself over and over "this isn't really happening" during the sexual episode. Passive resistance and dissociation of feeling seemed to be among the few defenses available in an overwhelming situation. Later, this carried over into relations with others.

The sense of distance and isolation which these women experienced was uniformly painful, and they made repeated, often desperate efforts to overcome it. Frequently, the result was a pattern of many brief unsatisfactory sexual contacts. Those relationships which did become more intense and lasting were fraught with difficulty.

Five of the seven married women complained of marital conflict, either feeling abused by their husbands or indifferent toward them. Those who were single or divorced uniformly complained of problems in their relationships with men. Some expressed negative feelings toward men in general:

> STEPHANIE: When I ride the bus I look at all the men and think, "all they want to do is stick their pricks into little girls."

Most, however, overvalued men and kept searching for a relationship with an idealized protector and sexual teacher who would take care of them and tell them what to do. Half the women had affairs during adolescence with older or married men. In these relationships, the sense of specialness, power, and secrecy of the incestuous relationship was regained. The men were seen as heroes and saviors.

In many cases, these women became intensely involved with men who were cruel, abusive, or neglectful, and tolerated extremes of mistreatment. Anne-Marie remained married for twenty two years to a psychotic husband who beat her, terrorized their children, and never supported the family. She felt she could not leave him because he would fall apart without her. "We were his kingdom," she said, "to bully and beat." She eventually sought police protection and separation only after it was clear that her life was in danger. Her masochistic behavior in this relationship was all the more striking, since other areas of her life were relatively intact. She was a warm and generous mother, a valued worker, and an active, respected member of her community. Lois was raped at age nineteen by a stranger whom she married a week later. After this marriage ended in divorce, she began to frequent bars where she would pick up men who beat her repeatedly. She expressed no anger toward these men. Three other women in this group of fifteen were also rape victims. Only one expressed anger toward her attackers; the others felt they "deserved it." Some of the women recognized and commented on their predilection for abusive men. As Sandra put it: "I'm better off with a bum. I can handle that situation."

Why did these women feel they deserved to be beaten, raped, neglected, and used? The answer lies in their image of themselves. It is only through understanding how they perceived themselves that we can make sense of their often highly destructive relations with others. Almost every one of these fifteen women described herself as a "witch," "bitch," or "whore." They saw themselves as socially "branded" or "marked," even when no social exposure of their sexual relations had occurred or was likely to occur. They experienced themselves as powerful and dangerous to men: their self-image had almost a magical quality. Kitty, for instance, called herself a "devil's child," while Sandra compared herself to the twelve-year-old villainess of a popular melodrama, *The Exorcist*, a girl who was possessed by the devil. Some felt they were invested with special seductive prowess and could captivate men simply by looking at them. These daughters seemed almost uniformly to believe that they had seduced their fathers and therefore could seduce any man.

At one level, this sense of malignant power can be understood to have arisen as a defense against the child's feelings of utter helplessness. In addition, however, this self-image had been reinforced by the long-standing conspiratorial relationship with the father, in which the child had been elevated to the mother's position and did indeed have the power to destroy the family by exposing the incestuous secret.

Moreover, most of the victims were aware that they had experienced some pleasure in the incestuous relationship and had joined with their fathers in a shared hatred of their mothers. This led to intense feelings of shame, degradation, and worthlessness. Because they had enjoyed their fathers' attention and their mothers' defeat, these women felt responsible for the incestuous situation. Almost uniformly, they distrusted their own desires and needs and did not feel entitled to care and respect. Any relationship that afforded some kind of pleasure seemed to increase the sense of guilt and shame. These women constantly sought to expiate their guilt and relieve their shame by serving and giving to others and by observing the strictest and most rigorous codes of religion and morality. Any lapse from a rigid code of behavior was felt as confirming evidence of their innate evilness. Some of the women embraced their negative identity with a kind of defiance and pride. As Sandra boasted: "There's *nothing* I haven't done!"

Those women who were mothers themselves seemed to be pre-occupied with the fear that they would be bad mothers to their children, as they felt their mothers had been to them. Several sought treatment when they began to be aware of feelings of rage and resentment toward their children, especially their daughters. Any indulgence in pleasure seeking or attention to personal needs reinforced their sense that they were "whores" and unfit mothers. In some, the fear of exposure took the form of a constant worry that the authorities would intervene to take the children away. Other mothers worried that they would not be able to protect their daughters from a repetition of the incest situation. As one victim testified:

> I could a been the biggest bum. My father called me a "big whore" and my mother believed him. I could a got so disgusted that I could a run

around with anyone I saw. I met my husband and told him about my father and my child. He stuck by me and we was married. I got to the church and I'm not so shy like I was. It always come back to me that this thing might get on the front pages and people might know about it. I'm getting over it since the time I joined the church.

Her husband testified:

> The wife is nervous and she can't sleep. She gets up yesterday night about two o'clock in the morning and starts fixing the curtains. She works that way till five, then she sleeps like a rock. She's cold to me but she tells me she likes me. She gets cold once in a while and she don't know why herself. She watches me like a hawk with those kids. She don't want me to be loving with them and to be too open about sex. It makes her think of her old man. I got to take it easy with her or she blows up.[27]

In our opinion, the testimony of these victims, and the observations of their therapists, is convincing evidence that the incest experience was harmful to them and left long-lasting scars. Many victims had severely impaired object relations with both men and women. The overvaluation of men led them into conflictual and often intensely masochistic relationships with men. The victims' devaluation of themselves and their mothers impaired development of supportive friendships with women. Many of the victims also had a well-formed negative identity as witch, bitch, or whore. In adult life they continued to make repeated ineffective attempts to expiate their intense feelings of guilt and shame.

Therapy for the Incest Victim and Her Family

Very little is known about how to help the incest victim. If the incestuous secret is discovered while the victim is still living with her parents, the most common social intervention is the destruction of the family. This outcome is usually terrifying even to an exploited child, and most victims will cooperate with their fathers in maintaining secrecy rather than see their fathers jailed or risk being sent away from home.

---

27. · Weinberg, pp. 151-52. See n. 5 above.

We know of only one treatment program specifically designed for the rehabilitation of the incestuous family.[28] This program, which operates out of the probation department of the Santa Clara County Court in California, involves all members of the incestuous family in both individual and family therapy and benefits from a close working alliance with Daughters United, a self-help support group for victims. The program directors acknowledge that the coercive power of the court is essential for obtaining the cooperation of the fathers. An early therapeutic goal in this program is a confrontation between the daughter and her mother and father, in which they admit to her that she has been the victim of "poor parenting." This is necessary in order to relieve the daughter from her feeling of responsibility for the incest. Mothers appear to be more willing than fathers to admit this to their daughters.

Though this program offers a promising model for the treatment of the discovered incestuous family, it does not touch the problem of undetected incest. The vast majority of incest victims reach adulthood still bearing their secrets. Some will eventually enter psychotherapy. How can the therapist respond appropriately to their needs?

We believe that the male therapist may have great difficulty in validating the victim's experience and responding empathically to her suffering. Consciously or not, the male therapist will tend to identify with the father's position and therefore will tend to deny or excuse his behavior and project blame onto the victim. Here is an example of a male therapist's judgmental perception of an incest victim:

> This woman had had a great love and respect for her father until puberty when he had made several sexual advances toward her. In analysis she talked at first only of her good feelings toward him because she had blocked out the sexual episodes. When they were finally brought back into consciousness, all the fury returned which she had experienced at the age of thirteen. She felt that her father was an impotent, dirty old

---

28. H. Giarretto, "Humanistic Treatment of Father-Daughter Incest," in *Child Abuse and Neglect—the Family and the Community*, ed. R. E. Helfer and C. H. Kemp (Cambridge. Mass.: Ballinger Publishing Co., 1976).

man who had taken advantage of her trusting youthful innocence. From some of the details which she related of her relationship to her father, *it was obvious that she was not all that innocent.* [Our italics][29]

Not surprisingly, the client in this case became furious with her therapist, and therapy was unsuccessful.

If the male therapist identifies with the aggressor in the incest situation, it is also clear that the female therapist tends to identify with the victim and that this may limit her effectiveness. In a round-table discussion of experiences with incest victims, most of the contributing therapists acknowledged having shied away from a full and detailed exploration of the incestuous relationship. In some cases the therapist blatantly avoided the issue. In these cases, no trust was established in the relationship, and the client quickly discontinued therapy. In effect, the therapists had conveyed to these women that their secrets were indeed too terrible to share, thus reinforcing their already intense sense of isolation and shame.

Two possible explanations arise for the female therapist's flight. Traditional psychoanalytic theory might suggest that the therapist's own incestuous wishes and fantasies are too threatening for her to acknowledge. This might seem to be the most obvious reason for such a powerful countertransference phenomenon. The second reason, though less apparent, may be equally powerful: the female therapist confronting the incest victim reexperiences her own fear of her father and recognizes how easily she could have shared the victim's fate. We suspect that many women have been aware of, and frightened by, seductive behavior on the part of their own fathers. For every family in which incest is consummated there are undoubtedly hundreds with essentially similar, if less extreme, psychological dynamics. Thus the incest victim forces the female therapist to confront her own condition and to reexperience not only her infantile desires but also her (often realistic) childhood fears.

---

29. R. Stein, *Incest and Human Love: The Betrayal of the Soul in Psychotherapy* (New York: Third Press, 1973), pp. 45-46.

If the therapist overcomes this obstacle, and does not avoid addressing the issue with her client, another trap follows. As one therapist put it during the round-table discussion: "I get angry *for* her. How can she *not* be angry with her father?" Getting angry for a client is a notoriously unsuccessful intervention. Since the victim is more likely to feel rage toward the mother who abandoned her to her fate than toward her father, the therapeutic relationship must provide a place where the victim feels she can safely express her hostile feelings. Rage against the mother must be allowed to surface, for it is only when the client feels she can freely express her full range of feelings without driving the therapist away that she loses her sense of being malignantly "marked."

The feminist therapist may have particular difficulty facing the degree of estrangement between mother and daughter that occurs in these families. committed as she is to building solidarity among women, she is bound to be distressed by the frequent histories of indifference, hostility, and cruelty in the mother-daughter relationship. She may find herself rushing to the defense of the mother, pointing out that the mother, herself, was a victim, and so on. This may be true, but not helpful. Rather than denying the situation or making excuses for anyone, the therapist must face the challenge that the incestuous family presents to all of us: How can we overcome the deep estrangement between mothers and daughters that frequently exists in our society, and how can we better provide for the security of both?

Beyond Therapy

For both social and psychological reasons, therapy alone seems to be an insufficient response to the situation of the incest victim. Because of its confidential nature, the therapy relationship does not lend itself to a full resolution of the issue of secrecy. The woman who feels herself to be the guardian of a terrible, almost magical secret may find considerable relief from her shame after sharing the secret with another person. However, the shared secrecy then recreates a situation similar to the original incestuous relationship. Instead of the victim alone against the world, there is the special dyad of the victim and her confidant. This, in fact, was a difficult issue for all the participants in our study, since the victims once again were the subject of special interest because of their sexual history.

The women's liberation movement has demonstrated repeatedly to the mental health profession that consciousness raising has often been more beneficial and empowering to women than psychotherapy. In particular, the public revelation of the many and ancient sexual secrets of women (orgasm, rape, abortion) may have contributed far more toward the liberation of women than the attempt to heal individual wounds through a restorative therapeutic relationship.

The same should be true for incest. The victims who feel like bitches, whores, and witches might feel greatly relieved if they felt less lonely, if their identities as the special guardians of a dreadful secret could be shed. Incest will begin to lose its devastating magic power when women begin to speak out about it publicly and realize how common it is.

We know that most cases do not come to the attention of therapists, and those that do, come years after the fact. Thus, as a social problem incest is clearly not amenable to a purely psychotherapeutic approach. Prevention, rather than treatment, seems to be indicated. On the basis of our study and the testimony of these victims, we favor all measures which strengthen and support the mother's role within the family, for it is clear that these daughters feel prey to their fathers' abuse when their mothers are too ill, weak, or downtrodden to protect them. We favor the strengthening of protective services for women and children, including adequate and dignified financial support for mothers, irrespective of their marital status; free, public, round-the-clock child care, and refuge facilities for women in crisis. We favor the vigorous enforcement (by female officials) of laws prohibiting the sexual abuse of children. Offenders should be isolated and reeducated. We see efforts to reintegrate fathers into the world of children as a positive development, but only on the condition that they learn more appropriate parental behavior. A seductive father is not much of an improvement over an abandoning or distant one.

As both Shulamith Firestone and Florence Rush have pointed out, the liberation of children is inseparable from our own.[30] In particular, as long as daughters are subject to seduction in childhood, no adult woman is free. Like prostitution and rape, we believe father-daughter incest will disappear only when male supremacy is ended.

---

30.   Shulamith Firestone, *The Dialectic of Sex: The Case for Feminist Revolution* (New York: Bantam Books, 1970); Florence Rush, "The Sexual Abuse of Children: A Feminist Point of View," in Connell and Wilson.

The authors gratefully acknowledge the contributions of the incest victims themselves and of the therapists who shared their experience with us. For reasons of confidentiality, we cannot thank them by name.

———————— **Chapter 11** ————————

CHILDREN NOT SEVERELY DAMAGED BY INCEST WITH A PARENT*

ATALAY YORUKOGLU, M.D. AND JOHN P. KEMPH, M.D.

O ften referrals to child guidance clinics are made by courts
when they suspect that a child has been subjected to incest
by a parent; in most cases it has been found that the children
were seriously affected by incestual relations with either parent.
More often than not these children show defects in their ego
functioning. Apparently in our culture the incest taboo is so
strong that when parent-child incest occurs, it is psychologically
traumatic to the child involved in the act; therefore, it is not
surprising to find that either boys or girls may become psychotic
after they have had incestual relations. A study by Fleck et al.
(1959) on the intrafamilial environment of the schizophrenic
patient provides evidence that parent-child incestual acts and
fantasies play a much greater role in the development of
schizophrenia than had hitherto been assumed. Rascovsky and
Rascovsky (1950) reported that it was common to find family
disorganization, alcoholism, depression, and sexual maladjustment between parents in the families where incest was consummated between father and daughter. Usually the child escaped
into homosexuality as a characteristic outcome of incestuous
relations. In cases of father-daughter incest, the psychopathology
of the daughters ranged from severe personality disorder and
sexual maladjustment to manifest psychosis.

—————

*From *Journal of the American Academy of Child Psychiatry*, 5:111-124, 1966.

In the cases of mother-son incest, the sons, according to various reports, were found to be seriously emotionally disturbed. Wahl (1960) and Guttmacher (1962) each reported a case of incest in which the son developed psychotic episodes following incestuous sexual relations with his mother. In another family studied by Brown (1963) murder occurred as a result of incestual relations. Since most cases of incest come to the attention of courts and psychiatrists as a result of family disintegration or severe emotional disturbance rather than because of the act itself, it may be assumed that there are many cases of incest that are undiscovered either due to lack of family disorganization, lack of recognized psychiatric illness, or due to the fear of scandal. In order to avoid scandal many families keep the parent-child incest a secret as long as possible. Furthermore, it seems to be the consensus of opinion (Masters, 1963) that incest between brothers and sisters occurs more frequently and produces less psychic damage than incest involving a parent.

We here studied two children with apparently healthy ego functioning who had incestuous relations with a parent; we sought to determine why they were relatively unaffected by the incest. The two cases which are reported in this chapter involve children who have had prolonged sexual contact with the parent without being at least manifestly seriously disturbed emotionally. In one of these, mother-son incest took place and in the other father-daughter incest occurred. Only pertinent material will be extracted from these case studies.

Case A

Jim, a thirteen-and-a-half-year-old, tall, good-looking boy with mild manners appeared older than his chronological age. When he was twelve years old, his mother was arrested for gross indecency related to acts of homosexuality with another woman. At this time it became known that his mother had been having sexual relations with him and with his sister, two years his junior, as well as with many suitors, both male and female. His mother was sentenced to one to five years in a house of correction on these charges, and her children were taken into court's custody. Jim and his sister were placed in a receiving home. There Jim upset other youngsters, stole some pigeons, brought fire in a can into the kitchen, broke a number of windows, ran away, etc. His behavior with girls was at first aggressive; if the girl tended to become aggressive with him, he would run away. Jim had participated in mutual masturbation with different boys when they would get together in bed. He was said to have exhibited himself to younger boys and to have formed a strong attachment to a boy two years his senior who was also in the receiving home. He was described as manipulative and smooth. He became sulky and unpleasant if he felt he was not being well treated. From the description of Jim's sister's behavior in the receiving home, it would seem that she also had difficulty controlling her impulses. On numerous occasions she became involved in sexual activity with younger girls in an exploratory way. She was described as a very aggressive girl in this area, though compliant in most other areas.

Jim was finally transferred to the detention home because of his unmanageable behavior. In an interview with the psychiatrist at that time he referred to himself as having been "a bad boy" and he expressed dissatisfaction with his current situation. He felt that he was responsible for his incestuous actions which he had "confessed" to the police when they had questioned him. He seemed to be well aware that he and his sister were placed in the receiving home as a result of his mother's "fight with a lady" (who had told the police about the mother's incestual behavior), but he had no knowledge of her homosexual activities. At this time psychological testing revealed some degree of depression and self-destructive tendencies. For example, he replied in sentence completion tests, "Sometimes I feel I might kill myself." He drew a picture of a family which consisted of three figures, all shown with their hands crossing over the lower region of the trunk. This passive self-protective stance was interpreted as indicating his guilt over sexual impulses and his fear of castration. In response to direct questioning, he indicated that the boy in the drawing was most afraid of girls, while he hoped to marry a nice young lady. Asked to make three wishes, Jim spoke of returning to his mother and then wished for another little kid, a child to adopt from the orphanage. He told psychiatrists and psychologists, as well as others, that he would prefer to go back to his mother, if she would stop doing what she did with him.

While waiting to be admitted to the University of Michigan Children's Psychiatric Hospital, he remained in the detention home where his behavior improved markedly. He no longer got into major difficulties. He showed no homosexual tendencies, but continued to be interested in girls. Jim, upon admission for inpatient treatment, assured his therapist that he would cause no trouble here because he did not want to go back to the juvenile home. When asked why he was brought to this hospital, he stated that he would be helped to get off his mind things that had happened between him and his mother.

He told his therapist that the sex acts between him and his mother had occurred for about two years, almost always after she had been drinking. Returning home late at night from work his mother woke him up by getting into his bed. She played with his penis and instructed him to use his mouth on her genitalia. She also placed his hand on her genitalia while he was sucking on her breasts. Some time later Jim's sister took part in their sexual activities. There had been episodes in which the boy would suck on one breast and the girl on the other. On one occasion Jim's mother used a vibrator on her genitalia while the two children were sucking. He claimed that his sister engaged in these sexual orgies only on a couple of occasions; when he and his mother had sexual intercourse, they were always alone. He felt all along that there was something terribly wrong with the whole affair, but he was curious about these sexual activities and after awhile he did not resist his mother's invitations. At times he thought since his mother saw nothing wrong in this, it must have been right to do these things. At other times he felt he was bad to sleep with her and said to himself and to his mother that she was doing this because she was drinking heavily and didn't know what she was doing. He claimed that his mother has always been a good mother to them; when she was sober she always treated them alike. She didn't seem to change in any way toward Jim after they began to have sexual relationships. He professed aggressively that he wanted to have nothing to do with drinking, it was a waste of money, that you could die from it, it could become a habit, and it could make you do things you have never done before. He added that when he last saw his mother at the police station she acted as though she didn't know what it was all about because his mother didn't know what she was doing under the influence of alcohol. When asked if he felt he could have avoided these activities, he commented, "I don't know, I was too scared, I don't know. I just didn't want to do it with her. First I didn't know what this was all about." He repeatedly wanted the therapist's assurance that no one would discuss this with his sister.

During the stay in our hospital Jim handled himself very well. He cooperated fully, and participated in all activities. He verbalized his satisfaction with the hospital program, saying that the kids enjoyed much freedom here. The hospital had turned out to be a better place than he thought. He showed a good sense of humor. His school performance was average. His peer relationships were appropriate. He carefully avoided getting into trouble or participating in any gang activities, but in a subtle way he tried to establish pal-to-pal relationships. No bizarreness or any impulsiveness were noticed.

He showed some degree of embarrassment in psychotherapeutic interviews when the therapist brought up the subject of the incestuous aspect of his relationship with his mother. It was a great relief to him that the therapist did not take a critical, punishing attitude toward him. Although he was not evasive, he showed some significant memory gaps, blocked on many details of his unacceptable sexual behavior. He manifested no thinking disturbance or any neurotic symptoms.

Psychotherapy consisted of a supportive and ego-building type of approach, since he seemed to have put up adequate defenses against his guilt feelings and incestual impulses. An uncovering type of therapy was avoided since this might have stirred up a great deal of anxiety. For the same reason hospitalization was kept to a short time.

During the interviews with his therapist, Jim maintained a strong loyalty to his mother. The only fault he could find with her was her drinking. Psychological testing revealed that his mother's psychological impact seemed to present a Dr. Jekyll and

Mr. Hyde riddle to him. He condemned her for her physical seduction of him, but he also liked her as a friend. He was still trying not to hurt his mother in any way by talking against her. It was also apparent that he had warm feelings toward her. He had apparently been able to split his perception of her; seeing her as a proper mother when she was herself and as a frightening seducer when she was not herself. He missed the type of relationship he had with her before the sexual contact began. He thought that if he had a father figure in the home this earlier relationship could be resumed; her sexual aggressiveness toward him could be deflected by an adult man. Jim still experienced fear that something awful might happen to him. Each new day brought with it the possibility of calamity. He thought that sometimes terrible things happen; for instance, an innocent bystander is hit by a flying rock. Although neurotic intrapsychic mechanisms are obvious here, still no manifest neurotic symptoms were noted.

Jim's superego, while punitive in some areas, was strangely pragmatic in other aspects. Although he had not been able to repress the memory of the sexual involvement with his mother, he had been successful in using repression and denial to disown the pleasure of the affect associated with it, remembering only his fear, puzzlement, and a sense of being helpless. He was anxious to reunite with his sister who was sent to a home for children following brief hospitalization in a different institution.

The mother's history was obtained from her after her release from prison. She was the seventh of nine children. There was a wide gap in age between her and her next oldest sibling. She was the fourth daughter. She described her father as "a hell fire and damnation preacher." He was so concerned about church activities and "saving souls" that he neglected his own family, but at the same time ruled with an iron hand. She reported that neither her mother nor her father ever had time to talk with her or her sisters. Her sisters made hasty marriages and left home to end the control of the punitive father. An older sister was forced into marriage and herein lay, according to Jim's mother, the beginning of her own problems. She told that, at the age of twelve, she was raped by this brother-in-law. All of the family knew of this, and because of their position in the community, nothing was done about it. This was followed with what appears to have been a stormy adolescence finally culminating in submission to the father's demands for Bible reading and no heterosexual contact. She reported being whipped repeatedly for breaking the rules set by her father, and on one occasion the father made her read a passage from the Bible dealing with the whoremongers. It is interesting to note that she harbored more resentment, however, against her mother than she felt against her father because her mother did not intervene for her.

At the age of seventeen she began to date and became fond of a boy who was a member of a church of another denomination. Since this was not acceptable to the parents, she stopped dating him. On the rebound she turned to Jim's father, an army lieutenant, who was five years her senior and belonged to the same church. She married him three months later. She indicated that this was an attempt to escape from her home. There followed a very unsuccessful five years of marriage in which she and her husband were separated forty-three times. The husband was unfaithful, drank excessively, and was continuously in difficulty with the police. She left him after he had severely beaten her. She said that he had been very brutal during sexual intercourse, which she never enjoyed. She had continuously supported the children by her earnings without help from her husband following their separation. She told her children that their father was dead.

She stated that she had never trusted anyone and felt inadequate in her relationships with adults. She was married a second time for approximately one year to a professional man whom she described as a "mama's boy, a weakling." During the interview it became obvious that Mrs. A. had been under great stress during and after her second marriage. She underwent a hysterectomy during her second marriage, and then she increased drinking and became sexually promiscuous. In the three years following the breakup of this marriage, Mrs. A. consistently increased her pattern of drinking which had begun during this second marriage. According to her report, "I was two people—one at work in a bar [as a bartender] and a different one at home. I wanted to break away from the business, but it offered me a good living and

I knew of no other way to support myself and the children."
There was continued guilt about her way of living, growing out
of her earlier training. She said she worried constantly about her
work, finances, and baby sitters. She said that she was drunk
when she married for the third time. She didn't realize she was
married until she sobered up several days later and immediately
separated from this man.

In spite of this background history, Mrs. A. was a well-dressed,
attractive woman with poise and good manners. She had a good
vocabulary. She seemed to be eager to talk and make a good
impression with her polished and well-rehearsed life story. She
related her traumatic past experiences and sufferings, and stressed
her sacrifices to be a good mother to Jim and his sister. She stated
that it was extremely hard to lead two lives. This she had not
realized until now. She felt that she had recently awakened from a
daze in which she had been for years. She claimed that she had
done a lot of growing up in the past few years. She described her
early experiences, giving detailed accounts of the rigid up-
bringing and the incident of rape. She pictured herself as a
helpless little girl who was the victim of circumstances.

One had the feeling that by discussing the early events she was
avoiding the exploration of the most recent events and the more
painful happenings in the incestual relationship with her
children. She did not deny her homosexual relationship. Without
showing any feelings she gave different versions of some of the
events. She thought she was framed by a girl's lover who became
jealous of their homosexual relationship. She neither denied nor
confirmed her incestual relationship with Jim and Jim's sister,
saying that it must be true since Jim never lied. When it was
pointed out that on three occasions she contradicted herself and
had given a different story earlier, she sheepishly stated that at the
time she made up things because she was angry at one particular
female interviewer. She added that she had no faith in women
anyway. It was different with the psychiatrist because he was a
man! She also denied that she told her children that their father
was dead, showing mock surprise. Speaking of her parents she
said that recently they had begged for her forgiveness for the
wrongs they had done to her; she forgave them and now they are

her best friends. She painted a rosy picture of the future and said she was looking forward to having her children with her.

Mrs. A. had a hysterical personality. Typically she sexualized everything, including motherhood. She was a very intelligent, but an emotionally immature and narcissistic woman who used very poor judgment in her interpersonal relationships. She had poor impulse control. She had made genuine attempts to change her way of life. She stopped drinking, gave up a job that paid well, and joined a new church in order to regain a new identity. She was obviously using denial to a great extent when she painted a rosy picture of her future in a conscious attempt to get her children back.

In her case one cannot help but think of the revenge nature of her sexual involvement aimed against her parents. Mainly on an unconscious level she tried to get even with her parents who denied her the most innocent pleasures but maintained a shameful silence when she was raped. It is interesting to note that she repeatedly stated that she forgave them for the wrongs they had done to her and that now they were her best friends.

Discussion

In this case of mother-son incest there was genital sexuality between the parent and the child, and at the same time mutual warm feelings. There seemed to be an absence of sadistic elements in this relationship, in contrast to the typical father-daughter incest cases in which frequently the child is threatened by the parent.

Jim, in the absence of a father figure, was given an adult role in the family. This is clearly seen in Jim's attitude toward and his statements about his mother. He regarded her as a dependent little girl in need of protection against herself and against others. He formed an alliance with his mother against a hostile world. The family structure was similar to that described by Weinberg (1955) with the mother dominant, the father absent, and the mother the aggressor in the incest relationship. Although his sexual contact with the mother was probably pleasurable at times, at least to the extent that he maintained an erection, yet he was not able to achieve an orgasm. Thus his premature introduction to adult sexuality was not entirely gratifying. He felt that most of the time he was fulfilling his mother's desire by participating in these acts in which he was a passive partner. It is interesting that he came to realize the full gravity of his involvement in these sexual activities only after he was separated from his mother. As long as he was doing what his mother told him, there seemed to be no strong superego pressure. One might speculate that as long as he lived with her his guilt feelings stemming from oedipal conflicts were not overwhelming. He felt the full impact when society condemned their relationship. There was insufficient evidence to substantiate any particular psychodynamic formulation, such as superego lacunae or well-defended guilt. Possibly his passive feminine orientation and homosexual activities following his mother's arrest were aimed at denying his active role in this forbidden relationship. During the two-year period of incestuous relationship, Jim had no adjustment problem or any scholastic difficulties. This would suggest that he was not severely disturbed during that period. Several factors may partially explain this ability to tolerate the incest. Clinical material in general suggests that forbidden fantasies may be as disturbing as the real trauma. Jim could recall no sexual fantasies toward his seductive and promiscuous mother. Since she had forced him into having sexual relations, he may have felt little responsibility for the incestual behavior. We have also some reason to believe that he had relatively good mothering prior to his mother's second marriage, which took place when Jim was about five years old. Before that time, despite serious marital difficulties, Jim's mother had been a full-time mother to her children and, as she stated, she had nothing but those children. Until her second marriage she had not been promiscuous, nor had she begun to drink. This may account in part for Jim's ego strength. The reports that we have received a year after his discharge from the hospital indicate that he continues to do well in his academic work, and his adjustment was described as excellent.

Case B

Jean, a beautiful seventeen-year-old girl, was referred for an evaluation after it became known to the court that she had been having incestual relations with her father for a prolonged period of time. She recalled that the father began to show her more attention than usual when she was thirteen years of age and in the seventh grade at school. Both her mother and father had been in the habit of coming into her and her brothers' rooms at bedtime to kiss them good-night. Her mother would come first and her father would follow. As she began to develop into womanhood, her father would stay longer, and he began to feel different parts of her body. This practice became more and more prolonged each night until she began to sense that there was something wrong. She knew nothing about sex at the time because her mother had never given her any information about the difference between men and women or how babies were born as a result of sexual relations. She had picked up some information by hearing other girls talk at school, but she did not have a clear-cut idea as to what motivated people to have sexual relations. She sensed that her father was doing something that he shouldn't, but she felt also that she should do as he asked or she would be considered disobedient. He would occasionally lie down beside her in bed and this she felt was certainly wrong because she had heard that sleeping with men could get girls into trouble. Therefore, she began to reject her father's attentions and would not allow him to get in bed with her. Nevertheless, he persisted in trying to do this and continued to force his attentions upon her.

When Jean was in the eighth grade, she decided that her father's behavior was very much wrong and tried to escape his attentions; she told her mother who spoke to him about it. This only caused her father to become infuriated, to get drunk, be more vicious with her mother, her brother who was four years younger than she, and with herself. For the sake of the family, as well as her own self, she found it easier to allow him to have his way as briefly as possible. She was forced to lie in bed beside her father who would hold her close, feel her for long periods of time, and eventually would have intercourse until he would reach orgasm.

Additionally, he would sometimes use his fingers in her vagina. He was never brutal. Whenever her mother was in another room, he would take the liberty of feeling her body.

For the first few years that her father showed Jean this attention she found sex very repulsive and felt that her father was some kind of sexual pervert with too much interest in it. Although she told her mother several times about his behavior, her mother spoke to the father about it, but nothing was ever done. As a matter of fact, her mother realized even before Jean told her that there was something of this kind going on between father and daughter.

For several months prior to the court referral her father's attention began to be pleasurable to Jean. She stated that she would occasionally become excited when her father would have intercourse with her. She felt at the time that it was probably a natural reaction, that after all, she was human, and even though she didn't want to experience any pleasure, it happened anyway. She then began to have severe anxiety and insisted that her mother do something more drastic to prevent her father from having sexual contact with her. She wanted her mother to stay with her more of the time. When the mother refused, the child went to the school psychologist and told him. The school psychologist suggested that she contact the juvenile court. One of the court workers brought the case before the judge who placed the father in a state hospital and referred the child and mother for psychiatric evaluation. The child indicated that she felt much more comfortable after the father was out of the home, but even so she felt guilty about her part in placing him in the state hospital.

The father was found to have chronic undifferentiated schizophrenia and was given a course of electroshock therapy with little or no change in his behavior. He tried to get his wife and daughter to lie for him to get him out of the hospital. The child, having found that the father did not change, stated that she felt a sick feeling in her stomach just as she used to when he would come into her bedroom and force his attentions on her. She had decided that she would do anything to evade his attentions because she felt she would go crazy if this continued. For the past year she had been going steady with a boy in school. She stated that she had never had intercourse with him even though she intended to marry this boy as soon as she graduated from high school.

The mother was a beautiful woman with considerable narcissism and hysteria in her psychopathology. She had never experienced sexual pleasure with her husband or any other man, although she behaved in a seductive manner with most men. She actually appreciated those times when her husband did not insist on having relations with her. Both the mother and the daughter agreed that the mother had never understood her husband and that the daughter seemed to be able not only to understand, but to help her father over acute aggressive outbursts merely by talking with him. The mother had unconsciously encouraged the daughter's becoming the sexual mate to her husband. The daughter enjoyed being able to help her father whenever he was agitated, but preferred that she keep her role in this category. She recognized that she saw her father more as a sick child than as a father.

Psychological testing indicated that this child had a superior intellectual capacity with an almost compulsive drive for achievement. She displayed considerable conscious control of impulsivity, although there appeared at times to be some weakening of this control in the Rorschach examination. She saw herself personally involved in many anxiety-arousing situations, yet she had a well-developed set of defenses which helped her to overcome this anxiety. She would often resort to escapist fantasies effectively during unfavorable impact with reality. However, her contact with reality was excellent.

Discussion

There are some common factors in these children which set them apart from others who have had incestual relationships with a parent. Both of them had the ability to see realistically the parent as a seriously disturbed person; often both assumed parental roles. They were obedient to the parent, mechanically performing a procedure as directed by the parent. Although they knew that the act was wrong, they were able to utilize sufficiently strong defenses to prevent themselves from consciously becoming aware of their own gratification from these relationships. Furthermore, they were able to prevent the development of, or defend themselves against, any intense superego pressure. Possibly the reason they were not seriously affected is that they had developed adequate ego functioning including defensive functions along with the resolution of early conflicts and adequate psychosexual development prior to their having the incestual relations.

They did not consciously strive for sexual contact, and actual sexual fantasies involving the parent were not remembered. Perhaps their having successfully resolved their oedipal conflicts in early childhood allowed them, paradoxically, to be involved in an incestual relationship without experiencing the anxiety which ordinarily results from the unresolved oedipus complex.

It is well known that even oedipal fantasies may produce serious conflict and developmental arrest. However, incest did not seem to produce long-lasting psychic symptoms in the children reported in this chapter. Therefore, one might speculate that oedipal fantasies may be even more harmful than the actual physical consummation of either mother-son or father-daughter incest in cases where the child is merely performing the mechanical act of intercourse at the parent's request without fully experiencing the significance of this act. This explanation assumes that these children had resolved their oedipal conflicts successfully prior to their incestual experiences. The only basis for this assumption is the lack of evidence for psychopathology on psychological examinations, and in psychotherapeutic interviews and the historical information indicating that there were no symptoms or deviant behavior. In a personal communication, Dr. Irene Josselyn has proposed the possibility that there was a regression to (or fixation at) the prestructured superego of obedience to parents. Since there is inadequate evidence to support either of these explanations, they must be considered purely speculative.

Although both Jim and Jean are now functioning well with little evidence of intrapsychic conflict, it is possible that they may develop difficulty in later phases of development. For example, in marriage they may be unable to accept their roles as parents or as partners in heterosexual relations.

Summary

In two cases of parent-child incest, one mother-son and the other father-daughter, the children were not seriously or permanently impaired psychologically. It was thought that their ability to withstand this trauma resulted from their having developed healthy ego functioning prior to the incestuous experience.

REFERENCES

Brown, W. (1963), Murder rooted in incest. In: *The Patterns of Incest*, ed. R. E. L. Masters. New York: Julian Press.

Fleck, S., Lidz, T., Cornelison, A., & Terry, D. (1959). The intrafamilial environment of the schizophrenic patient. In: *Individual and Familial Dynamics*, ed. J. H. Masserman. New York: Grune & Stratton, pp. 132-139.

Guttmacher, M. S. (1962), *Sex Offenses: The Problem, Causes and Prevention*. New York: Norton.

Masters, R. E. L., ed. (1963), *The Patterns of Incest*. New York: Julian Press.

Rascovsky M. W. & Rascovsky, A. (1950), On consummated incest. *Int. J. Psycho-Anal*, 31:42-47.

Wahl, W. C. (1960), The psychodynamics of consummated maternal incest. *Arch. Gen. Psychiat.*, 3:188-193.

Weinberg, K. S. (1955), *Incest Behavior*. New York: Citadel Press.

Chapter 12
HUMANISTIC TREATMENT OF FATHER-DAUGHTER INCEST*
HENRY GIARRETTO

The incest taboo is found in all known cultures, ancient, primitive, or civilized. It is generally agreed among social scientists that the essential purpose of the taboo is to optimize the survival and expansion of social systems.[1] Incest rules remain the most sternly enforced regulations for sexual relations and marriage throughout the world. But as social systems differ so do incest rules. To this day, laws defining and penalizing incestuous relationships vary markedly among nations and in the United States. In England, the law regards incest only as a misdemeanor. The penalties for incest in the U.S. range from a $500 fine and/or 12 months in Virginia, to a prison term of 1 to 50 years in California.[2] In most but not all states, first cousin marriage is illegal. Rhode Island permits first cousin marriage only between Jews.[3] For the purposes of this chapter, incest is defined as sexual activity between parent and child or between siblings of a nuclear family. The focus will be on father-daughter incest, as treated by the Child Sexual Abuse Treatment Program (CSATP).

Dread of incest is buried deeply in the unconscious of man and evokes emotions that are volatile and unpredictable, among them, repugnance, uneasy fascination, fear, guilt, and anger. This confused state finds expression in obscene comments or nervous disinterest when the subject is brought up in conversation, or quickly erupts into hostile behavior when an incestuous situation is discovered. Professional helpers themselves are not free of the incest dread. Many react either evasively when a case is referred or irresponsibly by failing to comply with child abuse reporting statutes. Nor can criminal justice personnel

---

*From *Children Today*, July-August 1976.

claim immunity from the panic induced by incest since their effect on sexually abusive families usually adds up to either rejection of the child's plea for help, if the evidence is not court-proof, or severe punishment of the entire family if the offender confesses. Finally, social scientists must also be afflicted with the dread of incest. How else can we account for the paucity of studies on incest which, with few exceptions, are superficial in conception and scope?

Typically, the repertory of law enforcement officials in the handling of father-daughter sexual abuse is ineffective and unpredictable. In one instance, the police officer or the district attorney may simply drop the case because of insufficient evidence even though there is strong suspicion that the victim's accusations are based on fact. The emphasis on a provable law violation has the effect of the community's turning its back on both the child and the family, thus leaving them in a worse condition than before. The child feels abandoned and must now face her hostile father, mother, and siblings alone. Often the father, though he may not repeat the crime, uses subtle retributive measures such as restrictions, extra chores, ostracization, etc.

In another instance, the criminal justice system, seeking sound, indisputable evidence, descends on the child and family with terrifying force. From the clinically detailed police reports, it appears that the only interest in the child is for the testimony she can give towards conviction of her father. The entire family is entangled in the web of retribution. The child is picked up and brought to a children's shelter, often without the mother's knowledge. The father is jailed and the mother must place her family on welfare. In sum, the family is dismembered, rendered destitute, and must painfully try to find its own way to unification.

Neglect of the sexually exploited child by the American community is vividly dramatized by Vincent de Francis in a 1971 report presenting the results of a three-year study in New York. He stresses that, "the victim of incest is especially vulnerable. The child is overwhelmed by fear, guilt, and shame. Substantial damage to the point of psychosis may ensue." As a rallying cry for action he adds: "I firmly believe that no community, rural or urban, can say such cases are unknown to it. Suffice it to say the problem of sexual abuse is a real one! It is a problem of immense proportions! It is pervasive!''[4]

Incidence and Effects of Incest

De Francis's alarm may not seen justified in view of the small number of detected incest offenders recorded annually by western nations. Over the period 1907-1938, Weinberg[5] determined that detected incest occurred in about one to two cases per million people in the United States; in Europe, the number of detected incest offenders ranged from one to nine cases per million. These rates seem to hold up to 1960.[6] All writers agree, however, that the low figures are the tip of the iceberg, that the laws discourage detection, and that data gathering methods render comparative studies extremely difficult if not impossible.

In the United States some improvement in detection and treatment of child abuse is developing as a result of rising public agitation. One tangible outcome of this pressure was the passage in 1974 of the Child Abuse Prevention and Treatment Act, which led to the establishment of a National Center on Child Abuse and Neglect in the Children's Bureau. Douglas J. Besharov, director of the Center, clearly spells out the position of the new federal resource on the overall problem of child abuse and neglect:

> The reality of child abuse is so awful that a harsh, condemnatory response is understandable. But such reactions must be tempered if any progress is to be made. If we permit feelings of rage towards abusers of children to blind us to the needs of the parents as well as of the children, these suffering and unfortunate families will be repelled and not helped. Only with the application of objective and enlightened policies can treatment, research, prevention and education be successfully performed.[7]

Other hopeful signs are the expansion and bolstering of child abuse reporting laws by many states, the increased attention being given by the media and the growing number of hotlines, several offering 24-hour service exclusively to calls on child abuse. Though major interest has been on child battering and neglect, some attention is slowly turning to sexual molestation.

In a recent issue of *Children Today*, devoted entirely to child abuse, Sgroi[8] submitted an article in which she deduces that the above-mentioned developments had much to do with a sharp increase in reported incidents of child sexual abuse in Connecticut. The number of such incidents reached 76 in fiscal year 1973, and rose markedly to 172 cases in fiscal year 1974, apparently as a result of strengthened child abuse reporting statutes, the opening of a hotline, and a persistent public education effort.

The CSATP serves Santa Clara County, which has a population of 1,159,500 (December 1973). In 1971, its first year of operation, 36 cases were referred. The annual referral rate increased slowly over the following two years, but during fiscal year 1974 the rate accelerated sharply to 180 cases. This burgeoning rate can only be attributed to added coverage by the media and to growing confidence in the CSATP approach. Even the rate of 180 cases of recorded incest in a population of 1.1 million inhabitants does not provide an accurate estimate of the actual prevalence of incest in Santa Clara County. Although this is a large increase from the two incest cases per million estimated for this country by the writers cited above, the true incidence of incest has yet to be established. All available figures are at best educated guesses.

More telling than guesses on the number of actual cases is the social price paid for the neglect of incest, which is beginning to surface through recent studies revealing the effects of incestuous experiences on child victims. James[9] interviewed 200 prostitutes in Seattle and found that 22 percent of the women had been incestuously assaulted as children. For several years, Baisden[10] has studied Rosaphrenia: "An individual who cannot accept her own sexuality regardless of how she practices sex." He discovered that an inordinately high percentage of women so afflicted were raped as children. (Here, rape is defined as sexual exploitation of girls by much older males.) Concentrating on a group of 160 women, whom he tested for Rosaphrenia, he found that 90 percent had been raped during childhood, 22.5 percent by fathers or step-fathers.[11] The Odyssey Institute in New York interviewed 118 female drug abusers to ascertain their sexual history. It was found that 44 percent of the women had experienced incest as children. The 52 incest victims confided that the 93 different incestuous offenders, a total of 60, were in the parental generation, and of this group 21 percent were fathers or stepfathers.[12] It is notable that in each of these three studies of troubled women, a background of father-daughter incest emerged in over 20 percent of the subjects.

Father-Daughter Incest

Father-daughter incest is potentially the most damaging to the child and family. Certainly it is the form most frequently prosecuted by the courts. A typical father-daughter incestuous relationship imposes severe stresses on the structure of the family. The father, mother, and daughter roles become blurred and this engenders conflict and confusion among family members. The most bewildered is the daughter, who is at an age when her budding sexuality requires a clear and reassuring guidance. The familiar father has suddenly put on the strange mask of lover. She never knows which role he will play at any given time. Her mother, too, becomes unpredictable. At one moment she is the usual caring parent, at another she sends subtle, suspicious messages that can only come from a rival. The girl's relationships with her siblings are also adversely affected as they become aware that she has a special hold on their father.

Of course, each family has its own unique cast of personalities and the dramatic twists and turns which they enact are of infinite variety. But the following composite case history is fairly typical of the families we have been treating, and how the authorities reacted before CSATP.

Leslie

Leslie is ten years old when her father begins his sexual advances. She has always been close to her father. When he tentatively begins to fondle her, she finds the experiences strange but pleasurable. Slowly the sex play becomes more sophisticated as it progresses to mutual oral copulation and, at puberty, to intercourse. Their meetings, which at first were excitingly secretive, now become furtive and anxiety-ridden. Leslie is about to enter the difficult teenage years when the mounting tension within her becomes unbearable. Her father is now interfering unduly with her peer relations. She senses that his fatherly concern over boys who are paying her attention is tainted by jealousy. She no longer can tolerate body contact with him and tries to resist, but he refuses to stop. Ashamed to confess the affair to her mother, she turns desperately to an adult friend, who immediately calls the police.

Though the policeman tries to be kind, Leslie is frightened by the power and authority he represents. His probing questions are excruciatingly embarrassing. But an odd feeling of relief inter-mingled with exhilaration comes over her as she realizes that her secret has now been exposed and her father's power over her broken. Her anxiety returns when she is brought to a children's shelter. Despite friendly attempts by attendants to make her stay pleasant, Leslie feels alone and threatened. This is the first time she has been forcefully separated from the family. She is overwhelmed by mixed emotions of fear, guilt, and anger, and is convinced she will never be able to rejoin her family or face her friends and relatives. Since there is suspicion of inadequate protection by her mother, a foster home is found for her. But she will not adjust to the new family, as this confirms her fears that she has been banished from her own family. Though often told that she was the victim of the incestuous relationship, Leslie believes she is the one who is being punished. She enters a period of self-abusive behavior manifested variously through hostility, truancy, drug abuse, and promiscuity.

Jim

Jim, Leslie's father, a successful accountant, is in his mid-thirties when he becomes aware of deep boredom and disenchant-ment with his life. He feels stalemated in his job and his prospects for advancement are poor. There is growing estrangement between himself and his wife. She no longer seems proud of him;

in fact, most of her remarks concerning his ability as a provider, father, or husband are critical and harrassing. Their sexual encounters have no spark and serve only to relieve nervous tension. He fantasizes romantic liaisons with girls at work, but he has neither the skill nor courage to exploit his opportunities.

Jim finds himself giving increasing attention to Leslie. Of all his children, she has always been his favorite. She is always there for him, accompanies him on errands, snuggles close beside him as they spend hours together watching TV. (His wife has no interest in this pastime; at night she is either taking classes or studying with her classmates.) As Leslie cuddles beside him he becomes keenly aware of her warmth and softness. At times she wiggles on his lap sensuously somehow knowing that this gives him pleasure. He begins to caress her and "relives the delicious excitement of forbidden sex play during childhood," as one client expressed it. But this phase is soon engulfed by guilt feelings as the relationship gets out of hand and he finds himself making love to her as if she were a grown woman. Between episodes he chokes with self-disgust and vows to stop. But as if driven by unknown forces he continues to press his sexual attention on her. He now senses that she is trying to avoid him and no longer receptive to his advances. Though he doesn't use physical force he relies on his authority as parent to get her to comply. He becomes increasingly suspicious of her outside activities and the seemingly continual stream of boys who keep coming to the house. With a sinking feeling he notices that she is beginning to respond to one of the boys. He cannot control the feeling of jealousy the boy evokes or his craven attempts to force his daughter to stop seeing him.

Jim's trance is suddenly shattered one evening as he returns home from work. A policeman emerges from the car parked in front of his home and advises him that he is under arrest. Numb with shame and fear he is transported to the police station for questioning. Though informed of his constitutional rights, he finds himself making a fully detailed confession. Jim is eventually convicted on a felony charge and given a jail sentence of one to five years. His savings are wiped out by the lawyer's fee of several thousand dollars. He finds imprisonment extremely painful: from a respected position in society he has fallen to the lowest social stratum. His fellow inmates call him a "baby-raper." No one is more despicable. He is segregated and often subjected to indignities and violence. His self-loathing is more intense than that of his inmates. He gradually finds some relief in the fervent resolution that, given the chance, he will more than make it up to his child, wife, and family. A well-behaved inmate, he is released from jail in nine months. But he has lost his job and after weeks of job-hunting, settles for a lower position. Jim faces an uncertain future with his wife and family.

Liz

The explosive reaction of the criminal justice system leaves Jim's wife, Liz, in shock and terror. She is certain that her family has been destroyed. There are subtle hints that she may have condoned the incestuous affair in the questioning by police and even others she once regarded as friends. She has failed both as wife and mother. Her feelings toward her daughter alternate between jealousy and motherly concern. Her emotional state vis-a-vis Jim is also ambivalent. At first Liz is blinded with disgust and hate at the cruel blow he had dealt her and vows to divorce him. Her friends and relatives insist this is her only recourse. But the rest of the children begin to miss him immediately and she realizes that, on the whole, he has been a good father. Liz is also sharply reminded that he has been a dependable provider as she faces the shameful task of applying for welfare. Nagging questions, however, continue to plague her. If she takes him back what assurance does she have that he will not repeat the sexual offenses with their other daughters? Will her relatives and friends assume that she has deserted her daughter if she allows him to return home? Will the authorities ever permit her daughter and husband to live in the same home again? Is there any hope for their marriage?

It is evident that typical community intervention in incest cases, rather than being constructive, has the effect of a knockout blow to a family already weakened by serious internal stresses. The average family treated by the Child Sexual Abuse Treatment

Program is not at all like the incestuous family described in the literature. Weinberg, for example, reported that 67 percent of the families he studied were in the low socioeconomic bracket and that 64 percent of the incestuous fathers tested were below normal intelligence. He also noted that there was a disproportionate number of blacks in his sample.[13]

The 300 families who have been referred to the Child Sexual Abuse Treatment Program constitute a fair cross-section of Santa Clara County. The families are representative of the racial composition of the county, which is 76.8 percent white, 17.5 percent Mexican-American, 3.0 percent Oriental, 1.7 percent black, 1.0 percent other. The makeup of the work force leans towards the professional, semi-professional and skilled blue collar. Average income is $13,413 per household. The median educational level is 12.5 years.

The Child Sexual Abuse Treatment Program (CSATP)

In 1971, cases similar to the representative one described above aroused the concern of Eunice Peterson, a supervisor of the Juvenile Probation Department. She conferred with Dr. Robert Spitzer, consulting psychiatrist to that department. Dr. Spitzer felt that family therapy would be a good first step towards constructive case management of sexually abusive families. I was invited to undertake a pilot effort limited to ten hours of counseling per week for a ten-week period. Initial criteria were:
   1. The clients would be counseled on-site at the Juvenile Probation Department.
   2. The therapeutic approach would follow a "growth" model predicated on Humanistic Psychology.
   3. Conjoint Family Therapy as developed by Virginia Satir[14] would be emphasized.

It was soon apparent that the new approach held high promise of meeting a critical problem of the community. The initial effort expanded slowly due to meager funds. But the pressure of client needs was so strong that perpetuation of the new community resource was assured. As the program got underway, I quickly discovered that conjoint family therapy alone was inadequate and, moreover, could not be usefully applied during early stages of the family's crisis. The fundamental aim of family therapy—to facilitate a harmonious familial system—was not discarded. Incestuous families are badly fragmented as a result of the original dysfunctional family dynamics, which are further exacerbated upon disclosure to civil authorities. The child, mother, and father must be treated separately before family therapy becomes productive. Consequently, the treatment procedure was applied in this order: (1) individual counseling, particularly for the child, mother and father; (2) mother-daughter counseling; (3) marital counseling, which becomes a key treatment if the family wishes to be reunited; (4) father-daughter counseling; (5) family counseling; and (6) group counseling. The treatments are not listed in order of importance, nor followed invariably in each case, but all are required for family reconstitution.

Another important finding during early phases of the program was that traditional counselor-client therapy, though important, was not sufficient. The reconstructive approach would be enhanced if the family were assisted in locating community resources for pressing needs such as housing, financial, legal, jobs, and so on. This required close collaboration between the counselor and the juvenile probation officer assigned to the case. In 1972 another development adding to program productivity was the formation of the self-help group now known as Parents United. The insight that led to this step came when a mother of one of the first families treated was asked to make a telephone call to a mother caught in the early throes of the crisis. The ensuing conversation went on for over three hours and had a markedly calming effect on the new client. A week later, three of the more advanced mother clients met together for the first time, and after a few meetings, to which several other women were invited, Parents United was formally designated and launched. The members meet weekly, and after a brief conference to discuss progress in growth and effectivity, the members form various groups: a couples group; an intense couples group size-limited to five pairs; a men's group; a women's group; and a mixed group. A separate organization, self-named Daughters United and composed of teenaged girls, meets earlier in the evening.

Objectives of the CSATP

1. Provide immediate counseling and practical assistance to sexually abused children and their families, in particular to victims of father-daughter incest.
2. Hasten the process of reconstitution of the family and of the marriage, if possible, since children prosper best in normally functioning families headed by natural parents.
3. Marshal and coordinate all official services responsible for the sexually abused child and family, as well as private resources to ensure comprehensive case management.
4. Employ a treatment model that fosters self-managed growth of individuals capable of positive contributions to society, rather than a medical model based on the vagaries of mental disease.
5. Facilitate expansion and autonomy of the self-help groups, initiated by the program known as Parents United and Daughters United; provide guidance to the membership, such as training in co-counseling, self-management, and intra-family communication; and in locating community resources —i.e., medical, legal, financial, educational.
6. Inform the public at large and professional agencies about the existence and supportive approach of the program, especially to encourage sexually abusive families to seek the services of the program voluntarily.
7. Develop informational and training material to enable emulation or adaptation of the CSATP model by other communities.

Treatment Model

The therapeutic approach of the CSATP is based on the theory and methods of humanistic psychology, in particular the relatively new incorporation by the field of the discipline known as psychosynthesis, founded by Roberto Assagioli.[15] Other writers of importance to the CSATP are Carl Rogers, Abraham H. Maslow, Virginia Satir, Frederick Perls, Haridas Chaudhuri, and Eric Berne.

Assagioli agrees that many similarities exist between psychosynthesis and existentialist/humanistic views. Principal similarities are: (1) the method of starting from within, experiencing self-identity; (2) the concept of personal growth; (3) the importance of the meaning a person makes of his life; (4) the key notion of responsibility and ability to decide among alternatives; (5) the emphasis on present and future rather than regrets or yearnings for the past; and (6) the recognition of the uniqueness of each individual. In addition, Assagioli stresses: (1) the will as an essential function of self; (2) the experience of self-awareness independent of immediate I-consciousness of the various parts of ourselves; (3) a positive, optimistic view of the human condition; and (4) systematic use of didactic and experiential techniques that follow an individuated plan for psychosynthesis, the harmonious blending of mind, body, and spirit around the unifying essence— the self.[16]

Central notions in the treatment model are: the building of social responsibility; the realization that each of us is an important element of society; the belief that we must actively participate in the development of social attitudes and laws or be helplessly controlled by them. Chaudhuri gives firm emphasis to this imperative: "Since psyche and society are essentially inseparable, one has to take into account the demands of society. . . . One may criticize society or try to remold it. But one cannot ignore society or discard it."[17]

Major Premises

1. The family is viewed as an organic system; family members assume behavior patterns to maintain system balance (family homeostasis).
2. A distorted family homeostasis is evidenced by psychological/physiological symptoms in family members.
3. Incestuous behavior is one of the many symptoms possible in troubled families.
4. The marital relationship is a key factor in family organic balance and development.

5. Incestuous behavior is not likely to occur when parents enjoy mutually beneficial relations.
6. A high self-concept in each of the mates is a prerequisite for a healthy marital relationship.
7. High self-concepts in the parents help to engender high self-concepts in the children.
8. Individuals with higher self-concepts are not apt to engage others in hostile-aggressive behavior. In particular, they do not undermine the self-concept of their mates or children through incestuous behavior.
9. Individuals with low self-concepts are usually angry, disillusioned, and feel they have little to lose. They are thus primed for behavior that is destructive to others and to themselves.
10. When such individuals are punished in the depersonalized manner of institutions, the low self-concept/high destructive energy syndrome is reinforced. Even when punishment serves to frustrate one type of hostile conduct, the destructive energy is diverted to another outlet or turned inward.

Productive case management of the molested child and her family calls for procedures that alleviate the emotional stresses of the experience and of punitive action by the community; enhance the processes of self-awareness and self-management; promote family unity and growth, and a sense of responsibility to society. The purpose is not to extinguish or modify dysfunctional behavior by external devices. Rather, we try to help each client develop the habit of self-awareness (the foundation for self-esteem) and the ability to direct one's own behavior and life style.

Method

It is necessary to generate a warm, optimistic atmosphere before productive therapeutic transactions can ensue with families that have broken the incest taboo. They must be given hope and reassured that their situation is not as singular or as disabling as they have been led to believe. Feelings of despair, shame, and guilt must be listened to with compassion, as natural expressions of inner states. Awareness and acceptance of current feelings, without evaluation, allows the clients to assimilate them and to move on with their lives.

I know that I must continually work at developing this attitude within myself. When I met my first family, it was easy to maintain an attitude of acceptance with the child and her mother. But in preparing myself for the session with the father, I read the lurid details of his sexual activities with his daughter, which included mutual oral copulation and sodomy at the age of ten. The compassionate, therapeutic attitude which I can now write about so freely (perhaps pompously) completely dissipated.

I was forced to go into deep exploration of my unconscious for its own incestuous impulses and found that my early religious upbringing had done its repressive work thoroughly. After confronting the revulsion and anger that I was projecting on my client, I was able to assume a reasonable therapeutic mien. When I actually met with my client, my problem was much less difficult than I had anticipated. The raw feelings of despair and confusion had needed to be attended to, and my own hangups had become less intrusive. I cannot overemphasize the importance of self-work on the part of the therapist. This is the central theme of workshops I conduct for individuals who want to help incestuous families.

Self-Assessment and Confrontation

Once a working relationship has been established and the highly charged emotional climate subsides, the clients begin to take an inventory of personal and family characteristics. Initially, during this exploration, I underscore the positive traits. What does the girl, for example, like about herself? What does she appreciate in other family members and the family as a whole? Before she can be motivated to work actively for personal and family growth, she must be convinced that she and the family are worth the effort. From this positive stance, the clients can then proceed to identify weaknesses and maladaptive habits that need to be improved or eliminated. These might include uncontrolled use of drugs, food, alcohol and cigarettes; hostile-aggressive behavior that interferes with progress in family, school, and work-relations; sexual promiscuity; inconsistent study and work habits; and, typically, the inability to communicate effectively, especially with important persons in their lives.

As the clients gain confidence in their search for self-knowledge, they begin to probe the painful areas connected with the incest. In what may be termed a confrontation-assimilation process, I encourage the child, father, and mother, as well as other family members, to face and express the feelings associated with the incestuous experience. It is indicated that buried feelings (fear, guilt, shame, anger), if not confronted, will return as ghosts to harass them. The feelings cannot be denied; they will have their effect somehow. If confronted now, they will lose their power to hurt them in the future. With some clients, the pain-provoking memories can be dealt with fairly early in the therapy; with others I find it prudent to proceed more slowly.

Although I listen with compassion and understanding to the father's feelings, I will in no way condone the incestuous conduct or go along with pleas for mercy, such as that he is cursed and forced into incest by evil forces, or that he suffers from an exotic mental disease. He eventually is induced to admit the bald fact that he was totally responsible for the incestuous advances to his daughter. No matter the extenuating circumstances, including possible provocative behavior by his daughter, his actions betrayed his child and wife and their reliance on him as father and husband. Personal responsibility for the incestuous behavior is often objectively acknowledged by the men during group therapy and in sessions with their wives and daughters.

As a general rule, the mother will admit eventually that she was party to the incestuous situation and must have contributed to the underlying causes. Certainly, something must have been awry in her relationships with her husband and daughter. In order to relieve the daughter of feelings of self-blame and guilt for endangering the family, she is firmly told by her mother and, as soon as possible, by her father, that she was the victim of poor parenting. This step is also important for regaining her trust in her father and mother as parents. In time, however, she will confide that she was not entirely a helpless victim and is gently encouraged to explore this self-revelation.

Up to this point, the therapeutic approach is similar to that used by many humanist psychologists, particularly those of the Gestalt school.[18] The major objective of these first steps is to bring to awareness certain conscious and unconscious components of the individual personalities, as well as those that comprise the "personality" of the family. An important feature of the treatment is deliberate coaching in the techniques of self-awareness so that each individual can develop independently the skill of observing his own growth process and that of the family.

Self-Identification

The last two phases of the treatment program draw on the writings of Dr. Assagioli and others in psychosynthesis. A key notion during the later phases is that the self is a unique entity which is more than the changing functions of mind, body, and spirit. A strong sense of self-identity must be internalized by an individual before he can experience self-esteem. Developing this line of thought, the counselor points out that the self in each family member should be a relatively stable center, which is more than the roles each plays as daughter, student, mother, wife, father, husband, or worker; more than the transient feelings of hostility, guilt, shame, etc.; more than the changing body states of pain and disease. Further, it is indicated that the marriage and the family also have integrating centers that are also more than the daily drama enacted by the principals.

Self-Management

Once the idea of the self is entrenched and distinguished from the changing elements of personality, the concept of self-management is introduced. The assumption is that everyone can learn to control the way he behaves and ultimately the course his life will take. Each person in the family can behave purposefully to realize his potential and move deliberately toward self-actualization. The marriage and the family, conceptualized as separate organisms, can also be given purposeful direction. A major milestone is reached when the client acknowledges that all his past and current experiences are available to him for personal growth. He will assimilate all experiences, disown none.

A particular psychological school or discipline is not rigidly adhered to in attempting to satisfy the aims of the therapeutic model. Though the model roughly falls under the umbrella of humanistic psychology, other theories and methods, such as the psychoanalytic or the behavioral, are not denigrated or dismissed a priori. To avoid a mechanical, step-by-step approach, the last three phases of the therapeutic program are not developed in strict sequence. After initial efforts to bring about a good working relationship, I use an iterative strategy in guiding the client through the concepts and processes of self-assessment, self-identification, and self-management. They are developed more in parallel than in serial fashion.

A variety of techniques are employed in implementing the therapeutic model. None is used for its own sake; instead, I try to tune into the client and the situation and try to apply a fitting technique. In most instances, experiential techniques are called upon that elicit affective responses, however, cognitive and spiritual needs are not neglected. When indicated, I will briefly discuss the strategy and progress of the therapy and answer questions from the client. Certain clients who begin to internalize and practice the techniques at home report profound spiritual experiences. These clients are given special exercises that help them to expand and integrate the spiritual awakening.

Principal sources of the techniques comes from psychosynthesis, Gestalt therapy, conjoint therapy, psychodrama, Transactional Analysis, and personal journal keeping. To maintain continuity, exercises that can be done at home or at work between meetings are given to the client. Many of these techniques were described in detail in an earlier publication.[19]

Preliminary Results and Milestones

1. No recidivism reported in the more than 250 families receiving a minimum of ten hours of treatment and formally terminated.
2. Compared to preprogram outcomes the integrated, compassionate approach indicates that:
   (a) The children are returned to their families sooner; 90 percent within the first month, 95 percent eventually.
   (b) The self-abusive behavior of the children, usually amplified after exposure of the incestuous situation, has been reduced both in intensity and duration.
   (c) More marriages have been saved (about 90 percent) many confiding that their relationships are even better than they were before the crisis.
   (d) The offender's rehabilitation is accelerated since the counseling program is started soon after his arrest and continues during and after incarceration. Previous to CSATP, individual and marriage counseling, if any, occurred after release from jail.
   (e) In father-daughter incest, the difficult problem of reestablishing a normal relationship is more often resolved and in less time.
3. Parents United has grown from three mother members to about 60 members, of which half are father-offenders. Daughters United, comprised of teenaged victims of incest, has also grown substantially. Both groups are becoming increasingly self-sufficient; several of the older members act as group co-leaders.
4. In addition to self-help benefits, the Parents United formula is proving to members that they can become a strong voice in the community, a significant realization to those members who used to regard themselves as the pawns of civil authorities.
5. Offenders, who formerly would have received long jail or prison sentences, are now given suspended sentences or shorter terms due to increasing recognition of the CSATP by the judiciary as an effective alternative to incarceration.

6. The difficult goal of mobilizing typically disjointed and often competitive services into cooperative efforts is gradually being reached.

7. Due to the public education work, the referral rate has increased to about 180 families annually; about 60 percent of the referrals come from agencies other than the police or Juvenile Probation Departments, or directly from people heretofore fearful of reporting the problem.

8. The CSATP is receiving nationwide coverage by the media. Staff members and, more importantly, members of Parents United have appeared on several TV and radio programs, and the CSATP has been the subject of numerous newspaper and magazine articles.

9. Hundreds of informational packets have been sent to requestors throughout the country to abet the aim of having the CSATP serve as a model for other communities.

10. Several presentations and training seminars are conducted each year for professional groups by the writer and staff members. The presentations now include mothers, daughters, and fathers of the families treated for incest who are willing to answer questions from the audience—a significant breakthrough.

11. The CSATP is involving many volunteers and graduate students, who make valuable contributions while being trained.

12. The CSATP is unique also in that it constitutes the only substantive attempt extant to apply the principles and methods of humanistic psychology to a serious psychosocial problem. Currently the program is obtaining financial support direct from the California legislature.

Discussion

Current attitudes and laws regarding incest are myth-ridden and ineffective. Society is not attending responsibly to a problem vital to its own survival. The impact of civic authorities on incestuous families, particularly those in which the father is the offender, commonly adds up to either rejection of the victim's plea for help or disruptive punishment of the entire family.

I do not suggest that criminal laws in support of the incest taboo should be abolished and offenders should be dealt with exclusively by mental health workers. Reliance on the weekly therapeutic hour alone has not proved successful in the histories of several CSATP families. Typically, the mother had become aware that her husband was sexually exploiting their daughter and threatened to break up the marriage if he did not obtain psychiatric treatment. The offender complied but stopped going to the therapist after a few sessions. A month or two later he resumed the sexual abuse of his daughter. In two instances the fathers continued their offenses even while undergoing treatment. The motivating drive and/or therapy alone were not sufficient and the troubled family was left with its problem. In five other cases in which punishment alone was employed, the deterrent effect hoped for proved equally inadequate. After serving long sentences, the five men came to the attention of the CSATP for repeating the offense with other daughters or stepdaughters.

The CSATP works closely with the criminal justice systems of Santa Clara County and other local counties. The promising results would not have occurred without the cooperation of the police, probation officers, and the courts. The police and probation departments are major referral sources. A distraught victim, mother, or friend will usually turn to the police for immediate help since they are available 24 hours a day. It is now a common practice for officers who investigate the cases to refer offenders and their families to the CSATP.

For the offender the implication is that involvement in the CSATP is likely to be strongly considered by the judge and prosecuting attorney during court proceedings. His own lawyer will also urge him to join the CSATP. Though all offenders hope that their penalties will be softened by participation in the CSATP, many find it equally compelling to do so for the aid the program gives to their families. Usually each man soon realizes that the program will help him understand and control his deviant impulses and to reestablish sound relationships with his wife, the daughter he victimized, and the other children.

In all cases the authority of the criminal justice system, and the court process, seems necessary in order to satisfy what may be termed an expiatory factor in the treatment of the offender and his family. It appears that the offender needs to know unequivocally that the community will not condone his incestuous behavior and that he must face the consequences. The victim and her mother also admit to deriving comfort from the knowledge of the community's clear stand on incest. All family members, however, will do their best to frustrate the system if they anticipate that the punishment will be so severe that the family will be destroyed— that they, in turn, will become "victims" of the criminal justice system, including the child-victim herself.

No matter what the reasons may be for admission of an incestuous family into the CSATP, it is our responsibility to help the family reconstitute itself as quickly as possible, hopefully around the original nuclear pair. Even if the offender comes to the CSATP only for the purpose of saving himself, it is up to us to show him that he can reap more substantial benefits both for himself and his family from honest participation in the CSATP. Of course, the CSATP is not equally effective with all clients. About 10 percent of referrals will elude our efforts. They will not come in for the initial interview or will drop out soon after treatment has begun. Four couples were dismissed from the program because the father and/or his wife would not admit culpability and placed the blame entirely on the child-victim and her seductive behavior. In these instances extraordinary effort was required in the treatment of the deserted child. After many attempts, three of the girls successfully adjusted to foster homes. They are now married and apparently doing well.

The CSAPT is a growing community resource. Some of its objectives have only partially been achieved; others will be added, or dropped, or modified. But there is at least the beginning of a response to Vincent de Francis's clarion call to the American community to protect the sexually molested child.[20] Moreover, the CSATP complies with Besharov's request for enlightened intervention that considers the requirements of the entire family, the parents as well as the children.[21]

By working integrally with the criminal justice system, the

CSATP shows promise of developing into a model for other American communities. Each community must be given the opportunity to treat incestuous families in a manner that is neither permissive nor cruelly punitive. A national position should be taken on the incest taboo and laws enacted that are effective and consistent; the community must publicize these statutes and the penalties for violating them.

To prevent incest the public must be educated to become aware of predisposing conditions and to take appropriate action. Finally, comprehensive procedures similar to the CSATP must be established in each community to treat sexually abused children and their families in order to enhance their chances for reconstitution and to prevent future violations.

REFERENCES

1. Mead, M. "Incest." *International Encyclopedia of the Social Sciences.* New York: Crowell, Collier and Macmillan, 1968.
2. Caprio, F. S. and D. R. Brenner. *Sexual Behavior: Psycho-Legal Aspects.* New York: The Citadel Press, 1961.
3. Kling, G. *Sexual Behavior and The Law.* New York: Bernard Geis Associates, 1965.
4. DeFrancis, V. "Protecting the Child Victim of Sex Crimes Committed by Adults." *Federal Probation* (September 15—20) 1971.
5. Weinberg, S. K. *Incest Behavior.* New York: Citadel Press, 1955.
6. Master, R. *Patterns of Incest: Psycho-Social Study.* New York: Julian Press, 1963.
7. Besharov, D. J. "Building a Community Response to Child Abuse and Maltreatment." *Children Today* (September-October): 2—4, 1975.
8. Sgroi, S. M. "Sexual Molestation of Children." *Children Today* (May-June): 18—21, 1975.
9. James, Jennifer. Private communications.
10. Baisden, M. J. *The World of Rosaphrenia: The Sexual Psychology of the Female.*Calif.: Allied Research Society, Sacramento, 1971.
11. Baisden, M. J. Unpublished data.
12. Benward, Jean and J. Densen-Gerber. *Incest as a Causative Factor in Anti-Social Behavior: An Exploratory Study.* New York: Odyssey Institute, 1975.
13. Weinberg, op. cit.
14. Satir, V. *Conjoint Family Therapy.* Palo Alto, Calif.: Science and Behavior Books, 1967.

15. Assagioli, R. *Psychosynthesis.* New York: Hobbs, Dorman, 1965.
16. *Ibid.*
17. Chaudhuri, H. *Integral Yoga.* San Francisco: California Institute of
     Asian Studies, 1970.
18. Perls, F. S., Hefferline, R. F., and Paul Goodman. *Gestalt Therapy.*
     New York: Julian Press, 1951.
19. Giarretto, H. and A. Einfield. "The Self-Actualization of Educators."
     In Marcia Perlstein, (Ed.), *Flowers Can Even Bloom in Schools.*
     Sunnyvale, Calif.: Westinghouse Learning Press, 1974.
20. *Op. cit.*
21. *Op. cit.*

Chapter 13

INCEST POLICY RECOMMENDATIONS
LeRoy G. Schultz

Intervention

1. Current law and statute, and various governmental agency policy, do not reflect all the current views and values regarding incest in a changing democratic society. It is recommended that the appropriate agencies reevaluate current law and policy, with recommendations for modernizing both in terms of a multi-value-based society.

2. In most instances of incest, excluding those where continued danger to the minor children exists, separation of family members is to be avoided. Separation may doubly traumatize.

3. When feasible, families where incest has occurred should be treated as a unit, not each member separately. Individual therapy has both diagnostic and treatment limitations.

4. While the *Child Sexual Abuse Treatment Program* (Giaretto) has been used successfully with father-daughter abuse cases only, it is the one treatment showing the most promise at this time, and it should be further researched with national dissemination of results to all professionals in the field of social work.

5. There is a need to further expand Parents United throughout the nation in both urban and rural areas. Such group efforts should be federally supported through the appropriate HEW organization.

6. Since it is commonly accepted as principle that in treatment one should "start where the client is," professionals treating incest situations should avoid compelling clients to accept esoteric or moralistic explanations of the incest event, and

begin working with the rationale offered by the participants themselves.

7. Where the offender is isolated by court sentence from his family, behavior modification methods are recommended for the treatment of incest that are both effective and ethical.

8. Sex therapy should be made more available for all at public expense (tax supported), before and after the incest event, as one part of a preventive program.

9. Incest victims or those threatened with it need more runaway centers where they can escape both parents with the option of a permanent foster care arrangement on demand. Adolescent victims must be given the right to charge parents with "incorrigibility" and "sexually acting out."

10. It is recommended that society openly endorse more sexual outlets for married couples, those "living together," *and* for children and adolescents. Perhaps the most important condition required for incest genesis is that extrafamily sexual outlets be denied youth.

11. Since authorities attribute much of incest to general family breakdown (before the act of incest), more adequate parental role training is required through the formal educational system. Despite the incredibly serious nature of parenthood in a family centered society, there is little preparation for it. It may be easy to retort that society gets what it deserves, but it is the children who may suffer. More adequate AFDC grants geared to inflation, abundant family-planning services including state-funded abortions, more family refuge centers, more day care services, more adolescent hot lines, and more run-away centers are required.

Education

1. A responsible nonhysterical national effort is required to raise this nation's awareness of the incest problem, in direct proportion to other social problems with which it must compete for attention and funding.

2. Terming incest as a sin is no longer an acceptable or effective

mode of dealing with the incest problem. Religious institutions should address the finding that incestors have a strong religious concern.

3. A sex-education program, responsible and timely, must be instituted from grades K through 12. Night classes in sex education are essential for parents. Such education should stress the positive and health-enhancing aspects of sexual expression in keeping with the law, with consumer input as soon as the child or adolescent is able to make choices in his own interest. The requirement of permission slips from parents to allow their children to take part in sex education classes should be reevaluated after the child reaches a responsible age. Incestuous parents are unlikely to give such consent.

4. There is a need for professional education regarding incest and its solutions for psychiatrists, pediatricians, nurses, social workers, and all para-professionals in child-care institutions and programs. In-service training and workshops with federal funding with mandatory attendance are required.

Research

1. The psychosocial damages resulting from father-daughter incest may be partially repairable through the new "feminist therapy." Analysis is required of this mode of therapy as to definitions, process, ethics, outcome, and therapist-manpower.

2. The FBI should require all local police jurisdictions to report incest cases as a separate category within the Uniform Crime Reporting System. Without some more reliable estimate of the offense, policy-making bodies have little data to support new efforts of control.

3. Research is required on the suitability of fathers raising children without a spouse in cases where the mother-wife is the offender, and for the gay household as well. Homemaker services may need expansion and more financial support within child welfare policy to meet these new

needs.

4. Research is required to spell out in realistic terms the damages cited as coming from the incestuous relationship, such as "betrayal of father trust," "loss of both parents," and "keeping it secret from mother." To date, there is little convincing data that these are traumatizing in the majority of cases coming to the attention of law enforcement or mental health professionals, and the literature reflects a simplistic outcome for all incest participants, irrespective of child's age, offender relationship, situational aspects, love versus force elements, child's ego strengths, child support network, etc.

5. Intensive research efforts are required to determine why most families are *not* incest-genetic. Herein may be the great impetus for preventive tactics that can be taught to all families or structured into family and children's policy.

6. One of the problems encountered in gaining access to victims is the lack of researcher's and helper's access to them within the privacy-bound family. Research is required to determine skills and methods needed to safely ferret out incest if it exists, but do no harm if it does not exist. Children report household crime differently than household adults do. (U.S. Department of Justice: *An Introduction to the National Crime Survey*, 1978, GPO, p. 26.)

7. Sibling incest, although perhaps the most prevalent type, has received scant attention from researchers, professional helpers, policy-makers, and families. It appears less immoral, less damaging, and less socially disruptive. This needs further clarification. The effects of differing types of incest (with whom, with what degree of force, at what age) on participants needs to be made public, if there are any.

8. It is very difficult to acquire sound data on so-called beneficial or neutral incest. The helping professions and researchers find such ideas professionally dangerous, and they refuse to remain open-minded until the evidence comes in. Others contend it is immoral, whether or not it does damage. Judgment should be suspended pending research publication of such results. Two such reports are due for

release in approximately 1981. If the research is convincing and damage is found to be nonexistent, our policy and programs and our concept of victim may need some alteration. The lack of damage need not be viewed as an endorsement of incest.

9. Almost all research on incest, necessarily, relied upon poor sampling techniques. Samples are usually drawn from court or social welfare agency records or rely upon victims' recall some ten or twenty years after the event, or the sample was drawn through newspaper advertisements, or events were solicited from the offender while he was incarcerated. Such samples raise question as to their generalizability. They may, in fact, represent only one or two types of victims. The literature reflects a parading of personal belief as fact or the misuse of data in the service of personal belief. The research truism holds: there is nothing that cannot be proven if only the outlook is sufficiently limited. Sample selection in the future must include social class, cultural, income, racial, age, sexual, and religious differences, as well as a control group. The standards of good research must be applied if believability is desired. Some professionals become upset when minors do not live up to their theories of cause and effect.

10. Iatrogenesis is the last frontier in professionalism. The literature on incest reflects the possibility that most incest events are short-lived in their effects. What is traumatizing over a long period of time may be the manner in which professionals (law enforcement and mental health) process the victim through their respective systems. Research is required on determining to what degree these systems of processing victims are themselves traumatogenic, and how this can be controlled.

Section IV

THE VICTIM AND THE JUSTICE SYSTEM

"One question which should always face the adult policy-maker is, would children make the same choice? An answer of "no" ought seriously to undermine almost any justification for supporting the particular policy process in that the question isn't asked, let alone answered affirmatively."

David S. Mundel: *Raising Children in Modern America.*
1976, p. 459.

Chapter 14

THE VICTIM AND THE JUSTICE SYSTEM— AN INTRODUCTION

LeRoy G. Schultz

Interviewing children and adolescents after an alleged sexual offense involves two different interests: the use of the victim as a witness for prosecution and the gaining of information necessary for victim welfare.

The American justice system requires the victim of an offense to come forward and make a defensable complaint that will withstand abrasive probing. The justice system may require the victim to relate the sexual event to perhaps some three or four different actors (police officers, grand jury members, prosecutors, and court members). The victim may also be expected to relate the sexual event to child welfare workers, mental health professionals, and emergency room staff. Thus, it would be possible for the victim to relate the sexual event to a wide range of strangers each claiming a set of special interests.

It is an assumption that repeating possibly unpleasant details of the sexual act to this large number of strangers, each with their own goals and values, creates psychic trauma. It is not an assumption that the process creates confusion and boredom for most victims. The young victim must use his/her own age-related concept of the event in an adult world where its proportion is exaggerated and where a short-lived event is adult-ized, dwelled upon over many months with excessive concern for boring details and swelled beyond the child victim's concept of reality. Some victims learn that their role is as justice system adjunct or vindicator of "good" parents (and adult behaviors) are not guided by the best interests of the child. All young victims have the constitutional right to remain silent and this option should be explained to the victim in clear language compatible with his intellectual stage and social class. Parents and professionals must be more accountable to the child and the child's choice.

Society's need to determine the details of the sexual crime and thus possibly traumatize the victim is of society's own creation. By making the death penalty the cost of child sexual abuse up to recent times, severe interrogation was required to make sure the right person was convicted and that a sexual offense actually took place. Foster and Ranum (1978) report on the great sexual detail in court records in fifteenth century France. Historically, youth have been viewed as distorters of reality, misperceivers, manipulators, fantasy-weavers, and instinctual liars, hardly the characteristics desired by the truth-searching process in an adversary setting. Bourdan, in his book *Lying Children* (1882), stated children become hysterical under stress and therefore untrustworthy and poor witnesses. In the classic professional textbook *Criminal Investigation* by H. Gross (in its 5th edition in 1908), young females were described as dangerous witnesses, particularly if they live dull lives and find attention in court as flattery. Gross thought the menstruating adolescent the most unreliable witness of all. He concluded that the child's perception of reality may be different from that of adults, with some adult perception completely outside the child's frame of reference, with numerous language problems between adults and children.

Not all children were viewed as liars, particularly if very young. Stone (1977) cites the case of a three-and-one-half-year-old in the 1880s testifying in a capital offense case of rape of a six-year-old, where she is described on the witness stand as witty and credible. G. Stanley Hall, the discoverer of adolescense, in his book *Children's Lies* (1890), claimed lying was closely related to children's play and naivete and children have a "mytho-poetic faculty" that finds truth and exactitudes tedious. The physician A. Moll, perhaps more than any other, codified much of the superstition and folklore of youth regarding sexuality and testifying. In his book *The Sexual Life of the Child* (translated into English in 1912), Moll contended that children, particularly girls, could easily fool lawyers and judges, particularly about sexual innocence. He demanded that "assumed" innocence be challenged and that alleged sex-victims be physically examined to ascertain virginity or sexual precociousness or if self-masturbation could account for vaginal irritation. He added a new dimension. He reported cases of charges of child sex abuse being placed as a method of discrediting one's political enemies following the Franco-German War. While Moll raised the prospect of legal process trauma, he was more concerned with child victimogenesis and culpability. Concern for controlling court-induced trauma was voiced as early as 1915 by the social worker C. Cartens, when he found that such court victims turned to prostitution following the sex event. He recommended that testimony be given once only; if the victim is female, a female interrogator was required.

This historical heritage has characterized the interrogation and interviewing process up to recent times and was based on outdated concepts of childhood and adolescence, sexuality and morality, which would seem to have little relevance today. Even so, this heritage is built into law today. A child sex victim is a presumptive victim until the offense is held to be proved, and the defense attorney has the duty of trying to discredit the alledged victim's statements. How then can society balance the need for a fair trial in which a suspect can face his/her accusor with the need to control legal process trauma?

Libai's contribution answers this question. It is a scholarly but practical address to the dilemma. He presents an excellent defense of legal testimony reform and proposes policy reformulation from a cross-cultural perspective. Flammang's chapter makes clear the importance of the police officer's role with child victims in stressing sensitive interviewing and acquiring the basic information necessary to make an arrest and a case. Since the police officer is usually the first professional encountering the victim, he/she is in a critical position in terms of creating psychotrauma and initiating the victim welfare system. Control over these elements defines effective police work.

The contribution by Stevens and Berliner makes clear that any professional involved with child victims should have some education and experience with the field of child development. Speaking from hospital and clinic experience, they present usable fundamentals. The victim's interviews can result in little information, or trauma, unless sensitively engaged in.

New methods aimed at preventing trauma while ensuring legality are being tried today. For example, in a murder trial, seven-year-old witnesses to the murder were taken to the courthouse well before the trial where they were to testify, and given ice cream, etc., in the courthouse, making for a more pleasant association. Witness waiting rooms can be made less threatening by providing play space and toys (*Newsweek* 6-27, 1977, p. 2; *Time* 6-6, 1977, pp. 13-14). Schultz has suggested mock trials to reduce fright (1975, pp. 257-273). A new concern with age-graded methods, children's rights, and new behavior modification techniques may make the police station and courthouse a safer place for youth in the future.

The Burgess and Laszlo contribution highlights the critical role that agency records play in court processing of sexual assault cases. While the article relates predominantly to the medical setting, its implications also apply to social welfare as well, or wherever the written work of professionals is used in justice settings. Clear concise writing is essential where the agency records are to be used in legal proceedings.

I have seen authority figures (police, parents, child welfare workers, nurses, teachers) who decried the molestor's capacity to negatively influence the immature mind of the child, only to use the same capacity themselves to influence the child to take roles in prosecution or treatment. Professionals must decide in each case whether the young victim has the ego strengths required for interviewing or interrogation, in both the justice system and the mental health system. If such strengths do not exist, or trauma is likely, it may be more humane to leave intact any compensating delusions that make the child's lot easier.

Chapter 15

INTERVIEWING CHILD VICTIMS OF SEX OFFENDERS*

C. J. FLAMMANG

With the continued increase of delinquency and youthful crime rates, one is prone to concentrate upon the juvenile in the role of the offender. Often overlooked within the day-to-day police operation are the numbers of youth who are victimized by other youth and adults. A significant amount of this victimization involves sexually oriented offenses directed toward children.

Even the mention of juveniles and sex invokes the traditional image of the incidence of statutory rape, with the victim being viewed as a co-participant. Thus, the concept of the juvenile as an offender continues to prevail.

While much has been written about interviewing, no significant amount of material is contained within the literature relating to sexual offenses directed toward children. Interviewing techniques are generally presented as a smaller segment of information dealing with interrogation. The interview, as such, has not received the attention that has been provided interrogation in police literature. As has been the case in many police functions, there is a question of misplaced priorities in relation to interviewing and interrogation. It is true that interrogation is highly important, but it is also true that the police do a disproportionate amount of interviewing. The skills necessary to conduct an effective interview are required tools of the police officer.

Interviewing is based upon a different objective than the goal of the interrogation. It requires a different approach, and these factors demand the utilization of a separate set of skills. The total

*From *Police*, *16(6)*: 23-28, 1972. Reprinted with permission of Charles C Thomas, Publisher, Springfield, Illinois.

setting of the interview is drastically altered in cases involving the young victim of a sexual offense. For the purpose of this article, the subject matter will be limited to those persons, usually under age fourteen, who have been subjected to a sexual encounter, and the subsequent police task of interviewing the child victim.

Range of Sexuality Encountered By Young Children

The term *pedophilia* is applied to that classification of persons who are prone to direct their sexuality toward children. While this group represents a large segment of the problem under discussion, child molest situations also involve youthful suspects committing sex offenses against youthful victims.

The incompetency felt by the pedophil individual toward the release of his sexual desires within a reasonably mature setting with persons of his own age is believed to be a large measure of the motivation to direct his attentions toward young children.[1] There are numerous other factors involved, including the *innocence perception*, in which the individual is attracted to the young child because of a shattered womanhood fantasy.

The youth who acts out his sexual drives by involvement with younger children is usually striving to release the tensions those drives have created. However, pedophilia is observed among adolescents, and in the event the tendencies are not discovered and corrected, that individual will probably carry them into adulthood.

Although sexual drives are an inherent part of the human needs response, sexual behavior is learned. As stated by Ullman and Krasner:

> . . . it is an area of taboo, an area associated with a primary source of positive reinforcement, and involves a complicated interpersonal relationship, it is not surprising that it suffers particular vicissitudes in our society. Emphasis is continually placed on sexual success as a measure of personal worth and therefore, sexual difficulties may, by generalization, be associated with many other role behaviors.[2]

---

[1] J. P. de River: *Crime and the Sexual Psychopath*. Springfield, Thomas, 1958, p. 160.
[2] L. P. Ullman and L. Krasner: *Case Studies in Behavior Modifications*. New York, Holt, Rinehart and Winston, 1965, p. 234.

While the actual incidence of sexuality directed toward young children is not known, the range of the offenses are commonly encountered.[3] Types of offenses run the totality of the continuum of the human sexual experience. The offenses include homosexuality, sodomy, incest, normally accepted acts of intercourse, various methods of oral copulation, and numerous incidents of sex play. The latter is most frequently encountered, due to the physical differences between the victim and the adult offender and the pain that is likely to occur during the act of penetration. The recognition of these facts by the adult participant tends to explain the often-heard statement by the suspect to the effect that the victim was not *hurt.*

Human sexual behavior is dependent upon a multiplicity of variables. Two of these are the interpersonal relationship and the circumstances of opportunity. It is because of these factors that so many police encounters with sex offenses directed toward young children tend to emanate from within the family or in the neighborhood setting. A great majority of the incidents are family oriented. These usually do not surface rapidly but, rather, represent long periods of chronic adult-child sexual activity.

The youngest victim to qualify as a witness and provide courtroom testimony against an adult suspect was a five-year-old girl. Admittedly, she was an exceptional child; however, children from seven years on should normally be able to perform the witness role.

Importance of the Child Victim as a Witness

The majority of sex offenses against small children occur in semi-secrecy and for obvious reasons. One of the major factors providing older suspects with a sense of confidence is the concept that the child will either not willingly testify or will be incapable of providing testimony. This concept is manifested by the suspect's statements or actions upon apprehension, that it is the child's word against his. Quite often the suspect is right. It is for this reason that the child victim is an important individual in the

---

[3]The American Humane Association, Denver, under the direction of Vincent De Francis, is studying the epidemiology of sex crimes against children.

investigation. A secondary reason for the importance of the victim as a witness lies in the need to establish the certainty of the corpus delicti before pursuing the investigation. The victim's description of the offense is the basis for accepting or rejecting the report of a crime in a child molest case in the absence of extensive physical evidence. Usually the offense is really a series of offenses that have occurred over a long period of time in a sheltered situation. These factors account for the small number of cases in which physical evidence of a meaningful nature is discovered.

The following examples will dramatize the importance of the child victim as a witness. During one four-hour period, the author successfully investigated and apprehended three different suspects, in three separate incidents, at three geographic locations, each remote from the other. One case involved acts of homosexuality being perpetrated upon elementary school boys while returning home from school. The second incident was an attempt to rape a young female while she was playing in a vacant lot. The last offense was a fondling of the private parts of a six-year-old girl adjacent to a recreation park. None of the victims had even seen the suspect before the offenses had occurred. The success attained in these investigations does not indicate an outstanding ability upon the part of the author, but rather reflects the capabilities of the children who were victimized to perform in the role of witnesses.

Another consideration of the child victim as a witness involves the importance of the child as a courtroom witness. Generally speaking, the suspect will often force the issue of the courtroom experience. This may be merely at the point of the preliminary hearing, but police officers should not be surprised if their victim is required to testify. In the event the case goes to court, the suspect is relying upon the hope that the victim will not make an effective witness. In addition, in the courtroom setting, the child victim is often the only vehicle for establishing that the crime, in fact, was committed.

In evaluating the several roles of the victim as a vehicle of information, one discovers three definite effects upon the totality of the investigative procedure. The first is the need for the victim to convince the officer of the actuality of the crime. The second is the utilization of the victim for information that will lead to the identification and apprehension of the suspect, in the event the suspect is unknown. The third is the necessity of viewing the victim in the role of the most important courtroom witness and predetermining the child's effectiveness at testimony.

The Elements of the Police Interview

Interviewing is a purposeful communication technique.[4] Its purpose is to seek information.[5] In the final analysis, it amounts to an interpersonal relationship. Because of the intimacy of the individuals involved, personalities play an important part in the interview. In large measure, the success of the interview depends upon the officer's ability to quickly interpret the personality of the person being interviewed and then to adjust the projection of his own personality to fit the needs of the situation. Most authorities agree that the initial contact between the interviewer and the person being interviewed is a crucial point in which a frame of reference must be established.[6]

The police interview is characterized by a degree of voluntariness on the part of the individual being interviewed.[7] It is not a situation in which the officer is the sole actor, but it requires the ability to listen and ferret out important information that is contained in the overall statements by the interviewed.

An interview has the elemental needs to establish rapport, to keep the person talking, to avoid long pauses or use them effectively, and to ignore or disregard some comments.[8]

The effective police interview has other properties, including the time factor. Interviews cannot be successfully conducted in a hurry. Haste must be avoided. They require preparation. No interview can be truly successful unless the officer has all of the

---

[4]C. J. Flammang: *The Police and the Underprotected Child.* Springfield, Thomas, 1970, p. 196.
[5]G. J. Dudycha: *Psychology for Law Enforcement Officers.* Springfield, Thomas, 1955, p. 68.
[6]*Ibid.,* p. 74.
[7]Flammang, *supra,* pp. 197-198.
[8]Dudycha, *supra,* pp. 74-78.

available information it is possible to have before entering the interview arena. Furthermore, the officer should plan the interview and know where he is to begin before the encounter. Included in the planning process should be reactions to the unexpected and the ability to adjust the thrust of the interview accordingly.

The nature of the interview requires the development of certain skills that are not a part of the interrogation or other communicative processes. The interview is but another example of the multiplicity of tasks involved in the police function.

Interviewing the Child Victim of Sexual Offenses

The interviewing of the young child is a sensitive situation. Police personnel often lose sight of the fact that a child is not just a small adult. If handled properly, children can provide very effective information.[9] In order to obtain solid facts from a young child, different skills must be employed than would be used in an interview involving an older person.

The nature of the offense is one in which parental and adult reactions are likely to be emotional and explosive. This fact has caused one authority to express the need for the officer to deal with the adult reactions as a primary function *before the interview.*[10] In order to control the interview of the child, the police must first take charge of the total situation in which the interview will occur. Usually by discussing the concept of *protection through innocence*, the parents will be brought to a realistic position. Protection through innocence suggests that the child victim of a nonviolent sexual act will not suffer greatly from the effects of the experience unless the child interprets the situation to be extremely wrong as a result of the reactions of the adults around him. Once parents and others are convinced of the harm that the adult reactions to the offense do to the child, the officer is in the position to move toward establishing the interview setting.

[9]H. Soderman and J. J. O'Connell: *Modern Criminal Investigation.* New York, Funk and Wagnalls, 1952, p. 34.

[10]M. Holman: *The Police Officer and the Child.* Springfield, Thomas, 1962. p. 109.

Where the interview occurs is not nearly as important as who may be included as observers. The only requirement for the setting of the interview is that the location provide a degree of privacy and that it limit interruptions from external sources. In the victim's home, a bedroom or the kitchen may be the best universal choices. The school may be a very effective place. Even the police vehicle may be successfully utilized. Naturally, if there is no emergency nature to the offense, an office at headquarters may be ideal.

Whenever possible, the child should be interviewed by officers only, with no observers. A word of caution: *a male officer should not interview a female victim without someone else present.* When it is necessary to have another person (not an officer) present, that other person should be a neutral party. Neutral in this context means a person free from excessive emotional reaction to the nature of the subject matter and a person who is willing to observe and not become engaged in the verbalization of the interview.

Determining the Child's Capability To Be a Witness

In the courtroom, the decision of whether or not to allow the testimony of the child is a matter that falls within the judicial discretion of the judge. In order to make that decision, the judge will question the child in an attempt to determine the youth's ability to observe the oath administered to witnesses. This ability can be predetermined by the officer, and this action can occur as a result of an important part of the interview. That part is the crucial opening of the conversation.

Beginning the interview with *icebreakers* that establish the child's ability to provide personal information places the interview into an immediate context of informality and friendliness. Children like to discuss themselves and show off their knowledge. Questions to be pursued include not only personal data, but also questions rating the child's development and maturity, establishing his concept of time, and relating to veracity.

EXAMPLES OF PERSONAL QUESTIONS—The questioning of the child about where he lives, the names of his parents, and information about other siblings in the home tends to bring about a responsiveness. If there are other children in the home, their names and ages should be secured from the victim, along with information about whether they are older or younger than the child being interviewed. (Later, this information can be used to determine the whereabouts of the siblings during the commission of the offense.)

The child should be questioned regarding school attendance, friends, and personal interests.

The child victim should be able to state the month or day of his birth. Either piece of information would be sufficient for a young child. The investigator should not disqualify a child on the basis of an inability to provide this information, especially in relationship to the year of the birth.

QUESTIONS RATING DEVELOPMENT AND MATURITY—It should be determined if the victim can tell time or answer general questions regarding community life which the particular child experiences, such as church attendance, recreational or educational opportunities usually open to children, and other areas of possible experience.

The officer should attempt to discover if the child can tie shoes or perform other motor control tasks normal for a child of that age.

QUESTIONS ESTABLISHING A CONCEPT OF TIME—These questions should be utilized throughout the interview, as it is necessary to demonstrate the child's ability to judge time, to some reasonable extent, in relation to the offense.

General questions aiding this procedure cover the subject matter of what days of the week the child attends school (or does not attend, a question with less answers that arrives at the same conclusion.) Having the child name the months or the time of year that he does not attend school provides a basis for the determination of the child's concept of a year period.

As the interview proceeds and the story of the offense unfolds, the child may be able to establish time periods in relation to childhood experiences. The daily television schedule provides the opportunity to direct the child's attention to the time of day. The same is true for eating habits; whether it was daylight or dark; if it occurred before or after going to bed or going to school. There are many routine daily functions in the life of the child upon which to relate the time element of the offense.

For broader time lengths, relating the incidents to various holidays, school vacation periods, important family activities, or other pertinent experiences will succeed in focusing the child's attention on a time period that delimits the vagueness.

QUESTIONS RELATING TO VERACITY—The child should be able to state in his own words what is meant by *telling the truth*. It is necessary for the child to make a negative connection to the act of lying and a positive one to the act of telling the truth.

The child does not have to explain the nature of truth. He merely has to indicate that he is aware of what is involved in the *act* of truthfulness. For the younger child, it may be helpful to frame the questions in reverse, such as, *what happens to a person who tells a lie?* The child must be able to show that he knows that telling the truth is good and that telling a lie is wrong.

The Child and Leading Questions

A tolerance exists to a minimum degree for leading questions directed toward children. This is an acceptable courtroom practice. The officer must remain aware of the suggestibility of the interviewee, and leading questions should be kept to a minimum, if not omitted entirely. The problem involved in the use of leading questions is the increase of the factor of inaccuracy. The purpose of the interview is to obtain factual information, and questioning forms that reduce the ability to achieve that objective are in opposition to the reason for the interview. Holman has warned against the officer putting words into the child's mouth and extends that admonition to include the act of parents being allowed to do the same thing.[11] This latter problem is best overcome by isolating the parents from the interview situation.

---

[11]*Ibid.*

Determining the Details of the Offense

The child being questioned must establish the facts of the crime. This requires the officer to pursue questioning that will elicit the details of the acts performed. Such details are not common experiential knowledge to a young child. Sexual activities cannot be described by young children, in a vivid way, unless the child has been exposed to the sexuality involved.

Because of the nature of the subject matter, the officer must use tact and discretion in formulating and stating the questions. He has to realize that the child will not have a vocabulary with which to express many of the facts. In those instances, it will be necessary to shift from one word or phrase to another, in an attempt to arrive at a verbalization of the event or item that is mutually understood. A very good method is to ask the child what term he applies to a certain body part or to describe a certain act.

Many children will not be able to provide a term that will describe an act of a sexual nature, while others may be found to be shockingly explicit. They all will be able to reach an understood agreement for terms that designate various portions of the body. Utilizing these body part terms, the officer can then question the child as to the mechanics of the act.

Some officers enter these interviews with preconceptions of how the act occurred. This is a fatal error. The deviations within the scope of human sexuality are close to infinite. The office should realize that in a situation where no penetration took place, the child may relate answers to questions concerning fondling, when in fact oral offenses also were included.

The term *child victim* can also be misleading, as it carries a connotation of passive participation. The realities are that a child may be stimulated pleasurably as a result of the sexual contact, and become an active participant. Thus, some questioning along the lines of what acts the child performed upon the person of the suspect may be in order. It represents a possibility that should not be discounted.

In entering into the main area of the interview, the officer should insure that the child understands the meaning of the victim role. The interviewer must recognize that there has been some excitement and reaction displayed since the child first allowed the situation to come to light. The fact of the presence of the officer indicates to the child that this is a more than normal situation. The child must not be allowed to believe that he is in trouble or that people think him to be *nasty*.

After quelling those types of fears on the part of the child and beginning the search for the details of the offense, the officer should conduct the interview with the recognition that it is an investigative process, not a course in sex education. Very sensitive areas may be encountered. If the child's reactions indicate that he is not aware of what the officer is talking about, and this lack of awareness is due to inexperience and not vocabulary, the officer should not pursue that course further. There is no need to teach the child facts that extend beyond the scope of the information-seeking goal of the interview.

Among adults who could affect the child by the adult reaction to what is stated is the officer. No police personnel should register any response to what transpires within the interview that could be misinterpreted by the child. Along this same vein, the officer should recognize that the child may be quite close to the suspect, beyond the sexual display. Therefore, the approach used by the police should omit any derogatory or other negative statements about the suspect in the presence of the child. Vindictiveness is not part of the investigative process.

Police Actions Related to the Interview, But Occurring Afterwards

Upon the completion of the interview, the police should explain to the parents that the child may have to repeat the story to others, including the prosecutor, and the act of testifying in open court. Officers should never state that the child will not have to testify or talk to others, if the case is to be pursued.

The parents should be cautioned against continued questioning or recounting the incident within the home. They should be encouraged to let the matter drop until the time that it is necessary to bring it out again. The child's emotional reactions and return to normalcy are given a better prognosis if the matter is allowed to lie dormant.

Later, if the case goes to court, the officer should be aware of the rapport that he established with the child during the interview, and that the child may have a close affinity toward the officer. Without going to extremes, the officer should be sure to recognize the presence of the child in and around the courtroom. He should take steps to alleviate the anxieties of the victim and to encourage the child's efforts at testifying. This is not intended to mean that the officer should react to the child while the latter is on the witness stand; rather, it refers to before-court sensitivity.

Conclusions

Police encounters with child victims of sex offenses are not unusual. The child represents an important vehicle in the investigative process, and the officer should approach the youth with that importance in mind. The interview of the child is a critical stage in the investigation, and the results of that interview will in large measure determine the results of the police action.

Chapter 16

THE PROTECTION OF THE CHILD VICTIM OF A SEXUAL OFFENSE IN THE CRIMINAL JUSTICE SYSTEM*

DAVID LIBAI

Introduction

The problems of juvenile offenders have won general recognition in Anglo-American countries, but those of juveniles who fall victims to sexual offenders have not. The juvenile offender is treated in a different manner from the adult offender.[1] In the pretrial period, juvenile offenders are interrogated by special police youth officers, and first offenders in particular can easily be handled without being brought to trial. Trials of juveniles are heard at different times and places than trials of adults, by judges who are specially appointed by the state to hear juvenile cases, in proceedings less formal than those conducted in trials of adults.[2] In addition, juvenile offenders may be assisted by probation officers or child guidance clinics, which combine the skills of the psychiatrist, psychologist, and social worker.[3] All of this must be done with a view to protecting the accused child without abridging his or her constitutional rights.[4]

---

*Reprinted with permission of Wayne State University Law Review, *Wayne Law Review* (Vol. 15, 1969), © Wayne State University Law School.

[1]*See generally* S. RUBIN. CRIME AND JUVENILE DELINQUENCY (2d ed. 1966); *In re* Gault, 387 U.S. 1 (1967).

[2]Mr. Justice Fortas, in *In re* Gault, 387 U.S. 1, 22 (1967), refers to "the commendable principles relating to the processing and treatment of juveniles separately from adults" and emphasized that they "are in no way involved or affected" by the decision in *Gault*.

[3]*See* C. VEDDER, JUVENILE OFFENDERS 160-162 (1963).

[4]Constitutional guarantees of due process cannot be traded for promises of rehabilitation, education, and salvation. Justice Fortas emphasized that therapy may well begin with protecting the essentials of due process, which leave on juveniles an impression of fair treatment, and that "the observance of due process standards intelligently and not ruthlessly administered, will not compel the states to abandon or displace any of the sub-

When a child victim is called to assist the prosecution of his accused assailant, he is treated in basically the same way as an adult witness. Parents who might wish to prevent their child from being repeatedly interrogated will find it difficult to withdraw their complaint against a child molester, even if it is the child's first involvement with the law, because the state regards its interest in punishing the offender as overriding the parents' interest in protecting the child. Child victims are generally interviewed by detectives who normally interrogate adult victims of sexual offenses, and child victims are required to testify in the same courts and in the same manner as adults. No special judges are appointed to hear child victims; the court's formal procedures make no allowances for their protection, and no expert in problems of children's mental hygiene is appointed by the state to support child victims.[5] The public conscience seems to have been awakened over the problem of juvenile delinquents because they are both children and accused. Yet, a child victim for the most part remains neglected by the state, a "forgotten child—a child whose presence, whose condition and whose cry for help is unrecognized or ignored."[6] The section of this chapter entitled **The Problem in Perspective** contains a brief description of the nature and magnitude of the problem created by this neglect. The kinds of harm associated with victims of sexual offenses are identified and the necessary preventative measures enumerated.

As will be shown, our knowledge of the child's mental condition after the offense gives rise to the question of whether the police are the most appropriate authority to interrogate child victims. **Pretrial Interrogations of Child Victims** of this chapter

---

stantive benefits of the juvenile process." *In re* Gault, 387 U.S. 1, 20-21 (1967). *See also* M. Paulsen, *The Child, the Court and the Commission,* 18 JUV. Ct. JUDGES J. 79-83 (Fall, 1967); Note, *Rights and Rehabilitation in the Juvenile Courts,*67 COLUM. L. REV. 281, 321 (1967).

[5]*But see* V. DE FRANCIS, PROTECTING THE CHILD VICTIM OF SEX CRIME 12 (1965) [hereinafter cited as DE FRANCIS]. DE Francis, the Director of Children's Division of the American Humane Association, reports on programs carried out in six American communities (under the auspices of Societies for the Prevention of Cruelty to Children), where social workers, in agreement with police and prosecutors, conduct interrogations of child victims. However, these practices are exceptional in the United States.

[6]*Id.* at 1.

conflict between the need for effective pretrial interrogation of child victims and the desire to protect them from any possible ill effects which police investigation might entail. Various practices devised in an attempt to reconcile this conflict by the United States, the Scandinavian countries, and Israel are presented, and an endeavor is made to evaluate each of these practices in regard to its capacity to meet the demands of both efficient pretrial investigation and the protection of the child victim.

The Accused's Rights and the Child Victim's Welfare, the fourth division of this chapter, is concerned with the conflict between securing the fundamental rights of the accused and protecting the mental health of child victims, which conflict is particularly sharpened whenever the child victim is called to testify against the accused. The well-being of some child victims, according to psychiatric opinions, may best be safeguarded by minimum and short interrogations, restricted cross-examination, avoidance of courtroom confrontation of the victim and accused, and shielding of the child victim from publicity. Yet, these characteristics of legal proceedings, which may contribute to mental trauma, are essential safeguards of fair trial for the accused in our adversary system. The choice is, therefore, between favoring one interest at the expense of the other, or somehow accommodating them. Some observations of the practices in Illinois are followed by a proposal to deal with the testimonial duty of child victims on an individual basis, while attempting to insure a fair and effective fact-finding process in trial. However, in the United States, any proposal to protect the mental health of child victims must satisfy the constitutional requirements for the protection of the accused's rights to due process of law. Accordingly, the last section, **The Accused's Rights and the Child-Victim's Welfare**, is devoted to discussing those constitutional safeguards and to proposing methods and practices for protecting child victims without abridging the rights of the accused.

The Problem In Perspective

In this chapter, the "child" refers to a girl or boy under fourteen years of age. The age of fourteen is often considered to be the dividing line between children who have not reached puberty and adolescents, and it is assumed that children under fourteen years of age are emotionally immature and incapable of making reasonable judgments concerning sexual relations with adults.[7] This age limit is fixed arbitrarily in order to simplify further discussions. "Adult" is a person who, according to the laws of the jurisdiction in which the crime was committed, is not eligible because of age to be tried by a juvenile court.[8] The term "child victim" denotes a child who is involved, or says he is involved, in a sexual offense.[9]

Psychiatrists, child experts, and commissions appointed by legislatures and governors frequently claim that child victims are

---

[7]*See* Ford, *Sex Offenses: An Anthropological Perspective,* 25 Law & Contemp. Prob . 225, 229 (1960); Halleck, *The Physician's Role in Management of Victims of Sex Offenders, 180 J.A.M.A. 273, 275 (1962).* See also the definition of "child" in Children and Young Persons Act (1963, c. 37§1; Laws of Evidence Revision (Protection of Children) Law 5715-1455 §1. 9 Laws of the State of Israel 102 (auth. trans. 1955).

[8]The modern tendency is to define a delinquent child as a boy under the age of seventeen or a girl under the age of eighteen. Thus, generally speaking, an adult is a person above seventeen years old. *Cf.* Pate, *The State Council and the Juvenile Court Act,* 18 Juv. Ct. Judges J. 20-21 (Spring, 1967).

[9]Child victims are further classified into three subgroups: (1) Coerced victims: those who were forced by the child molester to be involved in the offense. *See* P. Gebhard, J. Gagnon, W. Pomeroy & C. Christenson, Sex Offenders 54 (1965). In none of the studies of child victims did the percentage of "coerced victims" reach 5% of the total study sample; but among victims of incest or homosexual relations, the percentage of coerced victims increased to 10-15% in each of these categories. Neither bribery of any kind nor threats are regarded as "use of force" in this context. (2) Passive victims (sometimes called "accidental victims"): those who usually have only one noncoercive sexual experience, which they do not initiate. The molester is often a stranger, and the case is reported promptly by the child victim to the parents. *See A Summary of the Study of Child Victims of Adult Sex Offenders,* in California Assembly Interim Committee on Judicial System and Judicial Process , Final Report of Sexual Deviation Research , pt. C at 61 (Comm. Print 1954)[hereinafter cited as Cal . Final Report 1954]. (3) Participant victims: those who either have more than one sexual experience with adults (sometimes called "multiple accidental") or actively collaborate with the adult (sometimes called "collaborative victims"). There are many variations, but the typical participant girl victim is physically attractive and seeks to win the adult's approval either by her submissiveness or his pity. For the majority of participant victims, becoming a victim is a sign of emotional disturbance, family conflict, or broken homes. *See* T. Gibbens & J. Prince , Child Victims of Sex Offenses 7 (1963) [hereinafter cited as Gibbens & Prince]; Cal . Final Report 1954 at 59-61; Bender & Blau, *The Reaction of Children to Sexual Relations with Adults,* 7 Am . J. of Orthopsychiatry 510-13 (1937); Weiner, *On Incest: A Survey,* 4 Excerpta Crimin . 140, 146-49 (1964).

often profoundly disturbed, either by the offense or by the developments after its discovery.[10] It is generally agreed by child psychiatrists that the degree of psychic trauma is as much, or perhaps more, dependent on the way that the child victim is treated after discovery than at the time of the offense itself.[11] The need to protect child victims from damage to their future personality by the reactions of their parents and by police interrogations and legal proceedings in which they are involved has caused great concern among leading authorities on questions related to law and psychiatry in the United States,[12] England,[13] France, Germany, Austria, Switzerland, and the Scandinavian countries.[14]

Although the literature on child victims tends to agree that child victims are occasionally subject to physical harm, mental disturbances, and social maladjustment, the views are diversified as to the percentages and types of children affected by the crime or its aftermath. The "retrospective student studies"[15] of psychiatrists Landis[16] and Gagnon[17] suggest that at least one-quarter and

---

[10]See CALIFORNIA ASSEMBLY INTERIM COMMITTEE ON JUDICIAL SYSTEM AND JUDICIAL PROCESS, PRELIMINARY REPORT OF THE SUBCOMMITTEE ON SEX CRIMES 34-35 (Comm. Print 1949); ILLINOIS COMMISSION ON SEX OFFENDERS, A REPORT TO THE 73rd GENERAL ASSEMBLY 49-50 (1963); MICHIGAN GOVERNOR'S STUDY COMMISSION ON THE DEVIATED SEX OFFENDER 9 (1951); OREGON LEGISLATIVE INTERIM COMMITTEE ON SOCIAL PROBLEMS, A REPORT TO THE 52ND LEGISLATIVE ASSEMBLY ON THE CARE, TREATMENT AND REHABILI—TATION OF SEX OFFENDERS 35-37 (1962); DE FRANCIS, *supra* note 5 at 12-13.

[11]See M. Guttmacher, *Sex Offenses: The Problem, Causes and Prevention* 117-119 (1951).

[12]*Id.*: Halleck, *Emotional Effects of Victimization*, in SEXUAL BEHAVIOR AND THE LAW 684 (R. Slovenko ed. 1965).

[13]GIBBENS & PRINCE at 7, 18-23; W. CAVENAGH, THE CHILD AND THE COURT 39 (1959).

[14]*Das sexuelle gefährdete und geschädigte kind, 43* DEUTSCHE RICHTERZEITUNG 267 (1965).

[15]These are retrospective studies of experimental groups selected from students of colleges or universities, who acknowledged that they had been victims of a sexual offense in their childhood.

[16]Landis, *Experiences of 500 Children with Adult Sexual Deviation*, 30 PSYCHIATRIC Q., 91-99 (Supp. 1956). Dr. Landis studied a sample composed of 1800 university students from the "middle" and "upper middle" classes, mostly from urban families. Of the 1800 questioned by him, 500 students reported being child victims of adults. Among them 360 women (35% of all the women questioned) had had sexual experience while 140 men (30% of the total men questioned) had had sexual experience. Each of the 500 students was asked to give his evaluation of whether the experience caused damage to his emotional

perhaps more than one-third of the victims recognize the long-term ill effects of the sexual offense on their emotional development. Brunold concluded in his "witness retrospective study"[18] that "psychological injury of a *permanent* nature must be expected in about a tenth of the children concerned,"[19] which he considered "a serious number, which is still far too high."[20] Gibbens and Prince compared a selected "court sample" of child victims, who were involved in criminal proceedings, with a "random sample" of child victims and found that seventy-three percent of the "court sample" had behavior problems and overt disturbances, compared with only fifty-seven percent of the "random sample."[21] Some fifty-six percent of the child victims sample appeared to recover quickly, but only eighteen percent of the "court sample" managed to recover over the same period of time.[22]

All those who conducted studies of child victims may be regarded as pioneers in this field of investigation.[23] Inspection of

---

development, permanently, temporarily or not at all. Of the women in Landis' survey who asserted they were "shocked" by the offense, 17.8% said they had recovered from it in terms of days, 33% said from weeks to years were required for recovery, and 3.7% claimed they had never recovered. *Id.* at 100-101.

[17]Gagnon, *Female Child Victims of Sex Offenses*, 13 SOCIAL PROBLEMS 117 (Hall, 1965). Gagnon's sample was composed of 333 college educated females who had been selected from among 1200 female students interviewed by the staff of the Institute for Sex Research, founded by Dr. Kinsey, and who reported being victims of sexual offenses in their prepubertal life. Gagnon reports that the adult life of 5% of the child victims in his sample was "severely damaged," including some cases of prostitution, and criminal or mental hospital experience. *Id.* at 189.

[18]These are studies of substantial numbers of adults who, as children, were victims of sexual offenses and were involved in either police or judicial interrogations or both. The experimental group is selected ex post facto from official sources, particularly from the files of the police or district attorney, court records and social agencies. An empirical study of the Israeli system concerning child victims is being conducted now in Israel by the author and Judge D. Reifen.

[19]Brunold, *Observations After Sexual Traumata Suffered in Childhood*, 4 EXCERPTA CRIMIN. 6-8 (1964).

[20]*Id.*, at 7.

[21]GIBBENS & PRINCE. 18-23.

[22]*Id.* at 19. The differences were not attributed solely to court involvement, because much depended upon the child witnesses' previous maladjustment.

[23]The first published study of child victims was conducted by Augusta Rasmussen of Oslo. *See* Rasmussen, *Die Bedeutung Sexueller Attentate auf Kinder unter vierzehn*

the facts on which the studies are based, attention to the methodology used by the expert, the ingredients of each sample, and the fact that there is no generally accepted criterion for judging whether a child was *damaged* by the sexual offense or its aftermath[24] indicate that the results of the studies should be approached with care. Despite the studies' deficiencies, they do show that many of the child victims should be given preventive treatment such as medical care, psychotherapy, and social welfare services.

The vogue of ascribing the mental condition of a child victim subsequent to the sexual offense to any one particular cause is long past. To the psychiatrists, neither the child involvement in a sexual offense nor the single appearance of the child in court can be taken out of context to be diagnosed as traumatic.[25] What usually causes harm, in their view, is the need of a child victim to live for days, weeks, and months in a new situation at home, among friends, and school, and to adjust to it.[26] For this reason psychiatrists feel that the major factors determining the outcome of every experience related to the offense reside, to a large extent, in the previous personality development and family situation

---

Jahren Fur die Entwickelung von Geisteskrankheiten und Charakter-Anomalien, 9 ACTA PSYCHIATRICIA IT NEUROLOGICA 351-434 (1934).

[24]*E.g.,* the Rasmussen criterion for having little subsequent ill effects, as determined from study, was the capacity of the child victims to live in the community twenty or thirty years after the offense. By employing the test, Rasmussen could have regarded even shocking cases as being successful, once she learned—through correspondence—that the grown-up victim had already been released from a mental hospital and lived by herself supported by public welfare, or that she still suffered from hysteria, yet she was outside the institution. *Id.,* at 364, case 11; *Id.* at 365, case 12. L. Bender *et al.* evaluated the remote effects the sexual experience had on the child through the criterion of his responsiveness to social and clinical treatment. *See* Bender, *Offended and Offender Children,* in SEXUAL BEHAVIOR AND THE LAW, 687-89 (R. Slovenko ed. 1965); Bender & Grugett, *A Follow-up Report on Children Who had Atypical Sexual Experiences,* 22 AM. J. OF ORTHOPSYCHIATRY 825 (1952). As to the nature of Bender's control group, see Bender & Paster, *Homosexual Trends in Children,* 11 AM. J. OF ORTHOPSYCHIATRY 732-40 (1941).

[25]*Compare* GIBBENS & PRINCE 5 *with* CALIFORNIA ASSEMBLY INTERIM COMMITTEE ON JUDICIAL SYSTEM AND JUDICIAL PROCESS, PRELIMINARY REPORT ON SEXUAL DEVIATION RESEARCH 61 (Comm. Print 1952); *see* People v. Matthews, 17 Ill. 2d 502, 162 N.E.2d 381 (1959); People v. Martin, 380 Ill. 328, 331, 44 N.E.2d 49, 53 (1942); State v. Seanlon, 58 Mo. 204-205 (1874).

[26]GIBBENS & PRINCE 5-6.

existing as of the occurrence of the offense, when it was reported
to the police, or when it became the subject of court proceedings.[27]

The study of the damaging psychological effect of legal
proceedings, on a child victim, the so called "legal process
trauma," is exceptionally difficult, since subjects of this kind of
study are already suspected of suffering from a "prior personality
defect,"[28] "crime trauma,"[29] or "environmental reaction trauma."[30] Furthermore, for optimal validity, any study should
consist of an extensive and close examination of the child witness
from a time prior to his first confrontation with the police up to
the conclusion of the legal proceedings, and in appropriate cases,
for many years afterwards. Psychiatrists have identified compo-

---

[27]CALIFORNIA ASSEMBLY INTERIM COMMITTEE ON JUDICIAL SYSTEM AND JUDICIAL PRO-
CESS, PRELIMINARY REPORT ON SEXUAL DEVIATION RESEARCH 47, 52 (Comm Print 1953).

[28]*Prior personality defects:* even if mental trauma is observed immediately after the
occurrence of the offense, it may well be either a latent or an overt emotional disturbance
in the victim which existed prior to the sexual offense. CALIFORNIA SEXUAL DEVIATION
RESEARCH (1952), *supra* note 25; Gagnon, *supra* note 17 at 188; Schultz, *Interviewing the
Sex Offender's Victim,* 50 J. CRIM, L.C. & P.C. 450 (1960).

[29]*Crime trauma* is the psychological damage directly resulting from the offense. Some
factors which are involved in a sexual offense are more likely than others to cause mental
trauma to the child victim, *e.g.,* the use of force against a victim. It is evident from the
studies of Landis, Gagnon, and Brunold that serious sexual assaults on children have a
very high incidence of physical or mental damage, resulting in long-term institutionaliza-
tion. According to Landis and Gagnon, 80% of the coerced victims suffered permanent or
serious emotional damage. *See* Gagnon, *supra* note 17, at 188; Landis, *supra* note 16, at
101.

[30]*Environment Reaction Trauma* is a psychological ill-effect attributed to the reaction,
opinion, and behavior of adults not in official positions, and also of the victim's peers. A
common finding in studies concerning child victims is that sexual offenses which are
followed by disclosure of the facts to the parents are generally more traumatic than
offenses which have not been reported to anyone. Bender & Blau, *The Reaction of
Children to Sexual Relations with Adults,* 7 AM. J. OF ORTHOPSYCHIATRY 510-513 (1937).
In the Landis and Gagnon studies, a much higher percentage of children reported the
offense to their parents in the Landis sample. Landis also reported a much higher
percentage of damaged victims. *Compare* Landis, *supra* note 16, at 99, *with* Gagnon,
supra note 17, at 188-89.

Members of the family, neighbors, and friends are likely to react with surprise, anxiety,
fear, and hostility toward the offender. In many of these cases the reaction of revulsion
which the child sees around him upsets him more than the sexual experience itself.
Children from good environments and family backgrounds suffer less injury as a result of
sex offenses, especially when the environment continues to be good afterwards. Brunold,
Observations After Sexual Trauma Suffered in Childhood, 4 EXCERPTA CRIMIN 7 (1964).

nents of the legal proceedings that are capable of putting a child victim under prolonged mental stress and endangering his emotional equilibrium: repeated interrogations and cross-examination,[31] facing the accused again,[32] the official atmosphere in court,[33] the acquittal of the accused for want of corroborating evidence to the child's trustworthy testimony,[34] and the conviction of a molester who is the child's parent or relative.[35]

The four categories of trauma noted above are not isolated concepts. They are offered to facilitate analysis in the following discussion, not to suggest that they are mutually exclusive. A victim of a sexual offense may well suffer two or more of the said mental trauma in proportions that are not quantifiable. It makes little difference that a child whose experience exposed him to law enforcement activities suffers from one particular kind of trauma or another—as long as his mental health is injured, special consideration should be given by the law to the disturbed child victim. The fact agreed upon by psychiatrists, that a child may be affected only by the events subsequent to the offense (which itself did not affect him), or that the ill effects of the offense may be aggravated by those reactions, calls for further inspection of the relations between the child and the authorities. What counts for the system of criminal justice is the complex process a child victim must undergo and the chances of his being "damaged" at any stage of the offense-verdict period.

This chapter assumes that a state, through its legislative, executive, and judicial powers, must care for the well-being of all its children, particularly where parents fail to do so. This chapter further assumes that social services cannot solve all the problems of child victims without the cooperation of and coordination with law enforcement officials who are involved in the child's

---

[31]*See, e.g.*, Cross v. Commonwealth, 195 Va. 62, 77 S.E.2d 447 (1953).

[32]GIBBENS & PRINCE, 17.

[33]C. MULLENS, CRIME AND PSYCHOLOGY 192 (4th ed. 1949).

[34]Savage, *Corroboration in Sexual Cases*, 6 CRIM. L.Q. 282 (1964); Williams, *Corroboration—Sexual Cases*, 1962 CRIM. L. REV. (Eng.) 662. *Cf.* E. RADIN, *THE INNOCENTS* 158, 165-70 (1964).

[35]*See, e.g.*, Kaufman, Peck & Tagiuri, *The Family Constellation and Overt Incestuous Relations Between Father and Daughter*,[24] AM. J. OF OOTHOPSYCHIATRY 266, 272-274 (1954).

case. Progressive states have recognized that police detectives and formal court proceedings are capable of playing a destructive role in the lives of children, and consequently, have adopted the rehabilitative goal for juvenile delinquents and established police youth divisions and juvenile court procedures. Legislatures also are expected, inasmuch as conflicting policies allow, to act on behalf of and for the sake of the protection of child victims. The great significance of the studies conducted on child victims, in spite of all their authors' reservations and possible criticism, is that they indicate that there are justifiable grounds for judging each child victim on the merits of his personality traits and family surroundings, on the kind of offense, and on his vulnerability to legal process damage. A clear need emerges for personal care and treatment of the child victim and his family, some of which must be undertaken by the legal authorities who are obliged because of the offense to interfere with the child victim's life and home. If the public is to be protected, the child victim must assist law enforcement agencies, but this assistance may well be severely traumatic. The resolution of this conflict is the subject of the remainder of this chapter.

Pretrial Interrogations of Child Victims

Police investigation is the automatic response to the report of a sex offense.[36] Our knowledge of the child victim's mental condition after the offense raises the questions of whether the police are appropriate interrogators of child victims of sexual crimes. The core of this question is the conflict between the need for the effective interrogation of child victims and the desire to protect children from possible ill effects of such interrogations. Either within or without the police framework, different practices have been devised by the United States, the Scandinavian countries, and Israel in an effort to reconcile this conflict. The

---

[36]In some jurisdictions, police investigation is supplemented where certain offenses are involved by committal proceedings which are carried out by a judge or grand jury. Both the preliminary hearing and the grand jury hearing are excluded from this discussion, since they are considered in the context of the accused's right to be confronted with the witnesses against him.

essential feature of these attempts is that they entrust the function of interrogating the child victim to someone other than a regular detective. In Chicago this function is performed by the Youth Division; in Copenhagen and Stockholm by specialized police-women; and in Israel by youth interrogators who are not members of the police force. The wisdom of these practices is here considered in the light of their capacity to accomplish efficient investigation and the protection of the child victim.

Police Officers as Child Interrogators

The procedures employed in Chicago, Copenhagen, and Stockholm[37] designate specific police officers who, either by themselves or with representatives of other police divisions or social agencies, are put in contact with the child victim. While Copenhagen and Stockholm are almost identical in that respect, they both differ substantially from Chicago in the categories and functions of the special officer, the manner in which the child's interrogation is conducted, and the quality of the officers' reports.

The Chicago police force has a formal division of powers in matters of interrogating child victims, which, however, may not be observed in practice. Initially, according to the Chicago "Training Bulletin," youth officers are the proper persons to take care of both juvenile offenders and child sex victims.[38] The establishment of a separate Youth Division in the police force is a response to the specific problems of children who are involved in law enforcement proceedings. The designation of youth officers derives from the assumption that youth officers are more qualified to deal with child victims by virtue of having a better

---

[37]Police practices in the large cities of individual countries do not necessarily reflect their practices in the rest of the state. *E.g.*, Copenhagen uses a different system concerning child victims than the other urban and rural areas of the state. While the Danish procedure outside Copenhagen is similar to that in Norway, the Copenhagen system is almost identical to that of Sweden. *See* BOLVIKEN, AVHRING AV BARN I STRAFFESAKER LOV OG RETT 193-219 (1966) [hereinafter cited as BOLVIKEN].

[38]*Interviewing the Juvenile Sex Victim and Offender,*[5] CHICAGO POLICE DEPT. TRAINING BULL. No. 25 at E. 25 (1964).

understanding of child problems. In addition to the experience with children they acquire as youth officers, they also receive detailed directions and guidelines as to suitable approaches to children. The experienced youth officers adopt a special and careful orientation toward problems of interrogating a child,[39] such as the child's powers of narration, his veracity, and his vulnerability to mental trauma. Another distinct advantage of the Youth Division over other investigative divisions of the Chicago police force appears in the form of policewomen's service in this division.[40] Sometimes it is easier for a girl to talk about the offense with a woman, and some young children can be handled by women with more skill, tact, and care. Ideally, in order to fulfill specific needs for interrogators of a specific sex, a youth department should be comprised of both female and male interrogators.[41]

Contrary to the underlying intent of the written rules, child victims in Chicago are customarily first approached by a patrolman in uniform.[42] He is the first policeman to interview the child, and if any urgent steps are required in the detection of the suspect, he will deal with conditions and situations as he finds them. His "case report" is a summary of his preliminary investigation. It is transferred to the Detective Division for further investigation. Neither "beatmen" nor detectives have any training for dealing with special youth problems or with the mental health of child victims. It is up to them to request the cooperation of either a youth officer or a policewoman. Often they undertake a second interrogation of the child victim, making the youth officer

---

[39]Youth officers in Chicago insist on the distinction between an "interrogation" and an "interview" of a child victim. For a clarification of these terms, see O'Connor, *Interviewing and Interrogation,* in S. GERBER, CRIMINAL INVESTIGATION AND INTERROGATION 358-359 (1962). O'Connor emphasizes that many individuals tend to think of "interview" and "interrogation" as being the same thing, "which basically they are." The difference lies primarily in the degree of the policeman's control over his conversations with the victim. I do not make any such distinction between the two terms.

[40]No more than eighty policewomen are employed now by the Chicago Youth Division, which serves a city of three and a half million inhabitants.

[41]*See* W. CAVENAGH, THE CHILD AND THE COURT 197 (1959); A. MARTIENSSEN, CRIME AND THE POLICE 193-195 (1953).

[42]Description of the Chicago practice is based on private interviews with youth officers and detectives in the Chicago area during April-June, 1967.

in Chicago the third person in authority to approach the child victim, if he is notified about the child's molestation at all. Hence the present practices of the Chicago police result in repeated interrogations of the child victims, a fact easily capable of aggravating the child's mental problems.

In Chicago, the disparity between written police instructions and actual practice is the result of two combined factors. First, detectives are put in charge of investigating sexual offenses committed upon the children. Second, although the detectives should request youth officers to aid them in the victim's interrogation, they are not motivated to do so because they generally consider themselves as capable as youth officers to interview child victims.[43] The Chicago Youth Division is in fact composed of ex-patrolmen and ex-detectives and policewomen who are no more qualified or trained for interrogating child victims than the detectives. Every policeman who is interested in youth is eligible to serve as a youth officer. No specific educational requirement is needed to qualify as a youth policewoman.[44] Being acquainted with the qualifications of youth officers, detectives by themselves conduct the investigation of sexual offenses by adults against children, and cooperation between the Detective Division and the Youth Division of Chicago in such cases is rare. Whenever a youth officer is involved in the investigation, his function is merely advisory.

The function of interrogating child victims in Copenhagen and Stockholm is entrusted to special policewomen of advanced education, who are experienced in interrogation.[45] They alone

---

[43]The notification of the youth officer takes place in a haphazard manner, and since there is no requirement that he be notified, it is quite possible that the youth officer is not informed in a larger percentage of child victims' interrogations. This was my impression during my visit to several police stations in Chicago.

[44]Section 3 of the Policewoman Applicant Information Sheet states: "There is no specific educational requirement but high school graduation is desirable and is important as an aid in qualifying for police work."

[45]The Swedish system under discussion applies to children under fourteen years of age, and the Danish system to child victims under twelve. In Stockholm the interrogating policewomen are qualified nurses, who take special courses in psychology and psychiatry as well as special courses in police investigation. The description of the Scandinavian practices in this section are based on: (1) An interview with K. Lodmer and O. P. Stefanssen, at Police Headquarters, Stockholm, Sweden, on Sept. 18, 1969; (2) An inter-

have a mandate to interrogate the child, working without interference by investigators from other police divisions, because they are trained to exercise a high degree of care for the child's emotions and mental health in eliciting and tape recording the facts concerning the offense. However, due to their limited training in children's mental health, they do not assume the function of a psychiatric social worker or a child care worker.[46]

In summary, the chief distinction of status between the Danish or Swedish policewoman and the Chicago youth officer stems from the difference in their qualifications. The specialty of the Scandinavian policewomen is in the field of interrogating child victims, whereas Chicago youth officers have neither special training nor extensive experience in dealing with child victims.

THE METHODS OF CONDUCTING THE INTERROGATION — The methods by which police officers in Chicago, Copenhagen, and Stockholm conduct the child victim's interrogation are similar in that each endeavors to carry out the interrogation in an informal and relaxed atmosphere,[47] using terminology and vocabulary at the child's own level, being patient and sympathetic and letting the child do most of the talking.[48] The detailed techniques and their effectiveness vary, of course, from one interrogator to the other.

In other respects, the methods used in Chicago differ substantially from those used in Copenhagen and Stockholm. A unique feature of the Danish and Swedish systems is the tape recording of the child's evidence by a policewoman, which reflects the content of the child's story and the manner in which it is told much better than a written statement. The tape can detect whether the child's

---

view with Johannes Andenaes, Dean of the University of Oslo Law School, in Chicago, March 8, 1968; (3) BOLVIKEN. *supra* note 37.

[46]Consequently, the policy of protecting the child victims is supplemented in Sweden and Denmark by police cooperation with social agencies. BOLVIKEN. *supra* note 37, at 209.

[47]In Sweden, unless the child victim's parents insist on the child being interrogated at home, the child is invited to the police station, where his statement is recorded in informal surroundings. The Swedish experience indicates that the conditions for recording the child's statement are better in the police station than at his own home.

[48]*Compare* M. HOLLMAN. THE POLICE OFFICER AND THE CHILD 109-12 (1962) *with* Schultz, *Interviewing the Sex Offender's Victim*, 50 J. CRIM. L.C. & P.S., 448, 451-452 (1960).

narration was hurried or deliberate, angry or satisfied, calm or excited. Spontaneous statements can easily be distinguished from responses to leading questions,[49] and hesitant voices can be identified and compared with confident ones. The tape reveals whether the child is decisive or ambiguous, perhaps giving a vague account which can be needlessly harmful to the rights of the defendant.[50] Furthermore, a written statement does not convey the child victim's original story as authentically as a taped conversation. It provides the reader with indirect impressions of the child through the media of a third person and of writing, and may be an edited and amended version of the child's story. The more persons involved in the interrogation, the less authentic the recorded statement tends to be.

The specialization of the child interrogator and the method of recording the child's statement are two factors which determine how often the child victim must relive his ordeal. Police officers, the prosecutor, and various expert witnesses who require a direct impression of the child's story in order to form an opinion thereon will be reluctant to rely on a written statement taken from the child. As a result, according to the Chicago practice, the prosecutor invites the child into his office before the trial to rehearse his evidence, and a physician asks the child to repeat the details of the offense while he conducts the physical examination.[51]

---

[49]The policewomen try to avoid asking the child any leading questions. After the child tells his story, the interrogator might ask him to clarify some details.

[50]The child's self-consciousness at being tape recorded is no greater than his self-consciousness at the interrogator taking notes during the interview. The tape recorder may be hidden or shown to the child, according to the circumstances. The experienced policewoman may explain the recording to the child without causing him any anxiety. I was told by K. Lodner in Stockholm's police headquarters that the child victim is asked to speak loudly, and in a few seconds it seems that he or she forgets or ignores the tape recorder. Bolviken, who made an extensive study of the tape recording of child witnesses in Copenhagen and Sweden and who strongly recommends this technique, does not see any problem with regard to the effects of using a tape recorder on the child victim. *See* BOLVIKEN , *supra* note 37, at 204-11; *cf.* m. HOLMAN, THE POLICE OFFICER AND THE CHILD 92-93 (1962) (setting for interrogation).

[51]The evidence of physicians in court often asserts that "the child was frightened" during the medical examination. The presence of the child victim's mother or father cannot lessen the child's anxiety if the parents themselves are tense and upset. *See, e.g.,* Abstract of the Record 46-16, People v. Kolden, 25 Ill.2d 327, 185 N.E.2d 170 (1962).

Under the Scandinavian practice the child victims are generally saved from this continual repetition, because the tape recorded conversation can be used to acquaint the listeners with the child's evidence.[52]

QUALITY AND THE RELIABILITY OF THE REPORTS—The detectives' task is not only to "solve the crime" by the apprehension of a suspect, but to link the investigative authority to the prosecution and adjudication systems by providing evidence to prove the state's case against the offenders. For this purpose the accumulated evidence should be credible as well as admissible. With regard to credibility, efficient police investigation should endeavor to present its findings through persons whose reliability is most likely to be accepted by the courts.

In Chicago, Copenhagen, and Stockholm, certain evidence about the pretrial investigations is produced for the courts by police officers. Because of detectives' interest in concluding their investigation successfully, and the privacy and secrecy in which the police operate, courts are suspicious of police investigations. The gap in the court's knowledge of what really occurs in pretrial, nonjudicial interrogations leaves room for allegations of unfair police practice. Judges search for impartial evidence in support of one of the parties at the trial in regard to questions of admissibility and credibility of evidence recorded out of court. Since Scandinavian pretrial investigations are conducted with the expectation of presenting their findings to the trial court, pretrial investigations are supervised by legislatures, police authorities, and the judiciary in order to insure their accuracy and reliability.

Attention to the quality and accuracy of reporting pretrial interrogations in Copenhagen and Stockholm is illustrated by the procedure for recording the child victim's evidence by the special policewoman, who may support her sworn testimony by introducing in evidence the original tape recorded conversation itself. The court is thus acquainted with the child's authentic

---

[52]In the Scandinavian countries the pretrial recorded evidence is admissible in the trial itself.

story, without having to rely solely on the accuracy of verbal testimony of the policewoman.[53]

Another significant piece of evidence presented through policemen at the trial is the manner in which the out-of-court identification of the defendant was made. The courts worry more about accusations of unfair police practices during the identification process[54] than about inaccurate police reports of the child's extrajudicial statement. In principle, a child can be brought to testify in court, his in-court testimony having more testimonial weight than his earlier out-of-court statement, which may even be inadmissible.[55] But out-of-court identification of the

---

[53]In this section our concern is only with the correct transmission of an extrajudicial statement by the one reporting it; other legal complications involved, like the hearsay rule, demeanor evidence, and confrontation, are referred to in pp. 000-000 *infra*.

[54]By "unfair police practices" I refer primarily to the use by detectives of suggestive methods to obtain identification. It is demonstrated by a California case, People v. Evans, 39 Cal.2d 242, 246, P.2d 636 (1952), in which detectives showed the ten-year-old victim a picture of the defendant on the top of a pile of pictures. The child said she remembered having seen that person some time prior to the day of the offense, but was unable to remember where or when she had seen him. An hour after having been shown the defendant's picture, she was taken to a room where the defendant was alone and identified him as her attacker. *See* Simmons v. United States, 390 U.S. 377, 382-86 (1968). Another common suggestive method is the "show-up" where suspects are brought before the witnesses in handcuffs, or shown alone, in a police station to the children who identify them. *Cf.* P. WALL. EYE WITNESS IDENTIFICATION IN CRIMINAL CASES 27-41 (1965). In W. CAVENAGH. THE CHILD AND THE COURT 44-45 (1959), the author describes the case of a girl victim of six years who was taken to the scene of the offense in a police car. There were a number of unfinished houses, but the car was driven to one of them without hesitation and the two policemen got out. They disappeared into the house and almost immediately appeared accompanied by a builder's laborer. With this man between them, they came up to the car and asked the little girl something to the effect of: "Is this the man?" The child said that it was, and this person was indicted. When the same girl was asked in the courtroom to look around her and see if her molester was there, she pointed her finger not at the accused, but at the defense counsel's clerk. Acknowledging normal human fallibilities of perception and recollection as well as the power of suggestion, courts generally require the police to conduct a lineup and consider show-up identification unreliable. *See* Davis v. The King, 57 Commw. L.R. 170 (Austl. 1937); Rex v. Smierciak, 2 D.L.R. 156 (Can. 1946); R. v. Cartwright, 10 Crim. App. 219 (Eng. 1946); R. v. Williams, 8 Crim. App. 84 (Eng. 1912); J. WIGMORE ,3 EVIDENCE § 786a (3d ed. 1940) [hereinafter cited as WIGMORE].

[55]This is the rationale of the hearsay rule, and states which admit as evidence a tape recorded conversation with the child would also admit that oral testimony before the court generally has more testimonial value. Thus, they admit taped evidence instead of the oral evidence as a compromise between the conflicting interests discussed pp. 000-000 *infra* in the text.

defendant by the victim generally has more testimonial force than in-court identification.[56]

A positive out-of-court identification may have the effect of reducing the issue of the offender's identity in the trial itself "to a mere formality."[57] Only by considering all possibilities of unfair practices, as well as bona fide mistakes, may the trial court avoid miscarriages of justice due to erroneous identification. For this purpose the trier of fact should be informed about factors which may affect the particular child victim's credibility. He should also know how the accused was first identified by the child as the molester, which he may learn from the police, the victim,[58] the suspect, his counsel,[59] and persons who participate in the lineup. All of these factors are somehow involved in conducting the identification or sharing the interests of the defendant or the prosecution.

The Chicago practice provides the court with an additional source of information—the youth officer. The Chicago Training Bulletin instructs that "the presence of the youth officer gives the child support and confidence apt to minimize the harmful situation as far as possible."[60] Occasionally, a detective in charge of a "showup" or "lineup" asks a youth officer or policewoman to be present at the identification. The participation of youth officers in the identification process, however, does not satisfactorily answer the problem of "knowledge gap"[61] because youth

---

[56]*See*[4] WIGMORE, § 1130, at 208.

[57]United States v. Wade, 338 U.S. 218 (1966).

[58]Some child victims go so far as to report on clear suggestions and even directions from law enforcement officials which cause them to identify an innocent person as the offender, to wit: When a girl victim, six years old, was taken to the police station about a week after the alleged sexual offense, she was confronted with the defendant, and was asked if he was the man who had molested her. She told the police twice that he was not. Thereafter the policeman and her mother and the states' attorney told her to say that he was the man who molested her. All this became evident to the court when the girl testified that although she did not think he was the man until the policeman told her to say he was, she was not positive of her identification. People v. Martin, 380 Ill. 328, 44 N.E.2d 49 (1942).

[59]On the right to counsel in a "lineup", *see* United States v. Wade, 388 U.S. 218, 231, 235, 237 (1966); WALL, *supra* note 54, at 43;[3] WIGMORE, § 786a.

[60]5 CHICAGO POLICE DEPT. TRAINING BULL., No. 26 at E. 30 (1964).

[61]So far as the child's welfare is concerned, it is sometimes doubtful whether youth officers' efforts based on their private understanding, to support the child's confidence,

officers have the same credibility deficiencies as all other police-men.[62] Some other countries have impartial persons participate in the lineup, prohibiting police officers and suspects other than the defendant from standing with him,[63] so that persons who stand in the lineup may later testify in court about the event. Their names and addresses are recorded by the police and divulged at the trial. Furthermore, a series of photographs is taken during the identification process.[64] Nevertheless, neither these private persons, the defense counsel, nor the youth officer can guarantee the elimination of the innumerable dangers of suggestive influences on the child victim *prior* to the lineup. If any previous secret and unfair practices took place among the police, before the "official" pretrial identification, none of these persons is aware of it, minimizing the likelihood that it will be revealed to the court.[65]

Both the Chicago and the Copenhagen-Stockholm systems attempt to provide efficient interrogation and simultaneously protect child victims by designating special police officers to contact the child victims, but the designated personnel are not

---

are not as harmful to the child victim as the complete ignorance of the child victim's mental condition could have been. One youth officer told me that in order to make the child feel more secure he asks all the persons in a "lineup" to turn their faces to the wall, before the child is brought into the room. His assumption is that the child is not afraid of the suspects' backs as she is of their faces. Then, on the officer's order, all the persons in the parade are asked to turn their faces back towards the child. The officer is of the opinion that the sudden change in the person's position and possible surprise confrontation with the molester cannot mentally affect the child, because the police officer himself is already "standing behind the child" in order to protect her. "She knows that I am with her," said the officer, "Why should she be afraid?"

[62]The policemen testifying in Chicago courts in cases involving child victims are rarely asked about the police division they serve in. *E.g.,* Record at 58, People v. Chaten, 32 Ill.2d 416, 206 N.E.2d 697 (1965); the same "member of the Chicago police force" interrogated five boys and the defendant. Record at 101, 109, People v. Walker, 13 Ill.2d 334, 148 N.E.2d 748 (1958); the policemen identified themselves as "I am a city policeman." There is generally no distinction in the court between the youth officer and other policemen.

[63]*See* P. WALL, *supra* note 54, at 56. This is also the Israeli practice.

[64]*Cf.* Gardner, *The Camera Goes to Court*, 24 N.C.L. REV. 233, 242, 245-46 (1946).

[65]In Stockholm the lineup is conducted by the policewoman and a detective. The persons who stand in the lineup confront a "one way glass," and the child is told that these persons cannot see him. Defense counsel is allowed to be present. The policewoman is generally regarded by the courts as a reliable professional whose testimony in court can contribute to accurate findings of fact.

sufficiently qualified to adjust to the mental condition of the child victim. The greatest achievement of the Scandinavian system is the guarantee that child victims need make only one pretrial statement concerning of the offense—to a person trained in child victims' interrogation. Allocating special police officers to children's interrogations is inadequate for protecting child victims, for unless they have exclusive powers of examining the child, repeated interrogations inevitably ensue. The appointment and training of special police officers to deal with child victims can serve the three cardinal purposes of protecting the child's welfare, guaranteeing better methods of recording child victims' statements, and contributing to the quality and the trustworthiness of police reports before the courts.

Specialized Personnel as Youth Interrogators

An unprecedented experiment for dealing with the problem of child victims as witnesses was devised by the Knesset (Parliament) of Israel in 1955.[66] The two most dramatic innovations in the Israeli law affect pretrial investigations and court proceedings. The first is the vesting of pretrial investigative powers in impartial experts, called "youth interrogators," who are not members of the police force. The second is the exclusion of children under fourteen from the trial, absent the permission of the youth interrogator for the child to be heard.[67]

---

[66]Law of Evidence Revision (Protection of Children) Law 5715-1955 §4.9 LAWS OF THE STATE OF ISRAEL 102 (auth. trans. 1955). The material in this section is based on personal knowledge of the author, a former Chief Assistant to the Israeli State's Attorney, and on a study conducted by him.

[67]The youth interrogators are empowered by the law to discriminate between children whose mental condition enables them to appear in court and those who could not do so without danger to their mental health. Their final report to the police includes a decision, without explanation, as to whether the child may be heard in court, and this decision cannot be appealed, disputed or overruled. One effect of the youth interrogator's decision is to dictate by which of two sets of procedure rules the trial will be conducted: one in case the child may testify, and one if he may not. These trial practices are without the scope of this article. *See generally* Reifen, *Protection of Children Involved in Sexual Offenses: A New Method of Investigation in Israel*, 49 J. CRIM. L.C. & P.S. 222 (1959); Reifen, *The Sexual Offender and His Victim*, 12 INT'L. CHILD WELFARE REV. 109 (1958).

YOUTH INTERROGATORS AND ORGANIZATIONAL PROBLEMS —
The law is silent about personal qualifications of youth interrogators save that they are to be appointed by the Minister of Justice after consultation with an Appointment Committee.[68] In the spirit of the legislation, the Committee chooses interrogators who are trained in subtleties of dynamic human behavior and experienced in interviewing techniques: clinical psychologists, psychiatric social workers, psychiatrists, probation officers, and child care workers. They are instructed in legal procedure and rules of evidence, especially in matters relevant to sex offenses. Many of them are graduates of one of Israel's Institutes of Criminology or the School of Social Work.

The youth interrogators are not necessarily government employees. Some of them are, especially in the Ministries of Health, Education, and Welfare, while others are selected from the private sector. The determinative factors are their intention to serve as youth interrogators, approval of their candidacy by the committee, and official appointment by the Minister of Justice. A youth interrogator may either resign, or be dismissed upon adequate notice and a hearing to provide the proper opportunity to appear and present a defense.

Youth interrogators are paid a set fee by the Treasury for each interrogation, regardless of the time spent on it, and reimbursed for their expenses. In the event of an appearance in court, the court may order payment of further fees as "per diem," "compensation for loss of time," or "travel and lodging allowances." The Minister of Justice has fixed higher fees for youth interrogators than those ordered by the courts for other expert witnesses. Being a youth interrogator is therefore regarded as a second job, compensated severally for each assignment completed.

POWERS OF INTERROGATORS—The Protection of Children Law of 1955 transferred some traditional police powers to the youth interrogators[69]—the Knesset foresaw that the police might

---

[68]This committee consists of: (1) a judge, (2) a mental hygiene expert, (3) an educator, (4) a child and youth care expert, and (5) a high police official in charge of relations between the police and the youth interrogators.

[69]The Criminal Procedure (Evidence) Ordinance enacted in 1922 by the British mandatory government of Palestine is still in force in Israel. According to its provisions, when-

resist diminution of their authority by a new "foreign body" of expert interrogators outside their domain and control. With this new law in effect, detectives are restrained in their investigations not only by attention to the rights of defendants, as before, but also by legal restriction designed to protect victims. In order not to place the youth interrogators at the mercy of this anticipated police antagonism, the Knesset did not count on voluntary cooperation between police and youth interrogators, but entrusted the latter with almost exclusive powers of interrogation of child victims. The statute provides that a child shall not be examined as to an offense against morality[70] "save by a youth interrogator,"[71] except in cases of "questions put by the father, the mother, the guardian, the person having supervision or control of the child, or a physician," and "questions put at the time or immediately after the offense, or as soon as a reasonable suspicion arises that such an offense has been committed."[72]

These exceptions to the general rule reflect a very practical approach. Many offenses against children are discovered when parents, physicians, or teachers suspect that something has befallen the child, and question him about such suspicions. Natural expressions of legitimate interest and concern for the child are thus not proscribed acts.[73] This exception to the exclusive authority of questioning children by youth interrogators is also broad enough to permit police officers to question

---

ever an offense is committed, the police are authorized to hold inquiries into its commission, and to take down statements from any person who is supposed to be acquainted with the facts and circumstances of the offense. *See Israeli Criminal Procedure Law*, 13 AMERICAN SERIES OF FOREIGN PENAL CODES 126 (1967).

[70]"Offense against Morality" is defined by section 1 of the law as "any of the offenses enumerated in the Schedule," namely: rape, unnatural offenses, rape by deception attempts, illicit relations with unmarried girl (including incestuous relations between father and daughter), indecent acts, indecency in public, prostitution, solicitation, and indecent suggestions, etc.

[71]Law of Evidence Revision (Protection of Children) Law 5715-1955 §4.9 LAWS OF THE STATE OF ISRAEL 102 (auth. trans. 1955).

[72]*Id.*

[73]The exclusive authority of questioning children vested by the law in youth interrogators is also qualified by permission for the father, mother, guardian, any person having supervision or control over the child, and physicians to converse at any time about the offense.

the child victim immediately after the commission or discovery of the offense.

It should be noted that although the police are greatly limited in their authority to question child victims, they retain the powers of investigating sex offenses, even involving children under fourteen. However, police officers may exercise their limited right to question the child victim only when necessary for the detection of the suspect or for the collection of exhibits where any delay, such as the youth interrogator's arrival, might impede efficient investigation or prevention of further crime. In order to prevent exceptions from becoming common practice, the legislature entrusted the youth interrogator with two additional powers: first, to veto the admission at trial of any statement taken by the police from the child without his permission;[74] and second, to forbid the police from performing any act requiring the presence or participation of the child unless with the permission of a youth interrogator and in accordance with his instructions. These provisions prevent the Israeli police from circumventing the authority of youth interrogators as a reprisal for their enforced dependence on them. In this respect, the system of youth interrogators closes the lacuna of the Chicago system, according to which one police division investigates and another attends to the child's welfare, but where in practice, the investigative department can ignore the youth division with impunity. In Israel the investigative branch of the police cannot investigate and bring the suspect to trial without the full cooperation of the special staff of youth interrogators.

The youth interrogator need not choose between interrogating the child and subjecting him to participation in the identification parade or other stages of the investigation. More moderate choices are open to him. He may prepare the child and his family in advance for the sorts of actions required by law from witnesses; he may determine the time and form of the investigation, and he may accompany the child anywhere so that his presence and

---

[74]Law of Evidence Revision (Protection of Children) Law 5715-1955 §2(a), 9 LAWS OF THE STATE OF ISRAEL 102 (auth. trans. 1955) states: "Save with the permission of a youth interrogator . . . a statement by a child as to such an offense shall not be admitted as evidence."

understanding may give the child support, confidence, and comfort.

Indeed, the title of the Israeli law generally, "Law of Evidence (Protection of Children)," and certain sections of it specifically, provide that conflicts between the child's protection and law enforcement which cannot be accommodated without causing serious damage to the child's welfare are to be resolved in favor of the protection of the child.[75] Because the legislature relies fundamentally on the youth interrogator's experience and judgment to minimize the frequency and impact of such conflicts, the youth interrogators use their special training to evaluate the mental and social conditions of the victim and move immediately to calm the child and his family, transferring those who seem in need of treatment to appropriate agencies.[76]

INTERROGATIONS IN PRACTICE—In practice, police officers and youth interrogators work together to fulfill the intent of the legislature. Every police station has a list of youth interrogators available in the district. A detective contacts a youth interrogator, briefs him on the complaint, and upon request, provides transportation. In general, police officers easily adjusted to the propriety of interrogation by a qualified expert and they follow police regulations accordingly. Only in urgent cases, in order to elicit information required for quick action, will the police conduct an interview, and even then they speak to the child victim's parents rather than the child.

Youth interrogators never wear uniforms.[77] Regulations forbid the youth interrogator from questioning the child in a police station "unless there is no possibility to interrogate the child somewhere else," so as a rule, youth interrogators come to the child's home to interview him in private. They exercise full

---

[75]Law of Evidence Revision (Protection of Children) Law 5715-1955 §§2, 4, 7, 10.9 LAWS OF THE STATE OF ISRAEL 102-03 (auth. trans. 1955).

[76]*See* Reifen, *Protection of Children Involved in Sexual Offenses: A New Method of Investigation in Israel*, 49 J. CRIM. L.C. & P.S. 222 (1959).

[77]Regulations promulgated by the Minister of Justice forbid a youth interrogator to wear a police uniform while interrogating a child. The Minister was aware of the possibility that a qualified police officer may be appointed as a youth interrogator, as there is no legal prohibition of such appointments.

control over working conditions. They control the child's investigation, his medical examination, his presence and participation in the "process of identification," and his appearance in any other inquiry of judicial hearing, using their discretion in order to tailor efficient investigation to the specific requirement of the child's mental condition.

THE QUALITY OF THE YOUTH INTERROGATOR'S REPORTS—The earlier discussion concerned the need for interrogators who can conduct an efficient interrogation and report accurately and objectively to others on the pretrial investigation. The experiment with the youth interrogators indicates that they fulfill these requirements. They succeed in reducing the child's detailed statement to writing and supplementing the statement with a separate record of all their investigations, impressions, evaluations, and personal comments. Granted, written statements cannot reflect the nuances of the child's story and the course of the interrogations, as fully as tape recorded interrogations, without consequent costs to credibility. Youth interrogators in Israel are not equipped with tape recorders as are the policewomen in Sweden and Copenhagen.

The requirement of the youth interrogator's permission or instructions before the police may carry out any identification of suspects by the child means that detectives may not present a photograph or a suspect to the child without first consulting the youth interrogator, who should include the details of any such action in his records. The police are thus loath to contact the child when the youth interrogator is absent because the child or his parents may reveal the secret contact to the youth interrogator who can exclude the evidence. In this way the existence of youth interrogators fosters fairness in the identification process and constitutes a significant and reliable source of information for the courts.

At the end of the youth interrogator's investigation, the child's recorded statement and the interrogator's report are made available to the police. The head of the police investigation department reviews the evidence in the case, weighs the youth interrogator's opinion, and, with his own remarks, forwards the file to the prosecution.

SUMMARY—The Israeli pretrial practices guaranteed that: (1) the child need give evidence only once before the trial; (2) evidence is taken by an expert whose specialty consists both in treating children involved in sex offenses and in clinical interviewing techniques; (3) direct contacts between the police and the child are minimal; (4) the child completes his participation in police investigations soon after the offense occurs; (5) adequate mental care and social welfare are arranged for the victim by the youth interrogator immediately after the offense; and (6) the youth interrogator is authorized to forbid interrogation if the child's mental health might be jeopardized.

Implementation of the Israeli law did not create any noticable practical difficulties and was not met with any substantial criticism. The Knesset has not chosen since the enactment of the law in 1955 to amend any of its provisions which deal with pretrial practices. Judge Reifen, the Chairman of the Appointment Committee, summed up the experiment, saying: "In spite of the hesitations felt in many quarters, experience so far has shown good results."[78]

Conclusions and a Proposal

An analysis of pretrial interrogation of child victims, as practiced in Chicago, Denmark, Sweden, and Israel, indicates that the conflict between efficient investigation and children's protection can be greatly minimized. The conflicting policies in these two systems can be adjusted by the selection of persons, other than regular policemen, who are trained to reconcile the countervailing considerations. Chicago involves youth officers in addition to the beatmen and detectives in the child victims' interrogation. Sweden and Denmark add the services of child care workers to that of special policewomen, and reduce the number of children's interrogations to a minimum. Israel undertakes to combine these refinements in the person of one professional, the youth interrogator. In order to achieve successful child interrogation, he should possess in some measure the special character-

---

[78]Reifen, *supra* note 76, at 222.

istics of a youth officer and a child caseworker, the capacity to elicit a complete report of the offense from the child, objectivity for accurate recording and reporting of the investigation, and professional understanding of the mental health of child victims and their need for social welfare. Thus, the basic question of the role of persons most suitable for dealing with child victims of sex offenses can be answered satisfactorily by the employment of youth interrogators.

It is therefore submitted that child victims should be approached, investigated, and taken care of by "child examiners" who possess the same qualifications as those of the Israeli "youth interrogators."[79] They should not be controlled by police or dependent upon any organized official institution.[80] However, the child examiners would differ from the Israeli youth interrogators in two significant respects. First, instead of writing down the child victim's statement, they would adopt the Swedish and Danish system of tape recording their conversations with the victims, to be later referred to as "victims recordings." A better practice would be to video-tape the whole interrogation so that the child's appearance and demeanor may be seen as well as heard. There is room for speculation as to whether the child's appearance before the television cameras would embarrass him or would encourage him to talk; there is no data on this. It seems to be a more practical solution not to interrogate the child at home, and not to take television equipment there, but to escort the child to a pleasant room, where the atmosphere is informal and where hidden television cameras are permanently installed for such purposes. However, an indoor interrogation may require sufficient light, and an outdoor interrogation makes it difficult to

---

[79]While concluding that youth interrogators are fit to deal with child victims, we still have reservations about some aspects of the Israeli system. In order to differentiate between the Israeli "youth interrogator" and the person proposed by us to fulfill the series of functions answerable to the specific problems of child victims as witnesses, we shall refer to the qualified person as a "child examiner."

[80]The child examiners should be provided with the material assistance necessary for them to conduct the interrogation, such as tape recorder and tapes, by the chairman of the appointment committee, or a person appointed by him for this purpose. Transportation should be supplied to them by the police, and all their written communications with courts should be handled by the District Attorney's staff.

hide the camera from the child. Thus, the possibility of televising the child without his noticing it is negligible. Even if it could be accomplished, the cost might prove prohibitive unless the interrogation takes place in the *Child Courtroom*, which is discussed in the last section.

Second, to supplement the victim's recordings with information essential to determining his credibility or vulnerability, the child interrogator will prepare a written social profile covering the following:

1. The past history of the child, including full particulars about his family;

2. The state of health of the victim and the members of his family;

3. The child's intelligence, his behavior and achievement in school and in playing with his friends;

4. Any previous acquaintance of the child or members of his family with the accused;

5. Special personal circumstances, if any, which may affect the child's credibility or his involvement in sexual acts.

Although the profile may cast light on the victim's moral character, intelligence, and veracity, details or comments concerning the offense which caused the inquiry should not be included because the child examiner is not an appropriate person to pass judgment on the offense.

The contribution of child examiners to the criminal trial of child molesters, in the spirit of protecting the victims without neglecting due process of law for defendants, is discussed in the context of the broader issue of how to secure accommodation between a fair trial for the accused and a "healthy trial" for the child victim.

The Accused's Rights and the Child Victim's Welfare

When a child victim is summoned to testify in court, there is a tension between the policies protecting his mental health and the right of the accused to a fair trial. Because children, like adults, are not always scrupulously honest and accurate in their narrations,[81] courts are alert to detect fantasy and falsehood in any testimony, and child-victim complainants in sex offense cases, being children, raise special problems of their own.[82] As the best means of uncovering falsehood and inaccuracy, common law systems afford the accused in a criminal case the right to cross-examination of witnesses against him, to be conducted by defense counsel, in the presence of their trier of fact.[83]

In the United States the right of the accused to cross-examine an accusing child witness is protected by federal and state constitutions, and the child victim must appear in court to present his evidence, lest it be excluded as hearsay.[84] Because the accused is presumed innocent until proven guilty, the American procedural rules, asserted Mr. Justice Fortas, "are our best instruments for the distillation and evaluation of essential facts from the conflicting welter of data that life and our adversary methods present. It it these instruments of due process which enhance the possibility that truth will emerge...."[85] The history of procedure, wrote Mr. Justice Frankfurter, is "the history of American freedom."[86] Therefore, because loose procedures may deprive the accused of his liberty without due process of law, any attempt to

---

[81] For a discussion of children's credibility, see generally People v. Price, 33 Misc.2d 476, 226 N.Y.S.2d 460 (Ct. Spec. Sess. 1962); Record at 137, People v. Chaten, 32 Ill.2d 416, 206 N.E.2d 697 (1965); EVIDENCE AND BEHAVIORAL SCIENCE, 111-B-501 (A. Leyin ed. 1956); H. KALVEN & E. ZEISEL, THE AMERICAN JURY 180 (1966); J. PIAGET, THE MORAL JUDGMENT OF THE CHILD (M. Gahain trans. 1950).

[82] On legal attitudes toward child victims credibility, see People v. Chaten, 32 Ill.2d 416, 206 N.E.2d 697 (1965); People v. Nunes, 30 Ill.2d 143, 195 N.E.2d 706 (1964); People v. Price, 33 Misc.2d 476, 226 N.Y.S.2d 460 (1962); N.Y. PENAL LAW §130.15 (McKinney 1967); Note, *Corroborating Charges of Rape*, 67 COLUM. L. REV. 1137 (1967); R. v. Knight, 1 W.L.R. 230 (Eng. Crim. App. 1966) (credibility of the unsworn child victim); R. v. Trigg, 47 Crim. App. 94 (Eng. 1963); R. v. Campbell, 40 Crim. App. 95 (Eng. 1956); Andrews, *The Evidence of Children*, 1964 CRIM. L. REV. [Eng.] 769; Williams, *Corroboration—Sexual Cases*, CRIM. L. REV. [Eng.] 662, 665-666. *See generally* 2 WIGMORE §§ 505, 509; 3 WIGMORE §§ 924a, 938; 7 WIGMORE §2060.

[83] *E.g.*, Barber v. Page, 390 U.S. 719 (1968); Pointer v. Texas, 380 U.S. 400, 405 (1965). J. APPLEMANN, CROSS EXAMINATION (1963); J. MUNKMAN, THE TECHNIQUE OF ADVOCACY (1951); R. REDFIELD, CROSS EXAMINATION AND THE WITNESS 147 (1963); 5 WIGMORE §§ 1365-1365; F. WROTTESLEY, THE EXAMINATION OF WITNESSES IN COURT 94 (3d ed. 1961).

[84] *See* pp. 000,000,000 *infra*.

[85] *In re* Gault, 387 U.S. 1, 21 (1967).

[86] Malinski v. New York, 324 U.S. 401, 414 (1945).

protect a child by reducing his testimonial duty in a manner which infringes upon the constitutional rights of the accused must be unacceptable in the United States.

Nations without written constitutions have greater flexibility in reconciling conflicts between basic rights or interests, such as those of the accused and the child victim. Thus, even nations which tenaciously protect the accused's rights to confront and cross-examine witnesses, *e.g.*, Great Britain and Israel, can more easily make allowances for the protection of child victims. The Scandinavian states, observing few rules of evidence, no prohibition against hearsay evidence, and only the rudiments of cross-examination,[87] are relatively free to accommodate their rules of criminal procedure to the welfare of child victims without offending their concept of a fair trial. In fact, Scandinavian jurists regard their informal conduct of criminal trials as "a rational and reasonable way of finding out the truth and evaluating the conduct of the accused."[88]

Since the interests of the accused and child victims appear to be conflicting, each jurisdiction can either favor one interest over the other or strike some balances between them. Yet, in states which choose to protect either interest at the expense of the other, arguments are raised in support of better protecting the less favored interest. Moves to redress such imbalances are gaining support in many states, but not without posing constitutional problems. To illustrate the difficulty, the following discussion examines the practices of a typical American jurisdiction, Illinois, for taking the evidence of child victims in criminal trials, and proceeds with a proposal for dealing with the testimonial duty of child victims on an individual basis while attempting to insure a fair trial and effective fact finding.

Repeated Interrogations of Child Victim

The Illinois Criminal Code defines some sexual offenses

---

[87]Andenaes, *"The Legal Framework,"* *Scandinavian Studies in Criminology*, Vol. 2 (1968); p. 11.

[88]*Id.*

against children as "felonies",[89] which authorizes the courts to impose harsh sentences on child molesters in consonance with a policy of individual and general deterrence.[90] But in order to bring his felonious molester to justice, the complainant child must endure two additional stages of pretrial criminal procedure: the preliminary hearing, and the grand jury hearing. In the preliminary hearing the defendant is confronted by the child victim, whose testimony is usually essential for a showing of probable cause.[91] If the accused is held to answer to a felony charge, the case is sent to the grand jury.[92] However, there is no constitutional right to a preliminary hearing prior to the indictment or trial,[93] so that failure to hold the preliminary hearing is not considered a denial of due process of law.[94] Accordingly, child molesters may be brought before the grand jury without any previous preliminary hearing, which spares the child victim from ever confronting the defendant in court before the trial, since there are no confrontations between the accused and witnesses in grand jury hearings.[95] While the grand jury admits hearsay evidence, its general practice is to "hear" the child victim in order to determine whether the evidence constitutes "probable cause," excluding the accused and his counsel from the hearing. Thus, the child victim appears before a panel of grand jurors to narrate once again the same story he told the police and perhaps the judge in the preliminary hearings.[96] If

---

[89]Certain offenses against children [Ill. Ann. Stat. ch. 38 §11-4 (Smith-Hurd Supp. 1968)] fit within the definition of "felony" [ILL. ANN. STAT. ch. 38, § 2-7 (Smith-Hurd 1967)].

[90]*See* Andenaes, *The General Preventive Effects of Punishment.* 114 U. Pa L. REV. 949 (1966).

[91]The judge should determine whether it appears from the evidence that there is probable cause to believe that an offense has been committed by the defendant. The defendant can waive the preliminary examination. ILL. ANN. STAT. ch. 38, §109-3 (Smith-Hurd Supp. 1969).

[92]*See* Ill. Ann. Stat. ch. 38, §§109-3, 111-2, 111-3(b), 112-4 (Smith-Hurd Supp. 1969).

[93]*People v. Petruso,* 35 Ill.2d 578, 580, 221 N.E.2d 276, 277 (1966); *see* Ill. Const. art. 2.

[94]*People v. Petruso,* 35 Ill.2d 578, 580, 221 N.E.2d 276, 277 (1966).

[95]Ill. Ann. Stat. ch. 38 §112-6(a) (Smith-Hurd Supp. 1969).

[96]*Id.* § 112-4. In Texas the State's Attorney may present the transcript of the preliminary examination to the grand jury without calling the witnesses to give oral evidence. *See* TEX. CODE CRIM. PROC. ANN. art 20.03-04 (1966). In California, the State's Attorney is

there is no preliminary hearing, it is only after the grand jury returns an indictment that a trial is held. If the accused is charged with a misdemeanor, no pretrial hearings are required and the trial begins with an information or a complaint.[97] In short, Illinois guarantees the right of every defendant to confront witnesses against him, regardless of any adverse mental effect that such a confrontation may cause a child. In felony charges, the child victim must testify once or twice more in addition to various prior police interrogations.[98]

The Practice of the Negotiated Plea

The need to protect and assist child victims has won no notable official support in Illinois, despite the recommendations made in 1963 by the Commission on Sex Offenders.[99] However, the pattern of the negotiated guilty plea, a predominant feature of American criminal practice not limited to cases of child molesters,[100] does stand as one accommodation of both the welfare of the child and the protection of the defendant. In return for a defense plea of guilty, the prosecutor will either reduce a felony charge to a misdemeanor, reduce the number of charges in a multiple count indictment, or recommend that the court impose a more lenient sentence. The accused is told[101] that he will spare the child victim the ordeal of reliving his experiences in court, which will save the judicial machinery precious time and money, for which he will be kindly treated in return.[102]

---

authorized to sign an indictment after a judge in the preliminary hearing has found probable cause. CAL. PENAL CODE §§ 682, 739, 872 (West 1964). Consequently, there is no duplication in pretrial proceedings in those jurisdictions.

[97]ILL. ANN. STAT. ch. 38 §§ 102-9, 102-12, 111-2(2) (Smith-Hurd Supp. 1969).

[98]*See* p. 000 *supra.*

[99]*See* ILLINOIS COMMISSION ON SEX OFFENDERS, A REPORT TO THE 73RD GENERAL ASSEMBLY 11-12 (1963).

[100]*See* D. KARLEN, G. SAWYER & E. WISE, ANGLO-AMERICAN CRIMINAL JUSTICE 155 (1967). *See also The Negotiated Plea of Guilty,* in PRESIDENT'S COMMISSION ON LAW ENFORCEMENT AND ADMINISTRATION OF JUSTICE, TASK FORCE REPORTS: THE COURTS 9-13 (1967).

[101]On the role of defense counsel as "agent-mediator"and the motives for negotiating a "deal," *see* A. BLUMBERG, CRIMINAL JUSTICE 103-115 (1967).

[102]*See* AMERICAN BAR ASSOCIATION, PROJECT ON MINIMUM STANDARDS FOR CRIMINAL

The bargained plea seems to be supported by Vincent De Francis, Director of the Children's Division of the American Humane Association, who favors easing the problems of child victims without abridging constitutional safeguards. He praises the practice of some five or six East Coast communities in which a staff member of the local Society for the Prevention of Cruelty to Children, appearing in court with the child and his family as amicus curiae,

> will oppose unwarranted defense motions for adjournment; will seek to have the case heard in the privacy of the judge's chambers; may seek to have the general public excluded from the courtroom; and . . . will work the county prosecutor toward accepting a guilty plea from the offender. If a guilty plea is accepted, there will not be a trial and the child will be saved the ordeal of testifying in court.[103]

Undoubtedly, negotiated pleas are intended in part to minimize the damage wrought be court proceedings on child victims' future personalities, though basically they resolve to "bureaucratically ordained short cuts . . . in order to meet [the] production norms[104] of an efficient judiciary, serving less to do justice than to dispose of onerously large case loads and unknown risks, hopefully without doing injustice.[105] The agreement by the parties is taken as proof of the desirability of the "deal," but while there are favorable consequences to the child, the defendant is led to waive his constitutional right to a trial and may come to suspect that the law is something to be manipulated.

The judge, who may participate in the negotiations,[106] will ratify the bargained plea and lessened punishment. In Illinois,

---

JUSTICE, PLEAS OF GUILTY (1967).

[103]V. DE FRANCIS, PROTECTING THE CHILD VICTIM OF SEX CRIME 11 (1965).

[104]A. BLUMBERG, *supra* note 101, at 21.

[105]A trial is a "risk" for the adversaries because each is unwilling to lose his case, and sometimes it is a "risk" for the judge also, because a nonnegotiated verdict may be appealed and his conducting of the trial scrutinized by an appellate court. A negotiated plea relies on the assumption that the case ends in the trial court, and no other judge will examine it further.

[106]The role of judges in the "bargains" is affirmed by D. KARLEN, *supra* note 100; A. BLUMBERG, *supra* note 101, at xiii, 5, 131-37.

the simplest part of the operation is the replacement of a felony charge with misdemeanor, because the same *actus reus* and *mens rea* constitute the misdemeanor of "contributing to the sexual delinquency of a child" and the felony of "indecent liberties with a child."[107] The accused who is charged with one felony, or multiple felonies arising from the same event, must try for acquittal at the risk of being sentenced to the penitentiary, plead guilty to a felony charge and accept a light sentence, or plead guilty to a lesser offense carrying a lighter penalty in exchange for probation, a suspended sentence, or a short term.[108] The temptation to "bargain" is strong even for those who consider themselves innocent victims of the child or the circumstances rather than victimizers. Defenders of the guilty-plea system may discount this problem, but the pressures exerted to secure pleas of guilty must at least on occasion result in the conviction of innocent men. As the court and counsel employ what Blumberg calls a "bureaucratic due process" instead of "due process of law,"[109] the practice invites crippling of the constitutional rights of trial by jury, against self-incrimination, and of confrontation.[110] For all but a handful of cases in which a trial is futile and inhumane, justice itself may be sacrificed.[111]

The practice of the negotiated guilty plea is thus wholly unacceptable as a means of protecting child victims of sex offenses. It provides no care for children who are called to testify

---

[107]*See* ILL. ANN. STAT ch. 38, §§ 11-4, 11-5 (Smith-Hurd Supp. 1969). Each offense covers a wide range of sexual relations between adult and child, including "[a]n act of sexual intercourse," "[a]ct of deviate sexual conduct," and other indecent acts. Whereas reasonable but mistaken belief in the child's age is a valid defense in a felony charge, it is not in a misdemeanor charge.

[108]*See* ILL. ANN. STAT. ch. 38, §11-5 (Smith Hurd 1964).

[109]*See* A. BLUMBERG, *supra* note 101, at 21.

[110]*See* United States v. Jackson, 390 U.S. 570 (1968); *cf.* United States ex rel. Elksnis v. Gilligan, 256 F. Supp. 244 (S.D.N.Y. 1966) (constitutional problems presented when judge participates in plea bargaining).

[111]*See* Enker, *Perspectives on Plea Bargaining*, in PRESIDENT'S COMMISSION ON LAW ENFORCEMENT AND THE ADMINISTRATION OF JUSTICE. TASK FORCE REPORTS: THE COURTS app. A, 108-19 (1967).

in courtrooms, and it mocks the constitutional rights of defendants, tempting them to yield to the instruments and pressures promoting the negotiated guilty plea. Thus, the practice falls short of accommodating the conflicting interests of the accused and the victims. Still the pattern of bargains does remind the legal system that it ignores the child victim's welfare and that child witnesses deserve real and effective protection as witnesses.

Determining the Child Victim's Duty to Testify

Psychiatric opinions and studies emphasize that each child victim reacts to an offense and its aftermath in his own individual way. A case of incest is different from indecent exposure, a stranger-aggressor different from an offender whom the child knows, use of force different from willing participation, *etc.* Thus there can be no more justification for excusing all child victims from testifying[112] than for imposing the duty on all of them.[113] Each case merits its own individual decision.

Someone must decide whether a child is to testify. Submitting arguendo that the issue of the child's availability should be judged solely on the basis of his mental health before the trial and his vulnerability to "legal process trauma" and disregarding his credibility, the public interest in proving the charge, and the defendant's right to confrontation, there are three possible agencies for making the decision as to the child's availability.

First, the youth interrogator, as in Israel, is the most familiar with the mental and social background of the witness and therefore is the most competent to decide. However, the child examiner's opinion is open to the same criticism, as in any other psychiatric or psychological diagnosis. The child's vulnerability to "legal process trauma" is, after all, an imprecise and irresolved question, wide open to dispute. The second possibility is to treat the child's "unavailability" as a preliminary question of fact to be determined by the court. The child examiner's opinion should be respected by the court, unless serious evidence convinces it

---

[112]*E.g.*, the Norwegian and the Swedish systems.
[113]*E.g.*, the Anglo-American systems.

otherwise. A third option is a combination of the preceding approaches, having the judge decide whether to accept the child examiner's opinion or to transfer the matter for re-examination by a board composed of an appellate judge and two experts on child welfare. This is a more complicated mechanism but it spares the court from making a decision beyond its competence and from hearing further witnesses on this issue.

Considering the special circumstances of each child's case in view of these alternatives, it is apparent that child victims need neither testify fully in court nor be wholly prohibited from testifying. Several alternatives recommended by child experts can be made available to protect the child according to the special circumstances of his case, as limitations or conditions of their duty of testimonial attendance.

A. The *place* of the child's attendance may be:
    (1) the courtroom or the judge's chambers; or
    (2) an informal familiar place outside the courthouse such as a schoolroom, a youth club, or at home.
B. The child's attendance in a place mentioned in Section A (1) should be permitted for one or more of the following purposes:
    (1) giving regular oral testimony; or
    (2) submitting to a limited additional examination; or
    (3) being introduced, without being interrogated about the offense.[114]
C. The competent examiner(s) for the particular child victim may be:
    (1) the judge, the prosecutor, and the defense counsel; or
    (2) the child examiner, who might ask the child questions originated by the judge, the defense counsel, and the prosecutor; or
    (3) the judge only.

---

[114]In this case the child appears in court as "an exhibit," and none of his out-of-court statements are admissible. The child victim's personal appearance is of special significance in cases where his age or the defendant's reasonable mistake as to his age constitutes a material element in the case.

D. The *time* for conducting the child victim's examination may be:
   (1) the trial; or
   (2) a special session, prior to the trial.
E. The child should be totally unavailable for the legal process.
F. The accused's presence during his trial or during a "special session" [according to D(2)] is required, unless the child is submitted to "a limited additional examination" [according to B(2)] by the judge, the prosecutor, and the defense counsel [according to C(1)].

If the child is available for the legal proceedings, it is still desirable that the child examiner be present wherever and whenever the child is giving evidence, to advise the judge about immediate measures that should be taken to cope with unexpected developments.

An examination of these components of an individualized approach according to criteria of fair trial for the accused resolves to six basic solutions:

1. The trial of the child molester is conducted according to the standard procedure for criminal cases, and the rights of defendants are unchanged [see A(1), B(1), C(1), D(1)].

2. If the child victim is totally unavailable for the defense's examination [see E] and for the "limited additional examination" [see B(2)], none of the child's out-of-court statements are admissible at trial, since the accused had no opportunity to cross-examine.

3. If the child is "available" in person for the trial or the "special session" [see D(2)2], he must confront the accused, unless the system of the "Child Courtroom" proposed later in this article is adopted. Where such a confrontation is deemed too traumatic for the child, his pretrial evidence as recorded by the child examiner is admissible as an exception to the hearsay rule, provided that the defense and the prosecutor may examine the child [see F] in "a limited additional examination" [see B(2)].

4. If there are reasonable grounds to believe that defense counsel's cross-examination may be especially traumatic for the child, the "limited additional examination" [B(2)] may be conducted through the child examiner [C(2)]. Again, the term

"limited additional examination" assumes that the evidence recorded by the child examiner prior to the trial is admissible, provided the opportunity for additional examination in court is given to the defense.

5. Whenever the presence of a large number of persons in court or the court surroundings themselves may be regarded undesirable, the questioning of the child may take place in any of the places mentioned in section A(2), given prior public notice of the court's retirement to the chosen place and provided that the removal of the hearing does not deprive the accused of his rights to be present and represented by counsel.

6. Whenever a delay in the conducting of the trial may tend significantly to jeopardize the child victim's mental health, a "special session" may be convened [D(2)] to take the child victim's evidence, under courtroom rules governing his testimonial duty. A "special session" should not begin unless the court is satisfied that the accused has had sufficient time to prepare his defense.

It would be unwise to admit more than one of these limitations at a time, inasmuch as cumulating them must progressively increase the danger of depriving the accused of his right to fair trail. The court, proceeding carefully, may thus be satisfied upon hearing all the evidence that the protection of the child victim was not achieved at the expense of this fundamental right.

Since this proposal does not regard constitutional requirements of due process, these requirements must be examined and further solutions proposed to meet the dilemma of the child victim in court.

Proposals for Protecting the Child Victim and Attendant Constitutional Problems

In cases of sex offenses the defendant has an absolute right to counsel[115] "at every step in the proceedings against him,"[116] and

---

[115]Gideon v. Wainwright, 372 U.S. 335 (1963); Douglas v. California, 372 U.S. 353 (1963); Griffin v. Illinois, 351 U.S. 12 (1956). Although the sixth amendment right to counsel does not require the appointment of counsel in all misdemeanor cases, sex

to cross-examine adverse witnesses through counsel,[117] who alone decides how and whether to conduct such a cross-examination.[118] Thus, an attempt to deprive an accused of the effective assistance of counsel during confrontation with a child witness is a clear denial of sixth amendment rights to counsel and confrontation and fourteenth amendment due process of law.[119]

The right to confrontation, like the right to counsel, is "an essential and fundamental requirement for . . . fair trial," which has been made binding on the states,[120] as have the standards for the confrontation rule developed in federal cases.[121] The Supreme Court recently stated that "the right to confrontation is basically a trial right" because it includes "both the opportunity to cross-examine and the occasion for the jury to weigh the demeanor of the witness."[122] Effective confrontation therefore occurs at the trial, when the accused and his counsel confront the witness in the presence of the trier of fact. Any means of preventing the child victim from meeting the accused face to face at the trial, or limiting the scope of effectiveness of cross-examination, or having a child examiner conduct the questioning of the child, or permitting the introduction at trial of evidence given earlier by the child, must be closely scrutinized in terms of threatened infringements of rights of confrontation. Even more basic is the question whether the right to confrontation and the policy of child protection are reconcilable at all.

The sixth amendment specifies that "[i]n all criminal prosecutions, the accused shall enjoy the right to a speedy and public trial. . . ."[123] The Supreme Court has held that the right of public

---

offenses committed against children must be regarded as constituting "serious offenses" which do require the trial court to notify the accused of and protect his right to counsel. *Cf.* Winters v. Beck, 281 F. Supp. 793 (E.D. Ark. 1968).

[116]Powell v. Alabama, 267 U.S. 45 (1932).

[117]Pointer v. Texas, 380 U.S. 400 (1965).

[118]Brookhart v. Janis, 384 U.S. 1, 8 (1966) (separate opinion of Harlan, J.).

[119]*Cf.* Pointer v. Texas, 380 U.S. 400, 405, 410 (1965); Gideon v. Wainwright, 372 U.S. 335 (1963).

[120]Pointer v. Texas, 380 U.S. 400, 405 (1965).

[121]*Id.* at 405-406.

[122]Barber v. Page, 390 U.S. 719, 725 (1968).

[123]U.S. CONST. amend. VI.

trial is a fundamental element of due process of law, and thus applicable to and binding upon the states.[124] It must be determined whether a procedure designed to protect the child by taking his evidence with the public excluded from the courtroom, or in the judge's chambers or an informal place outside the courthouse, may operate as to deny the accused his right to public trial, and thus be unacceptable.

The accused also has the right to trial by an impartial jury, held binding on the states in "serious cases,"[125] whose presence is, however, likely to prove discomfitting to the child as he faces another large group of people in formal surroundings. Fulfillment of this right must be reconciled with relief of the child from its consequences.

This section examines several alternative proposals which seek to protect child victims without denying defendants these constitutional rights.

Proposal I: A Trial in the Child-Courtroom

The first proposal for protecting the child victim operates within the framework of the trial itself. The response to the constitutional difficulties previously referred to lies not in new legalistic formulations but in fashioning new techniques to resolve legal dilemmas. The price for protecting the child need not be infringement upon any of the accused's constitutional rights. The price which the states are called upon to pay for

---

[124]*In re* Oliver, 333 U.S. 257 (1948); United States *ex rel* Bruno v. Herold, 246 F. Supp. 363 (N.D.N.Y. 1965); *see* Washington v. Texas, 388 U.S. 14, 18 (1967). Almost every state, whether by constitution, statute, or judicial decision, requires that the accused be given a public trial. *See In re* Oliver, *supra* at 267-68 and nn.17-20. Mr. Justice Harlan has remarked: "A fair trial is the objective, and 'public trial' is an institutional safeguard for attaining it." Estes v. Texas, 381 U.S. 532, 588 (1965). In special circumstances exceptions may be made to the rule of publicity. *See* 6 WIGMORE. § 1835 (Supp. 1964).

[125]Duncan v. Louisiana, 391 U.S. 145 (1968), "[T]he right to jury trial in serious criminal cases is a fundamental right and hence must be recognized by the States as part of their obligation to extend due process of law to all persons within their jurisdiction." *Id.* at 154, "[W]e hold that the Fourteenth Amendment guarantees a right of jury trial in all criminal cases which—were they to be tried in federal court—would come within the Sixth Amendment's guarantee." *Id.* at 149, *see* Turner v. Louisiana, 379 U.S. 466 (1965).

protecting child victims while securing fair trials is money. Recent Supreme Court decisions indicate that states will do better if they spend a reasonable sum of money when necessary to secure constitutional rights than to save it "at the price of fundamental principles of constitutional liberty," because "that price is too high."[126] Furthermore, in some recent decisions, federal courts expressed the hope that the criminal justice system will utilize scientific and technological innovations.[127] The proposal submitted below seeks to implement this hope.

The proposal is based on the assumption that a state should not ignore the opinions of most psychiatrists, psychologists, judges, and parents that the mental health of the child victim should be given substantial consideration and protected where possible by the criminal justice system. The fact is that psychiatrists all over the world repeatedly warn that "legal proceedings are not geared to protect the victim's emotions and may be exceptionally traumatic."[128] The studies do not as yet demonstrate a clear causal link between the legal proceedings and the child victim's mental disturbances, but no psychiatric study has attempted to prove, or is likely to attempt to prove in the future, such a causal link. Psychiatrists agree that they cannot isolate the effects of the crime trauma from the "prior personality damage" or either of the foregoing from the "environment reaction trauma" or the "legal process trauma."[129] But psychiatrists do agree that when some victims encounter the law enforcement system, for one reason or another, the child requires special care and treatment.[130]

Recently, the Supreme Court, in discussing "a legislative finding" that sexual material defined by a New York statute as obscene is *"a basic factor* in impairing the ethical and moral development of our youth,"[131] the Court observed pointedly: "It

---

[126]*E.g.*, Bruton v. United States, 391 U.S. 123 (1968).

[127]*E.g.*, Virgin Islands v. Aquino, 378 F.2d 541 (3d Cir. 1967).

[128]*See* M. GUTTMACHER. SEX OFFENSES: THE PROBLEM. CAUSES AND PREVENTION 118 (1951).

[129]*E.g.*, GIBBENS & PRINCE 9.

[130]*See* pp. 000-000 *supra*.

[131]Law of April 29, 1955, ch. 836, §540 [1955] N.Y. Laws 1988-89 (repealed 1967) (emphasis added).

is very doubtful that this finding expresses an accepted scientific fact."[132] Mr. Justice Brennan, delivering the opinion of the Court, stated that the growing consensus of commentators is that "while these studies all agree that a causal link has not been demonstrated, they are equally agreed that a causal link has not been disproved either."[133] The Court held that in the absence of any "accepted scientific fact" concerning the mental or moral harm of "obscene" materials to children under the age of seventeen, state power to regulate material defined by it as obscene will be upheld where the Court can "say that it was *not irrational* for the legislature to find that exposure to material condemned by the statute is harmful to minors."[134] The need to protect child victims who were exposed to sexual acts, whether violent or nonviolent, is also likely to meet the Supreme Court standard of rationality, especially since the proposals in this section attempt to provide for protection while according to the accused his full measure of constitutional rights.[135] Bearing in mind that the United States was the first country in the world to bring forward the idea of protecting juvenile delinquents by establishing a special juvenile court,[136] one would expect that it would also do more for juvenile victims than it has.

PHYSICAL ARRANGEMENT OF THE CHILD-COURTROOM—In order to secure fair trial for the accused and a "healthy" one for

---

[132]*Compare* Memories v. Massachusetts, 383 U.S. 413, 431-432 (1966) (concurring opinion of Douglas, J.), *with id.* at 451-453 (dissent by Clark, J.).

[133]Ginsberg v. New York, 390 U.S. 629, 642 (1968).

[134]*Id.* at 641.

[135]While the care and nurture of the child is first of all the responsibility of the child's parents (390 U.S. at 639), the parents and others who share the primary concern for children's well-being, such as teachers and physicians, are entitled to the support of the state laws designed to aid them in the event that a child should fall victim to a sexual offense. The reluctance of American parents to cooperate with the police in cases of child molestation is a common finding of academic studies, state committees, and police authorities. (Only about 10% of sex offenses committed upon participant and passive girl victims below twelve are reported by parents to the police.) *See* M. GUTTMACHER, *supra* note 128, at 73; Gagnon, *Female Child Victims of Sex Offenses*, 13 SOCIAL PROBLEMS 177, 184 (Fall, 1965); Landis, *Experiences of 500 Children with Adult Sexual Deviation*, 30 PSYCHIATRIC Q. 91, 99 (Supp. 1956). Neither legislatures nor the Supreme Court can ignore parents' reactions in this area of their most basic concern.

[136]*See* S. ROBINSON, JUVENILE DELINQUENCY: ITS NATURE AND CONTROL 228 (1960).

the child victim, it is submitted that special facilities, a "Child-Courtroom," be established, the details and features of which are dictated by the conflicting requirements for protecting the assumed as well as the child victim.

The Child-Courtroom is designed to take a victim's testimony in an informal and relaxed manner, while the child can see only four persons around him: the judge, the prosecutor, the defense counsel, and the child examiner, who will all be seated in a "judge's room," arranged in a way which contributes to the security and psychological comfort of the child. The accused, the jury, and the audience should be seated behind a one-way glass, separating them from the judge's room, but enabling them to observe everything which occurs there. In this manner the defendant's right to trial by jury is secured and the jury can view the accused's demeanor while the child is testifying. In addition, the accused will have microphone and earphones by means of which he and his counsel, who is in the judge's room, will be able to communicate with each other. The proceedings are transmitted to the accused's box by suitable electronic methods which would not interfere with the accused's capacity to communicate with his counsel.[137] Of course, whenever the attorney requests a brief pause in the examination of the child to consult or advise his client, such requests should be granted by the judge. In addition, whenever the identification of the accused is at issue, he may be asked to enter the judge's room for a moment or two with several other persons for identification. All of these special arrangements should be in force for as long as the child gives evidence. Upon the conclusion of his testimony, the proceedings should be resumed in a regular courtroom.

The proposal secures the defendant's right to trial by jury in that the jury can observe from behind the one-way glass what is taking place in the judge's room without being seen by the child. It is desirable, and easily arranged, that the jury be capable of viewing simultaneously not only the witness, counsel, and judge, but also the accused's demeanor while the child is testifying.

---

[137]Such a method was in fact employed in the trial of Adolf Eichmann, which received worldwide attention. *See* G. HAUSNER. JUSTICE IN JERUSALEM 305-312 (1966).

The Child-Courtroom can be built as part of an existing courthouse or as a separate unit. In either case, an ordinary courtroom should be nearby so that, before and after the child testifies in the Child-Courtroom, the trial may proceed as usual in the normal setting. Also, it is essential to provide a suitable place where the child, his parents, and the child-examiner who accompanies them can wait for the trial without being exposed to undesirable company or a frightening or confusing atmosphere.

THE ACCUSED'S RIGHT TO BE PRESENT AT HIS TRIAL—It has often been suggested that the child victim's confrontation with the accused at the trial is a source of depression, anxiety, and fear for the child.[138] On the other hand, a study of the Supreme Court's decisions concerning the presence of the accused at this trial leaves no doubt that the confrontation clause requires the presence of the accused when witnesses testify at his trial. The Supreme Court has held that "the rule of orderly conduct of jury trial" entitles an accused "to be present from the time the jury is impaneled until its discharge after rendering the verdict."[139] Justice Cardozo wrote that "a defendant in a criminal case must be present at a trial when evidence is offered, for the opportunity must be his to advise with his counsel, and cross-examine his accusers."[140] Neither the desirability of the accused's presence at his trial nor the fact that his presence is "essential to the substance of a hearing" can be seriously doubted today. However, a question might be raised as to whether, due to counsel's regular presence at the trial and his significant role in cross-examining the witnesses, an exception to the general requirement of the accused's personal confrontation with each witness against him can be justified. The question has not yet been directly raised; the answer would seem to depend more on the meaning and nature of the right to counsel and effective confrontation than on any other constitutional right.[141]

---

[138]*See* p. 193 *supra*.

[139]Shields v. United States, 273 U.S. 583, 588-89 (1927).

[140]Snyder v. Massachusetts, 291 U.S. 97, 114 (1934) (citations omitted); *see In re* Hunt, 276 F. Supp. 112 (E.D. Mich. 1967).

[141]Also, the right of the accused to be heard and to offer evidence on his own behalf entitled him to be present at his trial, though absent the rights to confrontation and the

The apprehension which naturally arises in response to a suggestion of dispensing with the personal presence of a defendant, particularly in cases of sexual charges, is due primarily to the importance attributed to the cross-examination of the complainant in the presence of the accused, and secondly to the identification of the accused in cases where identity is at issue. For purposes of identification the physical confrontation could perhaps be limited, especially in light of the additional pretrial identification which is generally required. But for purposes of cross-examination, in its constitutional context, the accused must be given "a complete and adequate opportunity to cross-examination."[142] The Supreme Court has not yet defined "a complete and adequate opportunity." However, recent Court decisions dealing with the identity of the cross-examiner and his "adequate opportunity" provide some insights.

These cases emphasize the accused's right to be represented by an attorney who is provided with the opportunity to cross-examine. In *Pointer v. Texas*,[143] the accused personally confronted the witness at the preliminary hearing and had the opportunity to cross-examine him but failed to do so, although he did cross-examine other witnesses. The Supreme Court held that the introduction of the witness' preliminary hearing testimony as evidence at the subsequent trial was a clear denial of the right of confrontation, "since the statement was made without an adequate opportunity of cross-examination."[144] It is clear, however, that had Pointer been represented by counsel in the preliminary

---

assistance of counsel not necessarily during other witnesses' testimony, as long as he can have full knowledge thereof, for example, by means of transcripts of the evidence of witnesses available immediately upon its taking. However, in the series of cases in which the Supreme Court required an effective appointment of counsel in criminal cases, the Court considered the role of counsel only as "aid" and "assistance" to defendants, and never as a "substitute" for their presence and participation in the trial.

[142]Pointer v. Texas, 380 U.S. 400, 407 (1965).

[143]*Id.*

[144]*Id.* at 407; *accord* People v. Chapman, 380 Mich. 74, 155 N.W.2d 827 (1968); People v. Russell, 9 Mich. App. 44, 155 N.W.2d 691 (1967); Messmove v. Fogliani, 82 Nev. 154, 413 P.2d 306 (1966). The question whether the transcript of the witness' testimony would have been admissible, had the accused himself cross-examined the witness in the preliminary hearing, remained open in *Pointer. See* State v. Head, 91 Ariz. 246, 249, 371 P.2d 599, 601-602 (1962).

hearing, the confrontation clause would have been satisfied if he had been represented by counsel who had been given, at a full-fledged hearing, an adequate opportunity to cross-examine the witness. Thus, "a complete and adequate opportunity" of cross-examination is afforded through counsel; still, there is no sign that the Supreme Court might be ready to compromise over the physical presence of the accused while his counsel is cross-examining the witness.

One reason why the accused must be present in person during cross-examination conducted by his counsel is to insure that his attorney does not waive, against the accused's express desire, any of his constitutional rights.[145] The accused must be in a position to protest against the actions of his attorney and, if necessary, discharge him. Furthermore, the accused should be present to assist his counsel during the hearing concerning factual issues since it is conceivable that unexpected evidence might be introduced at the trial with which the attorney is unfamiliar. Because counsel's function is to give the accused "effective aid in the preparation and trial of the case,"[146] which includes effective cross-examination, it may be argued that the opportunity of both the accused and the attorney to communicate with each other during the cross-examination of an adverse witness is essential for an adequate and effective defense. If the state deprives an accused of an opportunity for such communication with his counsel at the trial by excluding him from the courtroom, there are valid grounds for the contention that such a restriction denies the accused effective confrontation. In addition, the accused may argue that some attorneys may be induced to perform more conscientiously if they must act in the presence of their clients.

In sum, the accused must be present when the child testifies against him, so that he may observe the proceedings, hear the child's testimony, and be able to communicate with his counsel. All this can be arranged in the Child-Courtroom without the ac-

---

[145]*See* Brockhart v. Janis, 384 U.S. 1 (1966). Honest mistakes of counsel, however, are usually binding on the client as one of the hazards of courtroom battle. Henry v. Mississippi, 379 U.S. 443, 446, 451 (1964).

[146]Powell v. Alabama, 287 U.S. 45. 71 (1932).

cused being seen by the child. The Child-Courtroom protects, by technological means, the essence of the accused's right to confront the child witness at trial. The accused can observe his counsel at work, communicate with him, and be aware of all the details of the court proceedings. He has the opportunity through counsel to cross-examine the witness against him, while the jury can simultaneously observe the child's demeanor and the accused's demeanor.

THE ACCUSED'S RIGHT TO A PUBLIC TRIAL—The right to a public trial, as generally interpreted, requires that the doors of the courtroom remain open. This allows persons unknown to the parties to come forward and offer evidence.[147] Furthermore, it is important not only that justice be done, but also that the public see that justice is being done. This reinforces public confidence in the judicial system and also affords the opportunity for the criminal trial to be subject to public criticism.[148]

However, a child is likely either to be confused and frightened by the presence of many persons, or impressed with his unusual opportunity for enthralling a large audience with his stories. In both cases the public's presence may serve to interfere with the child's powers of recollection and narration. In addition, psychiatrists have observed that "the victim naturally wishes to avoid publicity, the embarrassment which accompanies questioning by authorities, or courtroom experiences. Children in particular are often profoundly disturbed by this situation."[149] For these reasons, some foreign countries such as England,[150] and Israel[151]

---

[147]Tanksley v. United States, 145 F.2d 58, 59 (9th Cir. 1944).

[148]*In re* Oliver, 333 U.S. 257 (1948); *see* Radin, *The Right to a Public Trial*, 6 TEMP. L.Q. 381 (1932);6 WIGMORE, §1834.

[149]Halleck, *Emotional Effects of Victimization*, SEXUAL BEHAVIOR AND THE LAW 684 (R. Slovenko ed. 1965).

[150]The Children and Young Persons Act of 1933, 23 Geo. 5, c. 12, §42.

[151]Courts Law 5717-1957 §38 (b), 11 LAWS OF THE STATE OF ISRAEL 164 (auth. trans. 1955): "A court may deal with the whole or any part of a particular matter *in camera* if it deems it necessary so to do for the purpose of protecting morality or protecting the well-being of a minor." Law of Evidence Revision (Protection of Children) Law 5715-1955 §6 (a). 9 LAWS OF THE STATE OF ISRAEL 103 (auth. trans. 1955): "A person shall not publish anything calculated to reveal the identity of a child who has been examined as to an offense against morality or has testified in connection with such an offense before a court, save with the permission of court."

entrust the courts with powers to exclude the public from the courtroom when a child victim testifies.

The Child-Courtroom may do away with the need to exclude the public from the trial. The audience, like the jury, may be afforded the opportunity of observing the proceedings in the Child-Courtroom without being seen by the child victim by the use of the same technical devices described above. Furthermore, the right to a public trial does not require that a large number of seats be provided for the audience in the Child-Courtroom. This right is not an absolute or rigid one.

The minimum necessary to satisfy the public trial requirement has been stated, by Mr. Justice Black, to be that the accused is allowed to have his counsel, family, relatives, and friends present, regardless of the offense charged.[152] But as to the presence of other persons at the trial, both federal and state authorities agree that the defendant's right to a public trial is subject to limitations based on the following considerations:

1. Practical considerations related to the capacity of the place in which the hearing occurs: The public trial guarantee is not violated if an individual member of the public cannot gain admittance to a courtroom because there are no available seats.[153] There is no constitutional imperative that the trial be held in a place large enough to accommodate all those who desire to attend.[154] The right to a public trial belongs to the defendant, not the public.[155]

2. Considerations of orderly conduct of the trial: All spectators who are admitted to the place where the trial is conducted must observe proper decorum, and if their conduct tends in any

---

[152]*In re* Oliver, 333 U.S. 257, 272 (1948). *See also* 35 MICH. L. REV. 474 (1937).

[153]Tate v. Commonwealth, 258 Ky. 685, 693, 70 S.W.2d 817, 821 (1935): *see* Estes v. Texas, 381 U.S. 532, 588 (1965).

[154]United States v. Kobli, 172 F.2d 919, 923 (3d Cir. 1949). It is reasonable to assume, however, that the constitutional right to a public trial requires the courtroom to have enough room for a "reasonable" number of people.

[155]Estes v. Texas, 381 U.S. 532, 588 (1965) (concurring opinion). Although the sixth amendment right to public trial is the accused's right, and he may waive it, the right of the public to know must also be preserved. *See* Mueller, *Problems Posed by Publicity to Crime and Criminal Proceedings*, 110 U. PA. L. REV. 1, 2-10 (1961).

way to interfere with the administration of justice in the court-room, they may be removed.[156]

3. Considerations of protecting the morals of the young people among the spectators: In cases involving sexual offenses, young spectators may be excluded when the evidence is likely to involve the recital of scandalous or indecent matters which might have a demoralizing effect upon them.[157] If a judge concludes from the subject matter of the indictment that considerations of public morals require the exclusion of minors from the hearing, the defendant's right to a public trial is still safeguarded by the presence of interested adult spectators.[158]

Finally, considerations protecting the child victim of a sexual offense also limit this right. Child victims of "tender years" are protected in some jurisdictions by limited exclusion of the public from the hearing on the ground that a girl might be "seriously embarrassed in giving her testimony by the presence of spectators not concerned with the trial."[159] The ultimate reason given by courts for the removal of all members of the public not directly concerned with the trial is the prevention of a miscarriage of justice.[160] One state court summed up the issue in 1935, saying:

> It cannot be doubted that a trial judge . . . may protect a child witness, who, from the nature of the case must testify to revolting facts, by excluding morbid, prurient, curious and sensation-seeking persons from the courtroom, so long as he does not abuse his discretion and deprive the accused of the right to have his family and friends present as well as a reasonable portion of the public.[161]

---

[156]United States v. Kobli, 172 F.2d 919, 922 (3d Cir. 1949); People v. Buck, 46 Cal. App. 2d 558, 561-62, 116 P.2d 160, 162-63 (1941).

[157]United States v. Kobli, 172 F.2d 919, 922 (3d Cir. 1949); State v. Adams, 100 S.C. 43, 84 S.E. 368 (1915).

[158]See I. T. COOLEY. CONSTITUTIONAL LIMITATIONS 647 (8th ed. W Carrington 1927). State v. Holm, 67 Wyo. 360, 382-95, 224 P.2d 500, 508-13 (1950).

[159]United States v. Kobli, 172 F.2d 919, 923 (3d Cir. 1949). Relevant state statutes are collected in 6 WIGMORE. § 1835 n.2 (Supp. 1964).

[160]The audience is excluded not so much to protect the child but to enable her to testify without reservation. See State v. Callahan, 100 Minn. 63, 110 N.W. 342 (1907); Grimmett v. State, 22 Tex. Ct. App. R. 36, 2 S.W. 631 (1886). See also Hogan v. State, 191 Ark. 437, 86 S.W.2d 931 (1935); State v. Damm, 62 S.D. 123, 252 N.W. 7 (1933.)

[161]Beauchamp v. Cahill, 297 Ky. 505, 508, 180 S.W.2d 423, 424 (1944). Ordinarily, courts have required that the exclusion should expressly exempt counsel, representatives of the press, family, and friends of the accused.

Even the need for the presence of "a reasonable portion of the public" may be questioned in cases of child molestation. Insofar as the framers of the Constitution sought to avoid the risks of seventeenth century secret trials, [162] their aim for all practical purposes has been achieved. At the time of the Star Chamber, the accused needed, but was denied, a way to communicate with someone from his community. In the age of all-pervasive mass communication media, however, many criminal defendants and especially those charges with child molestation actually fear the hostile and relentless glare of publicity, and most of them probably do not even wish their friends and acquaintances to be informed of the charges.[163]

The argument that the actual presence of "the public" acts as a check on the judge, the jury, the prosecutor, and the witnesses seems also to have lost much of its force in modern times. In earlier times "all the town came to the courtroom to gaze at the proceedings."[164] Today, in most places, the observers consist mainly of the accused's family, young people who are truant from school, a few unemployed or retired persons, and occasionally a permanent court correspondent of the local newspaper or radio station.[165] The court, prosecutor, and the witnesses are more concerned with the possibility of there being one newspaperman in the audience than of the visible presence of a room full of other observers. The "public trial," as an institutional safeguard for obtaining a fair trial, cannot, therefore, be judged by the number of observers in the courtroom. Absent a realistic danger in a particular case that the denial of public access would injure the defendant, the Supreme Court might not forbid a reasonable limi-

---

[162]*See* I. J. STEPHEN, A HISTORY OF THE CRIMINAL LAW OF ENGLAND 350 (1883).

[163]Based on the author's impressions as prosecutor and defense counsel in Israel, and on visits to criminal courts in Illinois and California.

[164]Mueller, *supra* note 155, at 6.

[165]Fortunately, the press in the United States has adopted the practice of speaking under the self-imposed restriction of shielding from publicity and identification victims of rape and similar sex offenses, particularly children. There is no reason to suspect that this considerate self-restraint would not be extended to victims and witnesses in trials held in Child-Courtrooms, whether the purpose of the press report be to give a straight account of the trial or to inform the public of deficiencies or irregularities which should be brought to their attention as citizens.

tation upon access to the trial. The federal courts approach the right to a public trial with flexibility, and both federal and state courts have qualified the right by considerations of administrative convenience and public morality. In this process of weighing conflicting interests and factors, the protection of child victims should carry much weight. Because the primary purpose for excluding the public other than friends and relatives of the accused and the press from a trial conducted in an ordinary courtroom is to give an embarrassed child witness an opportunity to testify in conditions which lessen the danger of injuring his future development, the exclusion period is likely to be relatively short.[166]

CONCLUSIONS—The conducting of trials in the Child-Courtroom is only the first step proposed here for the protection of child victims. It should be regarded as the bare minimum which can be done for children without radically tampering with traditional criminal procedure and constitutional rights. It is a step forward in the sense that it is aimed at reducing the dangers of injury to the child inherent in his personal confrontation with the accused in the presence of the jury and audience in the formal atmosphere of a courtroom. Adding the innovation of the proceedings in the Child-Courtroom to the previous special care taken by a child examiner for the child victim and his parents may increase parents' trust in the state's ability to handle the problems of child victims, and should serve to safeguard child victims' future mental development far better than present practices. Yet some of the radical questions regarding the well-being of child victims remain unanswered. Should the child's appearance in the Child-Courtroom be one more repetition in a series of police interrogations and preliminary hearings? Should the criminal justice system wait for the trial itself in order to take the evidence of the child victim? After a brief examination of the constitutional

---

[166]Rarely is there eyewitness testimony in cases of child molestation. If there is such an eyewitness, I do not think his public evidence is likely to be as embarrassing to the child as his own testimony before an audience. Thus, I would not exclude the public as a matter of routine from this portion of the trial, but leave it to the discretion of the judge.

and evidentiary problems, a second proposal will be presented which attempts to deal with these questions.

The Extent of Flexibility in the Constitutional Safeguard of Confrontation

The major reason underlying the constitutional confrontation rule is to give the defendant charged with a crime an effective opportunity to cross-examine the witness against him through counsel.[167] Part of this effective cross-examination is the opportunity to compel the witness "to stand face to face with the jury in order that they may look at him, and judge by his demeanor upon the stand and manner in which he gives his testimony, whether he is worthy of belief."[168] To students of the child victim's in-court dilemma, the confrontation clause appears at first blush to bar in the United States an experiment to adopt a solution based on the opinion of child experts that it is better for a child victim and his family to repress the memories of the sexual offense as soon as is naturally possible, even before the criminal trial. This result is sometimes achieved accidentally in the United States, such as when the defense counsel makes no objection at trial to admitting a transcript of the child victim's testimony during a preliminary hearing,[169] or when the child witness is "unavailable" at the time of the trial through no fault of the state.[170] In such cases, as well as in cases in which the accused pleads guilty, the child is not bound to testify at the trial. But even in these cases the child victim may be waiting for "his day" in court until the day of the trial, not having any advance notice whether or not his testimony will be necessary. What is needed is a regular procedure whereby the child victims would be allowed to testify before the trial without violating the accused's right to confrontation.

The constitutionality of admitting the child's pretrial testimony as evidence at trial depends to a large extent on whether the

---

[167]*See* Pointer v. Texas, 380 U.S. 400, 406-07 (1965).

[168]Mattox v. United States, 156 U.S. 237, 242-43 (1895).

[169]*See, e.g.,* People v. Foster, 67 Cal.2d 604, 432 P.2d 976, 63 Cal. Rptr. 288 (1967). The victim was cross-examined at the preliminary hearing by defense counsel. *See also* People v. Stenchever, 249 Cal.App.2d 74, 57 Cal.Rptr. 207 (1967).

Supreme Court interprets the confrontation clause in a rigid or a flexible way. Although the Court has not yet fully articulated the federal standards required by the confrontation clause in various kinds of factual situations, the decisions indicate that the court has applied and will continue to apply the clause flexibly.

On two recent occasions, the Court has made it clear that considerations of greater speed, economy, and convenience in the administration of the law are not sufficiently important justifications for infringing the right to confrontation.[171] Where a witness, for example, is absent from the trial due to the inconvenience or expense which might be incurred in securing his appearance, either by himself or the prosecution, the witness cannot be considered "absent" or actually "unavailable."[172] Unless the prosecution can show that it has made every reasonable effort to produce the witness, the confrontation clause will be violated, even though the defendant had the opportunity to cross-examine the witness at a previous judicial proceeding.[173]

Similarly, the economic benefit and speed of joint trials will not justify violating the confrontation rights of one defendant by admitting into evidence the extra-judicial confession of a codefendant, despite an instruction to the jury that the confession bears on the guilt of the confessor only.[174]

However, where a witness is dead, seriously ill, insane, or there is a reasonable threat of danger to the life or health of an informer, and thus unavailability exists for reasons other than inconveni-

---

[170]*See, e.g.,* State v. Reynolds, 7 Ariz. App. 48, 438 P.2d 142 (1968).

[171]Bruton v. United States, 391 U.S. 123 (1968); Barber v. Page, 390 U.S. 719 (1968).

[172]*E.g.,* Holman v. Washington, 364 F.2d 613, 623 (5th Cir. 1966). The rule has been long settled that a living person may be "unavailable" at the time of the trial only in cases of insanity, illness, absence from the jurisdiction, or because he was kept away by the connivance of the other party. *See, e.g.,* West v. Louisiana, 194 U.S. 258, 263-64 (1904); Motes v. United States, 178 U.S. 458, 470-74 (1900). *See also* Comment, *Hearsay Under the Proposed Federal Rules: A Discretionary Approach,* 15 WAYNE L. REV. 1079-1101 (1969).

[173]Barber v. Page, 390 U.S. 719 (1968); Virgin Islands v. Aquino, 378 F.2d 541, 551-552 (3d Cir. 1967); State v. Weinrib, 140 Conn. 247, 250-251, 99 A.2d 145, 147 (1953).

[174]Bruton v. United States, 391 U.S. 123 (1968); *see* Note, *Admissibility of Codefendant's Admissions in Joint Criminal Trials,* 36 U. CIN. L. REV. 306 (1967); *cf.* Delli Paoli v. United States, 352 U.S. 232 (1957) (sufficiency of the instruction).

ence or expense, the Supreme Court allows the states greater leeway in introducing hearsay testimony against the accused, relaxing the confrontation requirement.[175]

In *Pointer v. Texas*[176] the Supreme Court reaffirmed the use of dying declarations as an exception to the right of confrontation. However, the temporary illness or inability of the witness to attend the trial is insufficient unavailability and the trial must be postponed.[177] Nevertheless, where the witness' condition, mentally or physically, is such that it is probable that he will be unable to testify, the witness is considered unavailable and his prior cross-examined testimony is admissible.[178] While the unavailability of the insane person is due to his incompetency to testify, serious illness is recognized as sufficient unavailability because the interest in the prospective witness' health overrides his duty to testify. Even the personal safety of an informer may cause sufficient unavailability provided the protection does not become a gross denial of the right to cross-examine.[179]

Thus, in certain circumstances the Supreme Court has not demanded rigid confrontation rights for the accused. In weighing the protection of the confrontation principal against another interest deserving protection, the Court's reluctance to allow an exception to rigid confrontation standards varies inversely with the protection offered the accused as a substitute for the lack of confrontation. Using as a yardstick the Court's attitude towards dying declarations, the unavailable witness, and their concern for the well-being of the child, a sound proposal which seeks to protect child victims without diluting the accused's rights shall now be advanced.

---

[175]*See* cases cited at note 172 *supra*.

[176]380 U.S. 400 (1965).

[177]Smith v. United States, 106 F.2d 726 (4th Cir. 1939); 5 Wigmore § 1406.

[178]Marler v. State, 67 Ala. 55 (1880); Williams v. State, 156 Ark. 205, 246 S.W. 503 (1922); Tanner v. State, 213 Ga. 820, 102 S.E.2d 176 (1958); State v. Wheat, III La. 860, 882-83, 35 So. 955, 963-64 (1903); Spencer v. State, 132 Wis. 509, 112 N.W. 462 (1907). *Contra* Commonwealth v. McKenna, 158 Mass. 207, 33 N.E. 389 (1893).

[179]Smith v. Illinois, 390 U.S. 129 (1968).

Proposal II: *A Special Hearing for the Child Victim*

The purpose of this proposal is to take the child victim's testimony in the Child-Courtroom after the accused has been apprehended and before the trial itself has begun, so that the child may testify and forget the offense as soon as possible. While the first proposal deals with the hearing of the child's evidence as part of the trial, this proposal sets out a practice of taking child victims' evidence prior to the trial, while protecting the accused's right to confrontation.

To satisfy the standard of effective cross-examination, the Special Hearing should not be confused with an ordinary preliminary examination, since the cross-examination at a preliminary hearing is usually narrowly confined, and the defense commonly conducts little or no cross-examination.[180]

Mr. Justice Marshall has pointed out that: "A preliminary hearing is ordinarily a much less searching exploration into the merits of a case than a trial, simply because its function is the more limiting one of determining whether probable cause exists to hold the accused for trial."[181] The increased attention recently given by the Supreme Court and lower federal courts to the distinction between the preliminary hearing and the trial, in the context of effective confrontation, has not yet brought any substantial change in the Supreme Court's policy concerning the introduction of transcripts of preliminary hearings at the trial where the witness is shown to be "actually unavailable" and the accused had a meaningful opportunity to cross-examine. But since the admissibility of prior testimony is justified on the condition, among others, that "the right of cross-examination initially afforded, provides substantial compliance with the purposes behind the confrontation requirement,"[182] it is likely that the Court will insist that any arrangement for cross-examination before trial may not fall short of effective confrontation.[183] Accordingly, the accused's counsel should not only be informed of the

---

[180]Virgin Islands v. Aquino, 378 F.2d 541, 549 (3d Cir. 1967).
[181]Barber v. Page, 390 U.S. 719, 725 (1968).
[182]*Id.* at 722.
[183]*See* People v. Gibbs, 255 Cal. App.2d 739, 63 Cal. Rptr. 471 (1967).

charge against the client, but should be given a transcript of the child's story as told by him to the child examiner before the Special Hearing. In addition, a copy of any other relevant evidence already in the possession of the prosecution or the police should be submitted to the defense counsel within a reasonable time before the convening of the Special Hearing.[184] Since the function of a Special Hearing, whether conducted as part of the preliminary hearing or not, is to take the child's testimony for submission as evidence at trial, the arguments for limiting cross-examination at a pretrial hearing will not have any force. Despite the opportunity for full cross-examination at the Special Hearing, however, a defendant many still legitimately complain that, had the child been present at the trial, his counsel could have cross-examined him in the light of recently discovered facts or witnesses, or new court decisions.[185] Such cases are likely to be rare, since once the child's evidence has been taken, there will usually be no reason to delay the trial itself[186] but a complaint that the accused has been denied effective cross-examination at the Special Hearing can be heard on motion before the trial judge. Whenever the judge has reason to believe that he could have conducted a more searching exploration into the child's credibility if post-hearing developments had been known to counsel, he may give special permission to conduct additional cross-examination of the child at the trial. Before granting such permission, the judge should be required to obtain an opinion from a child examiner on the effects the additional cross-examination may have on the child victim. By analogy to the procedure suggested in the concurring opinion in *Smith v. Illinois*[187] concerning informers, the trial judge would then ascertain the interest of

---

[184]The side effect of this proposal, therefore, is allowing full "discovery" for the defense in such criminal cases. Very little discovery is now permitted in the United States. *See* Traynor, *Ground Lost and Found in Criminal Discovery*, 39 N.Y.U.L. REV. 228 (1964).

[185]*Cf.* Holman v. Washington, 364 F.2d 618, 624 & n. 11 (5th Cir. 1966).

[186]After the Special Hearing, with the child's evidence before him, the prosecutor is likely to drop charges not likely to be proven, and the defense may plead guilty to accusations stated in a "clear and convincing" manner by the child. The Special Hearing is of particular significance for those cases where the child examiners urge a quick hearing to protect the child's well-being.

[187]390 U.S. 129 (1968).

the defendant in the answer and exercise an informed discretion in making his ruling.

To summarize, the accused should be given an adequate opportunity to cross-examine the child witness through counsel in the Special Hearing, and his counsel should be allowed sufficient time to prepare his cross-examination of this major witness whose testimony is ultimately to be used at the trial itself. To shorten the time for counsel's pretrial investigations and to give him a fair opportunity to cross-examine the child, the defendant's attorney should have access to all the evidence in the prosecution file, and in particular, he must be acquainted with the "child's recordings."[188]

A significant advantage of holding the special hearing in the Child-Courtroom is that a confrontation between the accused and the child can be had without the accused, the jury, and the public being seen by the child. Another technical advantage is that the child's evidence can be recorded on video-tape without interference with the normal proceedings in the "judge's room." All the technical devices are there, and they are hardly noticeable to a child. By taking the child's evidence in the Child-Courtroom prior to the trial, the jury and the public are excluded from this hearing. In a sense, the child's testimony in the Special Hearing can be likened to a dying declaration; it is evidence given in the absence of the trier of fact and the public which is nevertheless admitted in evidence at the trial as an exception to the hearsay rule. But while in the case of a dying declaration, the trier of fact has no opportunity to observe the declarant while he makes his declarations and the defense counsel has no opportunity to cross-examine the declarant, taking the child victim's testimony at the Special Hearing involves neither of these important shortcomings. The proposed situation is really more closely analogous to the use of evidence given at a former trial which may be admitted in a second trial of the same accused on the same charge under certain conditions. Even there, the jury cannot observe the witness' demeanor by video-tape. The two purposes of confrontation—effective cross-examination before the jury, and ob-

---

[188]The discovery of privileged matters is not within the scope of this article.

servation of the witness' demeanor by the jury—are achieved by means of video-tape. The case for admitting at the trial prior testimony taken in the new Special Hearing appears to be stronger than the case for admitting the written transcript of the testimony given in a prior trial. Therefore, it seems most unlikely that the Supreme Court would not accommodate the Special Hearing procedure into the confrontation clause. The Court still may be reluctant to dispense with the requirement of a public hearing which is present in the case of testimony given at a prior trial, especially since the public is invisible so far as the child is concerned.

Even after overcoming the constitutional difficulty of confrontation, trial courts may still entertain objections to admitting video-tape evidence at the trial based on the rule against hearsay. The answer to such objections is found in the conditions attached to the admissibility of the child victim's video-taped evidence: an opportunity for cross-examination was afforded to the accused, and the tape gives the trier of fact an adequate opportunity to observe the child's demeanor during his testimony and cross-examination.

Prior recorded testimony is admissible as an exception to the hearsay rule that, as in all hearsay exceptions, there is a necessity for the testimony and circumstantial guarantee of its trustworthiness. Specifically, the following conditions must be met: (1) the proceedings in the subsequent trial must be between the same parties; (2) essentially the same issues must be involved; (3) the party against whom the evidence is offered must have had a full opportunity to cross-examine the witness at the former occasion; (4) the witness must be unavailable to testify at the second proceeding so as to necessitate admission of the prior recorded testimony.

The Special Hearing not only meets these conditions, but by video-taping the testimony, even adds the element of demeanor evidence. As to the unavailability of the child victim to testify, a state statute may declare child victims to be unavailable witnesses for purposes of the trial unless a trial judge, in the specific case before him, rules otherwise. An alternative is to leave the question of each child victim's unavailability for trial to the discretion of a judge, who would determine the question prior to the use of the Special Hearing procedure, on the basis of expert evidence heard by him on motion.

A special hearing in the Child-Courtroom may reduce both the number of examinations for each child witness and may reduce the time during which he is expected to remember the details of the offense. In addition, conducting the Special Hearing in the Child-Courtroom should lend a relaxed and informal atmosphere to the proceedings which, insofar as the child victim is concerned, are conducted in the presence of only four persons: the judge, the prosecutor, the defense counsel, and the child examiner

The foregoing demonstrates that a genuine interest in the child victim's mental health may result in greater care and concern for him without significant dilution of the accused's constitutional rights. The Supreme Court will not permit rights traditionally considered fundamental to the American concept of fair trial to be violated. On the other hand, the fundamental right of a child to be protected against injurious state actions must also be respected. The proposals that a Child-Courtroom in the proper surroundings and atmosphere for the hearing of a child's evidence be established and that a Special Hearing be conducted, seek to advance the proposition so well stated by Justice Cardozo:

> But justice, though due to the accused, is due to the accuser also. The concept of fairness must not be strained till it is narrowed to a filament. We are to keep the balance true.[189]

---

[189]Snyder v. Massachusetts, 291 U.S. 97, 122 (1934).

Chapter 17

SPECIAL TECHNIQUES FOR CHILD
WITNESSES*

Doris Stevens and Lucy Berliner

I n recent years there has been much publicity about the ordeal
of prosecution for the rape victim. Many states have initiated
programs to address victims' rights, but it is too early to tell how
victim advocate programs and related legislation will affect the
rate of prosecution of rape and other sexual assault offenses.

It is not widely known that a significant number of sexual
assault victims are children. National statistics on the incidence
of sexual abuse of children are not kept. Many local jurisdictions
do not have systems for gathering such information either.
Incidents of child sexual abuse currently being brought to the
attention of police agencies are probably only the most unusual
or severely abusive cases. The number of child sexual assault
victims referred to the Sexual Assault Center for medical or
counseling services has been increasing steadily since 1973.
During the past year, over 25% of cases referred to SAC were
victims age 14 and under. Thirteen percent of our total cases were
age nine or younger. Twenty-one percent were sexually assaulted
by members of their immediate family. The majority of child
victims we serve are molested by an offender who is known to the
child (61%). Although child molesters are usually not violent in
the sense that forcible rapists are, child victims are usually
confused and frightened as a result of the abuse, and sometimes
physically injured as well. It has been our experience that child
molesting is often a compulsive behavior; therefore, if the

---

*From *Response*, December 1976.

offender is not prosecuted for his crime, a series of children will undoubtedly be exposed to his abuse.

If child molesters are prosecuted, child victims must endure the same processes as adult victims do, without benefit of special procedures or protection. This fact contrasts with the differential treatment which our society provides to minors in other areas of the criminal justice system. The United States was the first society in the world to establish separate criminal justice system procedures for juvenile offenders, based on the belief that children have experiences, capabilities, and vulnerabilities that are significantly different from adults. However, our society has not subscribed to protecting *all* children involved in criminal proceedings—only juvenile *offenders*. If a child is *witness* to a crime committed by an adult, that child is drawn into the adult criminal justice system procedures, where there is usually little allowance made for the child's limited ability to compete within an adult system. Two negative effects can result: (1) child victims and their families report being further traumatized by investigation and court procedures; and (2) prosecutions of child molesters are unsuccessful because the crimes are either not reported initially or the child witness is not able to convey the information necessary to corroborate the sexual offense charge in court.

If our society believes that sexual molestation of children is a serious crime, then it seems that special techniques must be adopted within the criminal justice system which not only encourage cooperation of child witnesses, but at the same time acknowledge the inherent limitations on a child's performance.

Although procedures for filing charges of sexual abuse and trial preparation are somewhat different in each jurisdiction, there are some common basic requirements. We shall assume that most systems necessitate several separate interviews in which the child witness is asked to review details of the assault; these are usually conducted by the police department and prosecuting attorney's office. (In Seattle, there is a minimum of three basic interviews.) The child is expected to recount the incident—as well as events preceding and following—in vivid detail. The child is also expected to provide to a series of strange adults additional accurate information on dates, times, sequences, and a description of suspect and location. Usually it is not possible for a parent or advocate to be with the child during these interrogations. The child may be required to identify the offender by picture or line-up, and there may be a preliminary hearing, during which the child again recounts details of the sexual abuse. If the suspect does not plead guilty, there will be a trial in which the child will testify again and also be subject to cross-examination in an open courtroom while facing the accused. The above process takes place over many months. (An average time for adjudication of these cases in Seattle is six months.)

It is no wonder that many parents and mental health professionals fear that the effect of criminal proceedings on the child will be more emotionally traumatic than the assault itself. At the Sexual Assault Center, we have observed on numerous occasions the negative effects of a child's involvement in investigation and prosecution proceedings. It is our opinion that the problems inflicted on child sexual assault victims in the criminal justice system result from (a) an inadequate understanding of children and their capabilities by system personnel, and (b) misconceptions held by those same personnel about the nature of the crime of child molestation. Without basic knowledge in both areas, criminal justice system personnel are ill-equipped to elicit necessary information from the victim or maintain her cooperation and that of her family.[1] Since the victim is usually the only witness, she is the prosecution's most valuable resource, particularly because there is rarely any corroborating evidence. Increased reporting of sexual abuse of children and improved conviction rates depend on changing those aspects of the legal system which inhibit victim cooperation. This chapter will present some general information about child development and child molestation. With this information as background, we will also suggest some different strategies for accommodating the child witness in criminal justice system proceedings.

---

1. Since ninety-three percent of child victims served by the SAC have been girls, we will use the female pronoun for the sake of clarity.

It is generally accepted that normal child development progresses in sequential, overlapping phases of increasingly complex learning. The child masters skills at one level and moves on to the next stage. Physical, intellectual, and social growth occurs in this fashion. Although there are many different theories of child development, the major theoretical frameworks all recognize similar phases, beginning with infancy and continuing through early childhood, preschool-age, school-age, and adolescence. Some of the major skills which the child must acquire are social relationship skills, language, conceptual thinking, and the ability to interact with an increasingly more complex societal framework. It must be remembered that each child learns at a different rate and generalizations are never strictly applicable to any one child.

Knowledge of the basic principles of child development has immediate significance for law enforcement personnel in investigating sexual abuse cases. Obviously the child cannot be a witness unless she has acquired verbal skills. In the case of the pre-verbal child who has been molested, another witness or corroborating evidence would be necessary in pursuing prosecution. A child establishes verbal language as the primary mode of communication between the ages of two and four. Although the preschool child (ages four through six) can talk well, she does not understand concepts well and, therefore, her verbal skills may imply a better comprehension than actually exists. The preschool child does not understand metaphors, analogies, or irony; she can memorize, but without comprehension. The narrative account of a four-year-old child tends to be rambling and disjointed, containing both relevant and irrelevent details. Children in the preschool-age group engage in intuitive thought; they can accept connections between events but do not understand causality. The preschool child entertains one thought at a time and cannot conceive of multiple thoughts as an integrated whole. Although she can vividly recall isolated events, often triggered by association with a familiar sight or sound, the memory is usually spotty and lacking in continuity and organization. For the four to six year-old, concepts of time, space, and distance are usually personalized and not logical and orderly.

Emotionally, the preschooler is an outgoing, spontaneous child with few internalized limits. She can be stubborn, quarrelsome, and scatological. The child spends most of her time in play, particularly dramatic, acting-out play. Although fantasy becomes an important element in the child's repertoire, she can easily distinguish fact from fantasy. When lying occurs, it is usually the child's attempt to make something look better or extricate herself from a problem situation. Children in this age group are unable to practice real deception because they still invest adults with complete authority and believe that adults would perceive any lie. In addition, the child still depends totally on her family to meet all physical and emotional needs. She has an egocentric perception of the world with only tentative awareness of any relationships which do not involve her directly. It is apparent that the abilities of the preschool-age child fall far short of the traditional requirements which the legal system has for witness performance.

The school-age child (ages six through eleven) is better prepared to respond to the expectations of an interviewer. This child is beginning the gradual shift from total reliance on family to a peer culture. She is aware of herself in different roles—as student, child, peer. But she still depends on parents for refuge and support. Girls and boys tend to group together in same-sex bands with separate interests. A group loyalty develops as the child seeks recognition from the group, with its rituals, traditions, and rules. It is at this point that children begin to practice deception and guile around adults as they establish a sense of separateness. Although they may become sullen, insolent, and taciturn with adults, they seldom lie about major issues. This is particularly true when relating to issues of justice and equality. They are very sensitive to any apparent unfairness or differential application of justice. They are often rigid and harsh on each other and become legalistic nit pickers with adults. Intellectually, school-age children have increasing mastery of language and symbols, can locate themselves in time and space, and gradually move from absolutism to relativism. Thinking still remains concrete rather than abstract, but they are voracious learners who are rapidly developing all skills and are intensely interested in understanding how things work.

The crime of child molesting—its characteristics and emotional consequences—can be examined within the framework of normal child development. Sexual abuse of children rarely involves physical injury and is perpetrated primarily by adult males who are known to the child. The child may readily submit to the known authority figure because she has been taught to respect and obey adults; therefore, the use of violence by the offender is generally unnecessary. Sexual abuse of the pre-adolescent child usually does not include sexual intercourse but consists of fondling, oral-genital contact, or manual penetration of the child's vagina or anus. The offender may have offered the child a bribe of affection, gift, or money. Unlike forcible rape, which is a single dramatic attack, sexual abuse may begin insidiously, progress to greater intimacy, and continue over a long period of time. This is especially true in cases involving family members, the most common of which is father molesting daughter. When the assailant is a stranger, it is far easier for the child to overcome her fear of "telling on" an adult because she has usually been asked by parents to report unusual behavior by a stranger. In the case of an offender who is known by the child (often a close family friend or family member), the obstacles to telling are much greater. This is a situation for which the child is not prepared; she is unclear about whether or not the act is wrong, and whether or not the people to whom she reports will believe her. If she has ambivalent feelings toward the molester, she may not want to cause trouble for him. If the adult molester denies the allegations, the child may be disbelieved and her tales of abuse characterized as "vivid imagination."

The specific emotional consequences of sexual abuse cannot presently be predicted, but the intensity of distress reported by child victims generally correlates with the reaction of the parents and authorities who become involved (doctor, counselor, policemen, attorneys). When the assault is nonviolent and occurs only once, it is clearly less traumatizing than the extremely violent or longer-term situation. If the child is not believed or is accused of provoking the incident(s), she will acquire additional negative feelings about herself. Too often parents who *do* believe their child's account can still be ignorant about the dynamics of child molesting; they may increase problems for their child by over-reacting and treating the child as if she has changed. The child often interprets this as blame. Even when the parent responds in a calm, appropriately supportive, believing manner, the activities of the criminal justice system will usually exacerbate the child's distress. Perceptual discussion of the sexual assault in repeated interviews over many months discourages rapid resolution of the assault-related trauma for both child and parents. The criminal justice system must address the conflict that exists between a child victim's emotional needs following a sexual assault and the requirements for prosecution of the case.

The first major issue in pursuing a sexual assault case is establishing the credibility of the child witness. Adults are extremely reluctant to believe a child over an adult, as all children well know. Popular mythology dictates that children often fabricate tales of sexual assault despite a lack of any research to substantiate this belief. Thus it is incumbent on the investigator, police, or prosecutor to dismiss such misconceptions and evalu-ate each case on its individual merits. Unfortunately, this task is usually made difficult because of the absence of corroborating evidence. Often the investigator must rely entirely on evaluation of the child's testimony. The inherent reluctance of a child to challenge adult authority and the possibility of retaliation which the child may be risking should be kept in mind when beginning an investigation. There are criteria which can be used to assess a child's statement. The words the child uses, the acts she describes, and the degree to which she is able to recount the event to a stranger can all be measured against characteristics of that child's developmental stage. If the overall adjustment of the child to family, school, and peers is satisfactory, it is highly unlikely that she would be deviant in one area of her personality development (i.e., producing an elaborate fabrication of sexual abuse).

There are many useful strategies for improving the investiga-tion of this crime by applying knowledge of children's behavior to the investigative procedure. Many of the following suggestions may seem obvious, but unfortunately these procedures have not been adopted in many jurisdictions. When the initial complaint is received, usual procedure is for the victim to be interviewed by a series of law enforcement personnel—uniformed officer, detective, and prosecutor—as well as by a doctor, and perhaps a counselor or Children's Protective Services worker. A child has a limited capacity to respond to repeated questioning, so in order to most effectively elicit information and maintain her cooperation, these various agencies might develop a coordinated approach. Joint interviewing could be established or preferably one person could be designated to take the victim statement. This should be done as soon as possible, following the assault because passage of time very significantly affects a child's ability to testify. The initial interview could be videotaped to afford the prosecuting attorney an opportunity to review her capability as a witness. One comprehensive statement should be adequate to file charges.

The setting of the interview and the manner in which it is conducted have significant bearing on the child's performance as a witness. The crowded, noisy, bare-walled precinct room or the formal attorney's office with a massive desk are not conducive to eliciting an easy flow of information from a child. She should be interviewed in a quiet, private room which allows the child some room for exploration. A child cannot comfortably sit still on a hard-backed chair for any length of time. Toys, books, crayons and drawing paper should be available to aid in occupying and relaxing the child so she can converse more easily. The younger child will need a parent or familiar person present to feel secure enough to talk during the interview, whereas the older child may be too embarrassed to talk freely if the parent is present. (Children generally develop a strong sense of modesty around the age of six or seven.)

The interviewer can alleviate the child's anxiety by establishing a personal rapport with the child. The interviewer should be relaxed and casual, and preferably not in uniform. Communication can be established by inquiring about the child's interests, family and friends, pets, school, and neighborhood, and by allowing her in turn to ask questions of the interviewer. A simple explanation of the function of the interviewer and the agency (police, prosecutor) will help the child understand and therefore cooperate with the proceedings. The language and the number and kind of questions used are the crucial aspects of the interview. Although it seems obvious that the level of language employed by the interviewer should apply to the child's level of comprehension, this rarely occurs. Attorneys are by far the worst offenders in this area. Children in the legal system are regularly subjected to legal jargon and terminology that even their parents do not comprehend. Much of the concern about credibility stems from the confusion which results when the child does not understand the question and therefore answers incorrectly or incompletely. Because the attention span of children is shorter than that of adults, the interviewer should carefully choose questions that elicit the most information. It is a waste of time to ask questions which the victim cannot answer. For example, a four-year-old who does not yet perceive time in a logical, sequential order need not be asked about dates and times of the abuse. Too often the interviewer is limited by his own fixed approach to investigation and does not adapt to the child's situation. The child may become frustrated and directly or indirectly refuse to discuss the incident further. The situation then arises where criminal justice system personnel, parents, or mental health professionals decide the child is not a credible witness or that she cannot "handle" the prosecution processes.

Time is an important element of the entire process. There is often a long delay between each subsequent step which can seriously limit a child's ability to testify. Whenever possible, the proceedings should be accelerated. A child's memory quickly blurs so that although she can remember the molesting incident, other details may become indistinct. It is usual in this jurisdiction for four to six months to elapse between reporting of the crime and a trial date. Even an adult has difficulty remembering accurately after this much elapsed time. In addition, children are often expected to sit for lengthy interviews on different occasions or to wait for several hours before testifying. This can damage the testimony also because of the child's limited capacity to wait.

Court appearances (preliminary hearing, grand jury hearing, or trial) are the most difficult encounter for the child witness. The courtroom is unfamiliar and intimidating to even the most secure adult. Astonishing as it may seem, children are generally required to testify while sitting alone on the witness stand; the child must speak into a microphone while facing the alleged assailant in an open courtroom which may be filled with spectators. Questioning may go on for hours with the child expected to sit quietly and respond without benefit of explanation or clarification. The prosecutor who initially interviewed the child may not handle the case for trial and usually additional interviews are conducted prior to trial. Even prosecutors who have managed to establish a rapport with the child find it impossible to transfer it to the trial setting because, once in the courtroom, they seem compelled to revert to legal terminology. When crossexamination occurs, it is usually unsympathetic despite the victim's youth, since the offender's attorney defends his client with the usual tactic of attacking the credibility of the victim. Prosecutors are often reluctant to object for fear of appearing too protective of the witness; judges hesitate to interject for fear of swaying the jury. Thus the child is abandoned to a set of abstract beliefs in justice, and we can ask if justice is indeed being carried out without the complete participation of the witness. One possible model to address this problem is assigning a legal representative to advocate for each child appearing as the victim/witness in a criminal matter. This person would be appropriately qualified with knowledge of child development and the law and could speak out in court when the questioning became inappropriate to the child's age, level of comprehension, or emotional state. The child victim advocate role would not interfere with the proceedings or abrogate the rights of the defendant.

Including the child's family throughout the process can provide a valuable aid to the child and to the criminal justice system in pursuing prosecution. It has been our experience that parents of the child victim are usually not informed of steps in the prosecution; yet at the same time, they are expected to cooperate fully with the investigation. Parents are asked to wait patiently while their child is interviewed. They pay for medical exams to obtain medicolegal evidence, arrange to take their child out of school, rearrange their own schedules for various interviews, and pay for parking, mileage, and babysitting costs. Throughout this lengthy, inconvenient process, parents are often not given opportunity to express their concerns regarding their child's involvement in the process. The parent who wishes to strongly pursue prosecution of the offender and is assertive about seeking information is labeled "too eager," and the reluctant parent is accused of obstructing justice. When parents are informed and educated realistically about the various proceedings, they can be invaluable in building a case. Their cooperation can be enlisted by treating them respectfully and involving them in decisions, consulting with them about their child, answering their inquiries, and patiently allaying their fears. We feel the opinion of the family should be gathered when the child victim cannot be involved (such as in making sentencing recommendations). Many parents find the experience with the criminal justice system so unpleasant that they vow never to report another crime. Families should be encouraged to participate not only when their own child is involved but as responsible citizens who believe the system can work.

In spite of the fact that the community at large is outraged by the crime of child molesting, the legal system has failed to develop mechanisms which support and encourage successful prosecution when the victim witness is a child. If criminal prosecution is the avenue society chooses to deal with this important problem, then there is an obligation to adjust the requirements of the legal system to conform to the special needs and abilities of children. These changes would clearly necessitate specialized training for all official figures involved with the investigation, as well as development of new and flexible procedures. Legislation should be explored to provide the legal foundation for special protection of the child witness.

Chapter 18

COURTROOM USE OF HOSPITAL RECORDS IN SEXUAL ASSAULT CASES*

ANN W. BURGESS AND ANNA T. LASZLO

Some victims of sexual assault whom nurses see in hospital emergency rooms may well become criminal court cases. There, the victim's hospital record, with or without testimony from the hospital staff who treated the victim, will become important and may be used to corroborate or weaken the victim's claim of rape or other sexual assault. The importance of care and precision in writing such records is obvious when one sees how both prosecutor and defense counsel use them.

Over a three-year period, we and other staff members of the Boston-based Victim Counseling Program have counseled over 500 victims of sexual assault. We have seen victims who were treated at the Boston City Hospital or were referred by the Boston Police Department and the Suffolk County District Attorney's Office. We also have accompanied through trial those victims who entered the legal process. The examples of courtroom dialogue included here are based on notes taken during some of those hearings or trials.

Recent judicial decisions have increased the importance of physical evidence in criminal prosecution. Physical evidence (also called trace evidence) is any fragment, particle, or remnant of any substance that can be examined microscopically or chemically to corroborate a crime. In cases of rape and sexual assault, physical evidence is of particular significance.

In some jurisdictions the victim's testimony must be backed by corroborative evidence. Although the corroboration requirement has been eliminated in a number of jurisdictions, juries have been reluctant to convict merely on the testimony of the complaining witness, and, in states which still require corroboration, the extent of that evidence has continued to be a point of debate(1).

The United States Court of Appeals of the District of Columbia affirmed the following opinion on corroborative circumstances:

> Among the "circumstances" we deemed corroborative are the following: (1) medical evidence and testimony; (2) evidence of breaking and entering the prosecutrix' apartment; (3) condition of clothing; (4) bruises and scratches; (5) emotional condition of the prosecutrix; (6) opportunity of the accused; (7) conduct of the accused at the time of arrest; (8) presence of blood or semen on the clothing of the prosecutrix and the accused; (9) promptness of complaints to the police; (10) lack of motive to falsify.(2)

The court's opinion, particularly its emphasis on medical evidence and testimony, has significant implications for the health care professional who sees the victim either immediately after the assault or at a later date. As prosecutors have noted, "Medical records haven't always been taken properly. The symptoms of trauma have not been indicated, and if evidence is not gathered quickly and completely, prosecution is difficult"(3).

The specific definition of rape varies from one jurisdiction to another. Recent amendments to rape statutes have substituted "sexual intercourse or unnatural sexual intercourse with a person" for the phrase "carnal knowledge of a female," thus including the male victim. The essential elements of the crime, however, remain constant: (a) penetration, (b) use of force, (c) without the consent of the victim. The prosecution carries the burden of proof, "beyond a reasonable doubt," of all elements of the crime.

Records which most accurately present the victim's state and best meet the procedural requirements of criminal justice are precise recordings of facts regarding the signs and symptoms of physical and emotional trauma(4). It is these four areas which will be discussed here.

Signs of Physical Trauma

A complete physical assessment of a rape victim includes inspecting the whole body for abrasions, bruises, swelling, lacerations, or teeth marks. Special attention is given to arms, legs, face, neck, breasts, and the inner aspects of the thighs. Gynecological examination includes careful inspection of the vulva, perineum, hymenal ring, vagina, and rectum for tenderness, redness, swelling, bruises, and lacerations.

Evidence of trauma should be noted and the victim asked to recall scratches and bruises. In court, she will be asked to recount her injuries and although the "hearsay rule" excludes the admission of extrajudicial conversations, the exception is the complaint of physical pain made to a physician(5).

In the following case the victim testified that the defendant hit her several times with his clenched fist, although she could not remember the extent of her injury.

DEFENSE. Where did he hit you?
VICTIM. On the right side of my face.
DEFENSE. Where you hurt?
VICTIM. Yes, I was bleeding.
DEFENSE. Anything else?
VICTIM. I don't remember. I was told he broke my jaw. I was in shock.
DEFENSE. You say the defendant broke your jaw and you don't remember whether you were in pain or not?

Upon reexamination, the district attorney read, at great length, both the emergency room record and the orthopedic surgeon's record regarding the victim's jaw surgery. This factual report was corroborative evidence of the degree of injury sustained.

The prompt and careful collection and preservation of physical evidence are crucial and cannot be overemphasized. Whenever possible, black-and-white photographs should be taken of the victim (with the victim's permission). We have observed that they provide strong corroboration. Color exposures are inadmissible in court, here, as they have been rule "sensational."

For example, photographs were effective in the case of a 21-year-old victim of a gang rape. The prosecution presented the photographs of the victim, showing multiple bruises and lacerations. "Gentlemen of the jury, I ask you to look at these photographs and ask yourselves, does a consenting woman look like this?" The jury convicted the defendants.

Laboratory evidence of physical trauma includes semen specimens, clothing, hair samples, and fingernail scrapings.

Semen specimens are obtained by using a swab on any suspicious stain on any part of the body such as abdomen or thighs. A swab is taken from the orifice which was penetrated; that is, the vagina, the mouth, or the rectum. A wet smear of the specimen, preferably with a drop of saline solution, is then examined for the presence of sperm.

If sperm are present, the examiner notes the quantity (rare, moderate, or numerous) and the presence or absence of motility. It is important to know that the absence of sperm does not rule out the possibility of recent intercourse, since the assailant may be oligospermic or aspermic or may have used a condom.

Testing the vaginal pool specimen for acid phosphates may be useful in indicating the time interval since the assault. A significant prostatic acid phosphate level is indicative of prostatic secretions and, although the level may decrease rapidly, it could remain positive for up to 18 hours(6). If the laboratory examination is going to be delayed, the acid phosphatase specimen should be frozen immediately. The Wood's light, which when passed over skin or clothing reflects semen stain, also may be used.

If the laboratory test is negative for sperm, the victim's statement on whether or not she bathed or douched prior to the examination and whether or not the assailant ejaculated should be included. In one case the physician accurately recorded that he saw no sperm on the slide. In court, the defense counsel used this fact in an effort to discredit the testimony of the victim.

DEFENSE. Do you know the word "ejaculation?"
VICTIM. Yes.
DEFENSE. Did he ejaculate?
VICTIM. Yes.
DEFENSE. Did you wash yourself off or remove any such substance?
VICTIM. No.
DEFENSE. Did you go to the bathroom?
VICTIM. No, they wouldn't let me.
DEFENSE. Did you bring all this to the attention of the authorities at the hospital?

VICTIM. Yes.
DEFENSE. Then how come the medical record says "no sperm?"
VICTIM. I don't care what the medical record says. He had intercourse with me.

Evidence of tears, stains, or soil marks on the victim's clothing are usually indicative of struggle and as many pieces of the clothing as possible should be given to the police for acid phosphate analysis. A change of clothing should be requested for the victim when notifying family or friends of the victim's admission to the emergency room. In all cases, the record should indicate what pieces of clothing were given to the police.

Broken fingernails also indicate some type of struggle and should be noted as should dirt under the fingernails, especially if the victim states that the assault occurred outdoors. Furthermore, skin scraping, removed from underneath the nails, may be analyzed at the police laboratories for evidence of struggle.

Loose hairs that adhere to the patient's body or clothing can become evidence and should be collected. Pubic hair combings are particularly important in the gathering of evidence. If possible, the victim may be given a comb and an envelope and instructed to comb her pubic hair and then place the comb in the envelope. The victim also is instructed to enclose a control sample of her hair. This sealed, properly labeled envelope can be given to the police officer.

In the case of a 12-year-old, pre-pubertal girl, pubic hair combings revealed three foreign hairs. The analysis, done at the police laboratory, typed the hairs as characteristic of a male of a different race. The prosecution introduced the evidence, which was contained in a sealed vial.

PROSECUTION. For the record, Commonwealth's Exhibit #1.
DEFENSE. Objection. There is no indication that these were taken from the victim at the time of the alleged assault.
PROSECUTION. Your honor, may the record show (reading from the hospital record) "Pubic hair samples sealed and given to the police investigator."

The prosecutor presented the record to the judge, who then admitted the evidence. However, under rigorous cross-examination, the defense counsel established that nine months had elapsed between the assault and analysis and thus raised the issue of possible disintegration of the hair. The defense counsel also established that "hair can be characterized but cannot be used as a positive identification of a person; that is, pubic hair is not analogous to the fingerprint." The defense counsel also successfully prevented a pubic hair sample being taken from the defendant for comparison.

All pieces of physical evidence should be accurately labeled and their disposition and time of disposition noted on the record. At trial, the "chain of custody" is an issue with respect to the integrity of the evidence. The chain of custody is important in determining whether the evidence has been opened, tainted, or destroyed between the times of collection and introduction into evidence.

Symptoms of Physical Trauma

When recording symptoms of physical trauma, the patient's verbatim statement on the nature of the physical assault should be included. Especially important is the description of the types of sex acts demanded and actually carried out, and the order in which the demands were made.

The victim of rape may be confused and in a crisis state and may not relate the complete details of the assault. Therefore, the nurse or physician may have to ask the victim if oral, anal, or vaginal penetration occurred.

One victim stated that she told the physician that she had been "assaulted." "When he threatened to kill me, I didn't fight anymore. I thought if you didn't fight, you couldn't call it rape. That's why I told the physician I was assaulted." It was only after the physical examination that the victim was asked, "Were you more than assaulted?" Because the victim is under stress, the professional needs to word assessment questions carefully to obtain accurate facts.

In the following case, the hospital record indicated the size of the young girl's vaginal orifice but not the victim's statement on the nature of the assault. In the cross-examination, the defense counsel argued that intercourse had not occurred.

DEFENSE. Isn't it true you said you were a virgin?
VICTIM. Yes.
DEFENSE. Did it really go in?
VICTIM. Yes, for a short time.
DEFENSE. Did it hurt?
VICTIM. Yes.
DEFENSE. But isn't it true it did not penetrate you?
VICTIM. It did.
DEFENSE. Were you bruised, bleeding?
VICTIM. No.
DEFENSE. Did the defendant physically hurt you?. . . Isn't it true you were too tight down there to have sex, that he could not penetrate you?
PROSECUTION. Objection!
JUDGE. Overruled.

The defense counsel repeated the question. The victim did not answer. In his summation to the jury, the defense counsel made the following contention:

I would like to argue this is not a case of rape. The girl was standing up, not lying down. Her pants were only down to her knees and yet she claims penetration. It clearly shows on the medical record that there were no abrasions, tears, lacerations, bleeding. It states that the uterus was not felt as the introitus was too tight to allow entry of more than one finger. . . Now I state that if one finger could not get into her how could there be penetration?

The jury acquitted the defendant. A more complete hospital record would have included the victim's account of the specific facts as to the genital contact of the assailant, which is important to corroborate penetration. Penetration, the crucial element of rape, need not be complete, but merely the slightest penetration (2).

Signs of Emotional Trauma

Signs of emotional trauma include the victim's behavior during the interview. A precise description of any concrete signs—sobbing, tears, trembling, hyperventilation, and signs of extreme quiet or withdrawn behavior—should be recorded. A courtroom example is as follows:

PROSECUTION. What did you observe about the victim?
WITNESS. She seemed very upset and frightened.
PROSECUTION. Did she look pale to you?
WITNESS. Yes, very pale.

Symptoms of Emotional Trauma

The victim's statements about the assailants threats and method of force also are considered symptoms of emotional trauma. Note should be made especially if the assailant used a weapon, including his hands or fists or both. One victim, for example, described the circumstances of the assault in the following manner:

He came up behind me, I think on the left side. I didn't see him follow me at all; suddenly he was just there. He grabbed my arm and said, "I just got out of prison three days ago and I wouldn't hesitate to kill you." I didn't see a gun or knife, but he had my arm and I wasn't about to question the truth of what he said.

The assailant had not been in prison, but the fact that the victim believed him was sufficient threat of force(7).

In a series of four rapes that occurred within several hours, all the victims stated that, after the assault, the assailant said to them, "I'm sorry it had to be this way." The police were able to arrest a suspect after reviewing the fourth hospital record, which contained the same notation as the previous cases. Police are able to use hospital records in such a manner only if the facts are carefully noted and the verbatim statements of the victim and the assailant are recorded.

Figure 18-1

Patient Record: Assessment and Formulation

Assessment

APPEARANCE: 62-year-old woman dressed in bathrobe, sitting in wheelchair during interview.

VERBAL STYLE: Answered all questions in detail and volunteered additional material.

EMOTIONAL STYLE: Identified her feelings freely—which were fear for her life, being scared and upset.

CIRCUMSTANCES OF ASSAULT: Patient states that around 3:30 A.M. today, while sleeping, a man broke into her room and jumped on her. He tried to strangle her by putting his hands around her throat. He hit her several times in the face, breast and back.

DESCRIPTION OF ASSAILANT: Never saw assailant's face, as pillow was held over her face during attack. Voice was of a young man.

CONVERSATION: "If you scream, I'll kill you."

SEXUAL DETAILS (DEMANDED AND OBTAINED): Patient states man put penis in her mouth and after that forced her to have intercourse. States there was complete penetration and ejaculation.

THREATS (PHYSICAL AND VERBAL): Assailant hit her and threatened to kill her.

WEAPON: Very sharp knife. Patient thinks it was a hospital scalpel. Patient was "stabbed in my stomach."

Formulation: Signs and Symptoms of Physical and Emotional Trauma

SIGNS OF TRAUMA:

PHYSICAL: *ENT:* Multiple bruises in face, especially lower lip and right frontal area with areas of swelliing. Erythema and hypertrophy of tonsils. Bruises around neck were prominent in right side. *Breasts:* Small bruises either side. *Chest:* 2 cm lacerations. *Back:* Multiple bruises. Palpation of ribs on either side is painful.

GYNOCOLOGICAL: Small 1/2 inch superficial laceration in posterior fourchette of introitus. No bleeding in vagina. No signs of other injury. Perineum very red.

PHYSICAL EVIDENCE: CUSTODY: Police Lab
SEMEN SPECIMENS. Wet slide shows multiple motile spermatozoids.

CLOTHING: None available.

NAILS: None broken—scrapings taken and sent to police lab.

HAIR SAMPLES: Three samples—labeled and given to police.

PHOTOGRAPHS: None taken.   NUMBER OF EXPOSURES: —

SYMPTOMS OF PHYSICAL TRAUMA: "I couldn't breathe when he put the pillow over my head."

SIGNS OF EMOTIONAL TRAUMA: Face flushed; deep sighing as she talked; pushing hair back from her face; wringing her hands.

CLINICAL IMPRESSION: Acute physical and emotional reaction to rape trauma.

Opinions or subjective impressions are recorded routinely on hospital records, most commonly as diagnoses. The defense counsel frequently uses this type of data to discredit the victim or to attempt to establish that the victim's character is such as to have permitted consensual intercourse(8). Consider the following case in which the defense focused on the amount of alcohol the victim had consumed prior to the rape in an attempt to imply that since she had been drinking alcohol all day as well as immediately before the assault, she probably consented to sexual intercourse.

DEFENSE. You'd been drinking that evening?
VICTIM. I was not drinking straight liquor. It was beer.
DEFENSE. Isn't it true that has alcohol in it?
VICTIM. Yes, but it doesn't make me high.
DEFENSE. But isn't it true you are an alcoholic?
PROSECUTION. Objection
DEFENSE. (reading from the hospital record) "History of chronic alcoholism."
PROSECUTION. Objection! That shouldn't be allowed.
JUDGE. Strike that from the record.

Although the court record was cleared, it is doubtful that the jury was able to disregard the secondary diagnosis, recorded by the physician on the patient's record. This diagnosis was not obtained from the patient, but was recounted by emergency room staff, who knew the patient from previous admissions to the emergency floor. The court case resulted in a hung jury.

In the following case, a defense counsel used the hospital record to emphasize the victim's use of a previously prescribed medication to control anxiety. He contended that the victim was taking drugs.

DEFENSE. Isn't it true that you were taking drugs?
VICTIM. No.
PROSECUTION. Objection!
JUDGE. Sustained.
DEFENSE. Isn't it true you were taking drugs on the day of the alleged incident?
VICTIM. No.

DEFENSE. (reading from hospital record) A drug, Valium, prescribed in the past. . .

The jury's interpretation might well be that the victim, under medication, was confused and could not accurately remember the incidents of the assault.

We have observed that a record, thoroughly and precisely written, is one of the strongest supportive documents of corroborating evidence to the victim's physical and emotional state. The records should report exactly what was observed; that is, the facts. Accuracy is essential and opinions as well as such value words as "normal, satisfactory, negative," or "positive" should be avoided. The diagnosis is a subjective judgment; however, it usually is based on factual material which can be found in the record, for example, in the history and the results of tests and examinations.

At a trial, if there is any discrepancy between the victim's testimony and the hospital record, hearers will assume that the record is correct. The juries we have observed do not seem to take into consideration that perhaps the record was hurriedly written or that the nurse or physician was reporting opinions rather than facts. What is most important, any recording error is likely to be used to discredit the victim.

The record may be introduced into legal proceedings even when the professional does not testify. We have observed this procedure, again to the disadvantage of the victim, specifically with regard to illegible handwriting.

In one case, the defense counsel focused on a medical term which was recorded, saying, "I don't want to say it out loud." This increased everyone's curiosity. The prosecutor and the judge inspected the record. None could interpret accurately yet the defense continued to use the word as evidence. The interpretation of the word in question was "gonorrhea" when actually the term scrawled on the record was "amenorrhea."

In another case, the prosecutor, in his summation to the jury, stated:

The Commonwealth will offer, with the consent of the defense counsel, a copy of the medical record with regard to Mary J. Since the handwriting is so difficult to read, I will repeat to you what I read. However, if when you look at it, what you read is different, it is your reading that is binding. . . . (reads the record). If you make anything different from this writing than I do it is your decision, not what I recounted.

The importance of the patient record in the legal process cannot be overemphasized. Our experience and observations impress on us the need for health care professionals to be knowledgeable of the role they may assume as witnesses in legal proceedings. The patient's record should include a brief, but inclusive, account of the incident, with as many of the victim's own words as possible. In addition, data should be listed and the assessment section should include complete coverage of the four areas of signs and symptoms of physical and emotional trauma.

REFERENCES

1. United States v. Jenkins, 436 f.2d 140 (D.C.Cir., 1970); Wesley v. State, 225 GA. 22 1969; People v. Augustine, 35 App. Div. N.Y.S. 2d 440(1970); Bakken v. State, 485 P.2d. 120 (Alaska 1971).
2. Allison v. United States, 409 F.2d 445 (D.C. Cir., 1969).
3. McLaughlin, Walter: Address to Suffolk superior court jury. *Juris Doctor,* 4:26, Dec. 1974.
4. Burgess, A.W., and Holmstron, L.L.: *Rape: Victims of Crisis.* Bowie, Md., Robert J. Brady Co., 1974.
5. McCormick, Charles: *The Law of Evidence,* St. Paul, Minn., West Publishing Co., 1969.
6. Alleged rape: an invitational symposium. *J. Reprod Med:* 12:133-144ff, Apr. 1974.
7. Baldwin v. State, 207 N.W. 603 (1973): Brown v. State 207 N.W. 602 (1973).
8. Hibey, Richard. Consent, corroboration, and character: a defense of rape. *Am Criminal Law Rev.* 11:309-334, Winter 1973.

Section V

THE CHILD SEX INDUSTRY

"It really didn't bother me that much. I felt GOOD. I felt warm, and like, I felt loved in a way."

(Boy Sex Film Star describing his role in films.)
CBS-TV. *60 Minutes*, 1977.

Chapter 19

THE CHILD-SEX INDUSTRY — An Introduction
LeRoy G. Schultz

As indicated in the first chapter, adult sexual interest in children and minors has been historically with us a long time. The invention of photography and later the motion picture simply made a universal voyerism more democratically distributed. The instant picture (Polaroid®) guaranteed the visual realization of each man's fantasy in economical terms. Today's concern for child protection in pornography springs as much from technology (making, printing, distributing films and magazines) as it does from the time-honored interest in children as sexual objects. Some European cities report a new crime in which adults call children on the telephone telling the child to masturbate while the adult caller listens (1). Books, describing the rape and seduction of minors, designed as sexual stimulants were published and sold between 1780 and 1800. (2). Photographs of minors engaging in sexual acts with other minors, adults, and animals were sold in Europe by 1862 (3). Even in the world of the pederast, the capitalistic principle of supply and demand holds. Why this demand? Richard Corless described it best:

> it's the appeal—the sexual or aesthetic—of the potential, the budding, the almost ready. It's the attraction of the mind and body struggling against cellular decay for a mind and body that can only become brighter, fuller, more. It's the desire to possess a child on the cusp of womanly self-consciousness, to mold the malleable flesh and sensibility like a sculptor-teacher. This is the perversion of all of (12 year old) Violet's sad-eyed suiters from her first client to Bellacq. The sexual experience life holds for (12 year old) Violet are no more pathetic than the lack of experience in the lives of these men. (4)

Most men are probably sexually stimulated by minors, at least in some situations, but do not act upon their feelings; some men do act on their feelings, and apparently a large group of men buy child pornography as a way of controlling their interest. One study has found that a liberal policy on pornography reduces child-molestation (5) and if this finding holds, policy-makers may be in a dilemma.

Anson introduces the problem of "kiddie porn" in this section with upsetting directness, highlighting the sleazy aspects of recruitment and film production. While the article generates social disgust, it should not create hysteria and prematurity in decision making. Carefully drafted laws, with reasonable time for deliberation, stand the best chance of avoiding First Amendment objections. Baker then presents a through dissection and analysis of all the legal issues on the problem, including new legislation. Concluding, Rossman presents unique material based on interviews with unconvicted child molestors and their mates, stripping away stereotypes and myths, making dishearteningly obvious just how complex the whole problem is.

REFERENCES

1. L. Boda and A. Szabo: *Kriminalistik, 22,* (8): 25-28, 1968.
2. M. Rugoff: *Prudery and Passion.* New York: Putnams, 1971, pp. 300-320.
3. A. Moll: *The Sexual Life of the Child.* New York: Emerson, 1912, p. 111.
4. *New Times,* May 1, 1978, p. 71.
5. B. Kutchinsky: The effect of easy availability of pornography and the incidence of sex crimes. *Journal of Social Issues, 29:* 163-181, 1973. Kutchinsky's findings are challenged by J. Court: Pornography and sex crime. *International Journal of Criminology and Penology, 5:* 129-157, 1977.

Chapter 20

THE LAST PORNO SHOW
ROBERT SAM ANSON

It was, as such films go, a rather tame affair. Merely two lovers in the midst of feigned passion, doing the things that people do in pornographic movies. No production values. No socially redeeming features. Not a dog or chain or bathroom in sight. Just average porn. With one exception. The stars were aged ten and eight. They were brother and sister. And the person who made the movie was their mother.

The lights snap on in one of the screening rooms of the New York City screening rooms of the New York City Police Department, revealing half a dozen beefy shapes, who have spent the better part of a sunny afternoon watching this and similar films. Usually, these are humorous occasions for vice cops. Some of the films are unintentionally hilarious, and the cops vie with one another to make smart cracks. But not this afternoon. As they move out of the room, they are quiet still, grim-looking, jaws set, bodies sagging. One of the cops walks to his desk and kicks an open drawer shut with a loud bang.

Something is happening today, and no one is quite sure what it is. Child pornography—"Kiddie porn" as it's called—is only part of it, a symptom of something much larger. Something so pervasive and elusive, something so quietly frightening, that people don't like to talk about it, don't like to think about it, don't even like to imagine it exists. It was there, in its grossest form, that afternoon in the police screening room. You hesitate to use the words that truly describe it, because they sound so old-fashioned, so moralistic. All you know is that something is terribly wrong, and that, suddenly, you need some air.

This is a story about children, little kids, eight, nine, ten years old, some as young as three, few over fourteen. It is a story about what is being done to them, and the people who are doing it. I wish I could tell you that it was a story about good and evil, dirty old men and innocent young children. But I can't. Because this is a story about what happens when concepts like good and evil lose their meaning. It is a story about today.

Times Square is as good a place as any to begin, and maybe better, if only because Times Square is the symbolic center of what is happening. On warm summer nights, you literally have to push your way past the battalions of pushers, hookers, hustlers and whores to get where you are going, which, on Times Square, invariably means to a massage parlor, prostitute or one of the live sex acts that have become the current rage.

There used to be a lot of kiddie porn in Times Square, sold right out in the open. Apparently, it had been there for some time, but only came to the attention of the police after the cops opened their own pornographic bookstore, in an attempt to make some contacts in the business. "It was sort of like picking out groceries in the supermarket," one of the cop-proprietors later recalled. "You'd tell the guy what you wanted, I mean, anything, you name it, and they would get it for you, usually within three days." The operation was so efficient that, for a time, some kiddie producers were running a studio on wheels, picking up kids in a van, photographing them on the spot, then putting them out on the street $200 richer. One well-heeled pederast, a prominent lawyer, used to arrive each week at the cop's porno store in his chauffeured limousine, and dispatch his manservant to pick up the goods. His tastes ran to little boys, and he could afford to be quite selective. There were books specializing in boys of virtually any age, race or description: long penises, short penises, circumcised or no, brothers, twins—like the cop said, *anything*. There were items for heterosexuals, too. Films, magazines and paperbacks by the dozens: one instructed fathers on how to insert locks in their daughters' labias "to keep them all for you"; while another provided step-by-step instructions for the would-be child molester, including instructions on ignoring a child's screams (merely a sign of pleasure, the book suggests); another advised on having sex with pre-teenagers who are "too small."

Most of the kiddie porn is gone now, at least temporarily, since, for the moment, the cops have been cracking down. (It's election

year in New York.) But you can still find an occasional peep
machine, like the one in the big porno shop on 42nd Street, two
blocks down from the police department substation. The film is
called "First Communion," and, to see it all, you have to drop in a
total of a dollar in quarters.

The first reel shows five eight-year-old girls receiving their first
communion, perfect innocents in the perfect ceremony of
innocence. Suddenly, a motorcycle gang breaks into the church.
Right then, you know what is going to happen, but you can't stop
from dropping in the second quarter. And here there is a surprise.
For, instead of immediately commencing to rape the girls, the
gang pauses to beat up the priest with chains. Then they crucify
him to the cross above the altar. Finally, by reel four, the sex
begins. You can actually see the little girls bleeding. All of them
are screaming. Except the movie is silent, and you can't hear their
cries.

Back on the street, the pimps and prostitutes and hustlers are
still there, but something has changed. Some sort of line has been
crossed.

The people who know about these sorts of things—cops and
shrinks and prosecutors—say it all began to happen a couple of
years ago, when the Supreme Court finally decided that it really
didn't know what was obscene, and left it up to "community
standards" to decide. That, they say, opened the floodgates.
Sure, they admit, there had always been some kiddie porn
around—Lewis Carroll, the author of *Alice in Wonderland*, was
an avid collector—but now it came pouring out, the really hard-
core stuff, little boys masturbating and little girls fellating and an
occasional priest getting nailed to a cross. A lot of the states, like
Illinois and Michigan, didn't have any laws against it, and many
that did, like New York, seldom, if ever, prosecuted. Porno and
sex were everywhere—15,000 obscenity and prostitution-related
arrests in Manhattan alone last year—so why just single out
children? A couple of months ago, before kiddie porn became a
hot issue, a Manhattan D.A. advised one anti-kiddie-porn group
that his office should spend its time "going after really dangerous
criminals, like muggers." Besides, the courts would just throw
the cases out. Always, it was the courts. They were to blame.

And, to an extent, maybe they were. What, after all, were the cops to do when child molesters routinely got off with probation, and a big operator like Eddie Mishkin, a New York porn dealer busted a few months back, was sentented to 27 *weekends* in jail? It certainly didn't stop Eddie. The third week into his sentence, he was busted again for the same crime. But there was something more to it. Someone had to be buying the stuff. There had to be a market, a taste, a demand, or there would not have been a supply in the first place. The reasons for that are a lot rougher to get at.

Porn is an industry, a service industry you might call it, and, like any industry, it has to constantly create a demand for new products, or else the market becomes stagnant. And, the fact is, until kiddie porn came along, the porn business was in trouble. Everything had been tried. People were bored. Why, *Deep Throat* was so chic you could take your wife or girlfriend to see it. So the great search commenced. First, explicit ejaculation. Then orgies. Then bisexuality. Then SM. Then urination and defecation. Then bestiality. And still, the senses were sated. What would happen to dear, sweet Hef, we debated. Would *Playboy* have to "go pink" to stay *au courant?* Could *Hustler* outgross *Playboy* and *Penthouse?* We held our breath, signed our *New York Times* ads (poor, persecuted Larry Flynt, it developed, shared the plight of Soviet dissidents), threw our cocktail parties for Harry Reems, and, as we did, the industry found The Answer, "the last frontier," as one "straight" porn producer puts it, the ultimate turn-on: kids.

It was not a barrier that was crossed in a day or a week or even a year. Only looking back, from the perspective of the little girls in their first communion dresses, do you see the signposts: the soft-focus pix that began showing up in *Playboy* a couple of years ago, the "art" photographs of preteenagers getting in and out of their leotards, while looking dreamily at one another; the progression of Jody Foster from spoiled, corrupting brat in *Alice Doesn't Live Here Anymore* to 13-year-old whore in *Taxi Driver*; the phenomenal success of *Show Me*, the explicit "sex education" book, showing little kids examining themselves and one another, giggling over an older brother's oral sex. Then, last November, *True*, the "man's magazine" it used to call itself, took the big step:

"32 Pages of Beautiful Pussy!" the cover headlined, the vagina in question belonging to a 14-year-old runaway.

A Little Child Shall Lead Them

Now kiddie porn is out of the closet altogether, and business, as you might expect, is booming. Yearly profits are in the tens of millions. For one things, the initial investment is low—often no more than an inexpensive home movie camera and the "cooperation" of some neighborhood children; and even the fact that "professionally shot" kiddie porn features can cost up to $50,000, as compared to a "one-day wonder" professional adult porn film, which comes in at $6,000, doesn't deter producers. They know they can recoup with rental and purchase rates five to six times higher. Nearly the same arithmetic holds for magazines: $7.50 for kids, a dollar and a half for adults. After a while, it begins to dawn on people: there is money to be made here.

And it is being made all over the country. Not just in major cities, but in middle-sized small towns as well. Quiet, unlikely places like North Bellmore, New York, out on Long Island, in the very bosom of tree-lined, buttoned-down suburban comfort. Gene and Joyce Abrams used to live in North Bellmore, and they were just as quiet and unlikely as the town they lived in. Gene was an aerospace engineer, and a good one: some of his inventions had been included in the first manned mission to the moon. Joyce was just the average suburban housewife, with a taste for the good things in life. Gene was anxious to please, so, to make his salary stretch, he placed an ad in Al Goldstein's *Screw*, offering "$200 fee for girl model, 8-14 (must have parents' consent), one-day photographic session." Before long, people started knocking on the Abrams' door, leading their kids by the hand. Some of the parents appeared in the pictures *with* their children, others merely allowed their children to have sex with Gene. One little girl, age 11, who ran crying from a bedroom after being told to have sex with a man of 40, protested. "Mommy, I can't do it. I won't do it." "You have to do it," her mother answered. "We need the money." And, of course, the little girl did.

By the time the cops arrived, some 18 children had had their pictures taken by or with Gene Abrams. Joyce no longer had to worry about Gene's salary. The porn operation was bringing in $250,000 a year, tax free. The material in the house alone filled an entire van: 4,000 envelopes prepared for mailing, 3,000 negatives of kids having sex and $70,000 worth of photographic equipment, not to mention orders from as far away as Trinidad, England and South Africa. Because Gene, with his precise, methodical, engineer's mind, had gone big-time. He had a deal with a New York photo studio, which processed and duplicated his film, and then passed it on to a mob-controlled company for distribution. From there, it was not long before it was on stands of porno shops across the country.

Quiet North Bellmore is just like quiet Yonkers, where a friendly suburban couple takes in runaways, houses and feeds them, then charges them "rent" in the form of appearing in pornographic films; and quiet San Jose, California, where a mother recently fell afoul of the law for appearing in a porn film with her son, age three; and quiet Winchester, Tennessee, and quiet Port Huron, Michigan, and quiet Security, Colorado, and a lot of other quiet, nice towns that have recently been the sites of porno exposés.

After a while, the stories take on a depressing similarity. There is the Boy Scout master in Santa Monica (not to be confused with the Boy Scout leaders in New Orleans), the boys' camp in Michigan (just like the boys' camp in North Carolina), the father who sells his sons in Illinois, the family who does the same in Colorado.

They are all such average folks, so relentless in the banality of their evil. Not at all what you expect and hope for: some stereotypical dirty old man in a semen-stained raincoat, lusting after a little girl. It would be more comforting, perhaps, to think that most child pornographers are like that. But that is the trouble: they are so normal.

That is what the people in Studio City, California, say about their neighbor, Ed Leja. You come to Los Angeles to meet people like Ed Leja, because, of course, L.A. has got to be the center of kiddie porn. It is only right. This, after all, is the place where the production of fantasies is the major industry, where the whole youth cult began. And you are not disappointed. The cops report that yes, indeed, L.A. is the center, with 3,000 kids and 17,000 adults actively involved in porn and prostitution. Ed Leja is one of those statistics. Four arrests, one conviction. Punishment: a $250 fine.

When, a year ago, Leja was arrested the latest time—for conspiring to endanger the welfare of a child—his neighbors professed shock and indignation. A number of them rallied to his support. Ed was not a pornographer; all you had to do was see his house, as well-kept as any house on the block, or meet his three fine sons, or know of his community activities. Why no, it couldn't be. The cops were merely out to get him.

And, true enough, in the flesh, Ed Leja seems just as nice and friendly and normal as any of his neighbors. To show you the kind of man he is, Ed subscribes to the Reader's Digest Condensed Books, and thinks that "the government is just one giveaway scheme after another. Why don't they make people work for a living?" Leja, burly-chested, bearded and 57, has reason to sound bitter. Although the judge threw out the case against him and his co-defendants—the parents whom Leja had paid for permission to photograph their children—a plague of misfortune has descended on him. First, an earthquake undermined the foundation of his house. Then his wife left him, running off, he says, with the associate editor of one of his magaines. Then there was the arrest and all the bad publicity, and legal bills amounting to more than $40,000. And, on top of all that, his magazines (Leja used to publish several of them) ran into financial trouble—trouble, Leja says, directly attributable to the "kiddie porn witch-hunt.

Ed Leja wants you to know that he is not a child pornographer. There is no explicit sex—not so much as an erect miniature penis—in the "Moppets" series he used to publish. He would like to get his hands on some of those pornographers, Leja says; they are ruining his business. What Leja, a former engineer, is, by his own description, is a photographer, publisher and practicing nudist.

"I know for a fact that nudism for children doesn't hurt them,"

Leja says. "Whether sex activity does or not, well, I don't know." He seems an eminently reasonable man, propounding an eminently reasonable, if somewhat eccentric, philosophy. *Moppets* itself seems reasonable—well, some of it, the part that shows the kids cooking hotdogs or frolicking down at the beach. It is when you reach the other part—the *Penthouse*-style spreads of open-crotched little grils looking longingly at the camera—that the uneasiness sets in. But Ed is constantly reassuring. "See," he says, pointing to an older woman cuddling her child. "That's her mother. A practicing nudist. All my subjects are practicing nudists."

Only later do you learn that two of the parents arrested with Leja are professional hard-core porn actresses, one of them a junkie and prostitute as well, and that the "nudist camp" turns out to have been Ed Leja's backyard.

It is about then that you begin to wonder about Ed Leja, whether he is so nice and warm and friendly after all. Because he never mentioned those things, never mentioned the testimony at his trial—like the part about the two-and-a-half-year-old girl being molested during one of his shootings—never mentioned where *Moppets* winds up after it leaves the racks of the adult bookstores. The police found a copy not long ago in the briefcase of a child molester, arrested outside a playground. Also included in the case were several other kiddie porn books, a few rubber dolls and one item essential to his line of work: a jar of Vaseline®.

Sergeant Lloyd Martin knows the child molester with the jar of Vaseline, and he knows the work of Ed Leja; he knows, too, how one leads inexorably to another. There are a lot of people in Los Angeles, including some within his own department, who think that Martin has become obsessed. For the last six months, he and his squad of five detectives have been working 16-hour days, almost seven days a week. It is back-breaking, frustrating work, filled with round-the-clock surveillances and leads that never pan out.

But Martin asked for it. There was no kiddie-porn squad in Los Angeles, or anywhere else in the country, until Martin thought it up. It was about 3 years ago, and Martin, then working Administrative Vice, helped bust a notorious pornographer named Guy Strait. Strait jumped bail, but the material he left in the hands of the LAPD sickened Martin.

Martin thought he had enough to keep investigating indefinitely. But there was resistance from within the department. Other crimes had higher priority. Martin was told to get back to work on his other cases.

But, in his spare time, Martin kept probing, kept pulling together material, until he had finally compiled a thick black looseleaf notebook, filled with kiddie porn, m.o.'s of the major purveyors and a detailed proposal for going after them. In September, the department gave Martin the green light.

Today, Martin and his unit operate out of a crowded warren of borrowed offices in the Juvenile Division. The phones ring constantly. The FBI wants to know about an upcoming raid. A police department in Michigan is looking for information. The D.A.'s office has a question about a search warrant. A plaque on Martin's desk reads: "Expect a Miracle." With the way things have been going, Lloyd Martin needs one.

There is a threat to cut off funds and shut the whole operation down. Not enough arrests, too few convictions, the homosexual community screaming about police harassment. But it goes deeper than that. Even now, people have a difficult time believing that Martin isn't making the whole thing up. "The only way to get to people is to really horrify them," he said to a friend not long ago. "But how do you horrify them if you can't show them the stuff that is supposed to do it?"

This morning, Martin makes an exception. He pulls out a portable file drawer, and begins talking. He is still talking, still showing pictures, two hours later. The briefing starts out slowly, with innocent-looking nude studies of young girls. Then boys. Then girls with boys. Then girls and boys awkwardly making love. Then children being sodomized by adults. Then bondage. And then finally, and most grotesquely, a series of pictures taken not by a professional pornographer, but by the children he had enticed, showing him smeared head to foot in his own blood, various torture devices sticking out of his body, nearly all of which require children to operate. The pictures lie on Martin's desk without comment, until, after several moments, he clears his throat: "Now this individual," he explains, in the most dispassionate police argot, "is a masochist. That is to say, he receives his sexual satisfaction from others hurting him, in this case, children. Now what do you suppose would have happened. . ." He pauses ". . . if he were a sadist?"

You don't have to suppose very long in Martin's business. Once you imagine the worst, it invariably happens, and, sure enough, it has already happened. Green plastic garbage bags keep turning up in and around Los Angeles, 18 of them so far in the last 18 months. Inside the bags are the dismembered, mutilated bodies of young boys, Mexicans mostly, some of the kids who Martin says are being smuggled across the border, sometimes in specially constructed compartments concealed in the floorboards and fenders of cars, to infuse fresh, exotic blood in the kiddie porn industry. Kiddie porn, though, has a constant appetite for young faces, the newer, younger and smoother-skinned the better. Disposal, then, becomes the chief problem.

As Martin talks, the image of a young New York hustler comes to mind. His name, he said, was "Jersey," and his occupation of the moment was servicing chickenhawks on East 53rd Street. He had been at it now for 12 years, ever since he was eleven. But he had been a kiddie porn star once, he claimed—before he got too old, maybe 15. Between tricks, he had talked matter-of-factly about the experience. "This guy Eddie took pictures," he had said. "At first, he was just going to go down on my Johnson for $55. But he came out with this pad, asking me all sorts of questions. Did I have any hair—you know, *that* kind of hair. Well, I really didn't have much, and they seemed to like that. They also wanted to know whether I had any scars. I made $80 that night. Put on white stockings, took them half-way down, scratched myself, played with myself. They wanted me because I have baby skin." But Jersey was luckier than the kids Lloyd Martin was talking about: he had gotten out. "They was getting into bizarre things, into freaky things," he had explained, "like whips and dildos and 18-year-olds with Teddy bears. I was leery at the time.

Now, Lloyd Martin was talking about the kids who didn't get out, the children in the plastic bags. There was one film reportedly making the circuit—supposedly it had been a big hit at an L.A. party a few weeks before—showing a boy actually being murdered. He had been one of Dean Corll's kids down in Texas, the story went. That had happened to a lot of Dean Corll's kids. By the time they finished digging them up, the Houston Police had come up with 27 of them. Police strongly suspected that a number of young porn stars were among Corll's victims.

You could begin to see why Lloyd Martin was obsessed, and when he talked about the chickenhawk rings that shuttled kids from one city to another, the kiddie porn key clubs where a member had to produce a photograph of himself having sex with a young boy to gain admittance, the mutilations and murders, it seemed not only eminently probable, but inevitable, even logical, given the business.

Where were they coming from, these kids? How was it happening? Who was doing it to them? "Go to the Cup," someone said. "Stay there for a night. Check it out. You'll know."

The Cup and the Rack

In Los Angeles, when people say "the Cup" they mean the Gold Cup Cafe, at Hollywood Boulevard and Las Palmas, first stop on what is called "the meat rack." The meat rack begins at the Cup, runs down Las Palmas, then turns right on Selma, goes on for a couple of blocks, then left on Highland to Santa Monica. It is not hard to find it. Simply follow the slowly cruising cars and look for kids lounging on the street. When the cars stop and the kids walk over, you're there.

On any night of the week, the Gold Cup is jammed: with kids, both boys and girls, menacing-looking black pimps, a few assorted lesbians and a sizable contingent of middle-aged chickenhawks. The atmosphere is a cross between a YMCA club and Dante's ninth circle. In the back of the Cup half a dozen teenage boys are playing pinball. A scantily dressed prostitute wanders in to watch the action. When she leans over one of the machines to see the score, one of her breasts flops out. No one looks twice. In the front of the cafe, three beefy chickenhawks sit in a booth, chatting, sipping coffee, and commenting on the passing merchandise. "Who's that sweet little blond?" one of them calls out, and blows a kiss to a boy sitting at the counter. The youth turns, smiles knowingly, and walks to the table. One of the chicken-hawks reaches out and fondles his crotch.

At 9:30, when the cafe closes for the night, the kids straggle out the door, some heading off for other well-known "chicken coops" in the neighborhood, others around the corner to the bookstall on Las Palmas (where one of the gay magazine features pictures of one of the boys who'd been playing pinball that night), and still others down the block to Selma Avenue. There they queue up for the cruising chickenhawks.

The girls are not being left out. One 14-year-old—call her "Ginny"—is nursing a badly split lip, received in an altercation outside the Cup two nights ago. She is originally from New York, she says, but the family moved to Hollywood when she was eight. She and her mother—the father left years ago—still live in the neighborhood. Going to the Cup for her is a nightly ritual. She first had sex at 11, and turned her first trick at 12—"But I ain't no pro," she insists. "I only do it when I need money, like for pinball or drugs." Twice she has been asked by passing motorists— "They were driving expensive type cars"—if she wanted to appear in films, but both times she turned them down. Some of her friends had not, however. "It's easy work," she shrugs. "You just fuck and suck a little and they give you fifty bucks."

Ginny more or less dropped out of school a little more than a year ago. She spends most of her days at home, sleeping, "or doing Quaaludes when I can get them," waiting for night to fall, and the chance to come to the Cup. The stupid question more or less pops out on its own: "Do you think your childhood is well, kinda different from other kids'?" "Like how?" she answers, genuinely perplexed. If there were ever a truly vacant face, it belongs to Ginny: "Well, yeah, I guess you could say I'm a little different," she says at last. "You see, most of my friends don't live at home. But I got a good relationship with my mom. She's real cool. I can talk to her. My mom's okay. What I want to do, that's all right with her. I told her about turning tricks and all, and she just kinda laughed. I don't think she likes it. I don't think she dislikes it. She's cool. And she's got her own boyfriend too, you know."

Ginny is about to say more, when a white Buick glides to the curb. The man inside gestures Ginny over. They talk briefly, and Ginny gets in. As the car pulls off, she waves goodbye.

She's cool. Everyone is so cool. On the Strip, they are still talking about Roman Polanski and the alleged rape of a 13-year-old. Polanski will get off, the betting goes. The chick was a pro. Part of a mother-daughter act. No big deal.

They come to Los Angeles by the tens of thousands, these kids. Runaways, some of them; others simply "throwaways," a million of them in the country, according to the best estimates. With no skills, no job prospects, there is only one way they can survive, Martin says. "Drop their pants or pull up their dress." First porn, then pros, then, well, no one knows. Somehow, though, they must grow up, get old, have their own kid. They must.

Like Serena. Serena has been in the biz a long time, a very long time. She's 20 now, a veteran. She ran away from home the first time at 12, was caught, spent some time in "juvie," as she calls it, then came home, just long enough to plan how to run away for good. It was her parents, you see; "working-class heroes," she calls them, her mother a waitress and semi-invalid, her father a bartender. She hasn't seen them in more than five years. The last time she did, her father yelled at her mother not to talk to "that whore." When she split the second time, she was, as she puts it, "kinda back and forth, bus rides, hitching. I just kinda floated out on that one." There was some more time in juvie, then picking pears in Oregon, bumming around Berkeley, and, finally, a steady fella. Money, though, was always a problem, so, at 14, she turned her first trick—"I needed money for cigarettes." By 16, two years under the legal limit, she was doing nude modeling. A career in hard-core films followed. She has remained in hard-core ever since, between occasional gigs as a stripper, such as her current engagement at the Cave in Hollywood, and as a performer in one of the Mitchell brothers' lesbian sex acts in San Francisco, where, as she describes it, "I make love to three ladies six times a day."

Serena, in short, has seen and done it all, and to hear her tell it (which, she politely informs you, will cost $30), there are no regrets, save an occasional wondering "what it would have been like to have been a real kid, you know, with proms and bubble baths and all that.

There is a break between her shows, and we are sitting in a Howard Johnson's, talking. Serena is drinking milk. She is blond, smooth-faced, strikingly attractive, and far younger-looking than her age. "That's some of my appeal, you know," she explains. She is reminiscing about growing up in Glendale, California, what it was like to discover she had a body that attracted older men, dropping out of school after the eighth grade, and being the best dancer in her modern ballet class. "I was really a precocious kid in dance," she says. "My teacher said I was the best she had seen, the way I moved so naturally. Not like a kid at all, but like a grown-up.

It is tough these days looking so young in Los Angeles, when you happen to work in Serena's profession. The heat is really on. Modeling agencies, which seldom look at IDs, are now demanding three proofs of age. Everyone is worried about Lloyd Martin and his cops. The other day they were hassling one of Serena's friends, a prominent porn photographer accused of taking hard-core shots of a 14-year-old. The police couldn't make the beef stick, but Serena knew it was true. "He was asking if I knew of any really young stuff. You know, *really* young. But he's okay. He only shoots kids getting it on with other kids. And what an artist he is. He is totally into his art. He really demands a lot from you.

What he demands doesn't bother Serena, "so long," she says, "as the kids can handle it." She has her own daughter now, just a year old, and already she can sense that "she is going to be a far-out, free little kid." Let her do porn, say at 10? "Kids are growing up so fast now, even faster than I was. I mean, I was fucking at 12, so she'll probably be fucking at 10. You know, that's how these things work." The child of one of Serena's friends is already doing porn, "and she is only five." So, it's possible. Everything is possible.

"You oughta catch my act," Serena says. It is an invitation impossible to resist. We go next door, and, in a few moments, Serena is there on stage, bathed in a red light, nude but for childish knee socks. The music scratches on, and Serena begins to dance, languidly, invitingly, an erotic ballet, tracing again the steps learned as a girl.

After an evening at the Gold Cup, a talk with Serena and Ginny, you no longer wonder where the kids are coming from. The talent pool is bottomless: the million runaways, the 2.4 million children of drug addicts, the 2.8 million children of prostitutes, the unnumbered children who can't be lumped under any group, but simply belong to parents who don't give a damn. Now the stories take on some meaning. Like the porn producer who operated, undetected, in Houston for more than 18 years, employing dozens of kids in the neighborhood, including one set of 12-year-old twin boys, who in turn recruited their younger sister, who in turn recruited a still younger brother. . .

"Let me tell you about kids involved in child pornography," a notorious porn producer said in a recent interview. "They are children of lawyers, doctors, policemen, preachers—who are attracted to older men because their fathers have no time for them. They are searching for a father. And no one jumps in front of a camera for money. These kids do it for ego. Take a youngster who has never been appreciated. You tell him he's good-looking enough to be in front of a camera and that people will want to see him and be interested. It's a great boost to his ego."

"I've helped a lot of kids," he added, "raised about 40 of them, although I didn't have sex with all of them. Some are 40 years old now. I put those in college who wanted it. I've given away bikes. I love to give gifts to children. I've spent a fortune on them."

It is a theme you hear over and over again about child pornographers: how much they love children, how they are giving them, as Martin says, "what they aren't getting at home, attention and affection, even a perverse kind of love." And there is love of a sort. One child pornographer operated in Santa Monica for a long time without detection, precisely because he was so loving, so caring about the children. He was their scoutmaster. There seemed to be nothing he wouldn't do for them. Take them on overnight camping trips, go-carting, expeditions to Disneyland. The parents, many of whom were divorced, didn't give his motives a second thought; they were glad to have the children off their hands.

The Santa Monica pornographer never threatened his children, never used force at all. He didn't have to. He was doing something for them, something no one else was doing. Such friends seldom testify against one another. In one recent case, an Illinois boy, 12, did; afterward, he committed suicide. More common, though, is the experience of Tennessee authorities, who have been having a rough time making a case against Reverend Claudius. "Bud" Vermilye, the 47-year-old Episcopal priest who was arrested for turning his "Boy's Farm" into a kiddie porno production studio. "These kids," says one cop, "have a strange sense of loyalty to him." Well, why not? As his lawyer, Joe Bean, puts it indignantly: "These boys had been kicked out of their homes and mental and penal institutions. They were what they were before they got there. They expect the defendant to have done what their parents couldn't do—reform the boys. Vermilye has done much good for humanity. He's a nice humanitarian, dedicated to doing good for the helpless and the wayward."

They are all such nice humanitarians, so interested in young people, so appreciative of their beauty. The mail-order ads for kiddie porno fairly gush in their enthusiasm. One 13-year-old is "a blond beauty," an 11-year-old "a cute little fellow with curly black hair." Their sexual prowess is only secondary. The ads exult when a child is not well-developed, when he performs clumsily and innocently. Forever young, the kiddie porno industry wants them. Let us all stay forever young. There is even an organized lobby in California—it calls itself the "Renee Guyon Society"—that wants to drop the age of sexual consent down to five. "Sex before eight," goes their motto, "or else it's too late." "In the springtime of childhood, sex doesn't seem very important—to an adult, but, to a child, it is the very mystery of life," one of Ed Leja's magazines rhapsodizes. "There is a faint stirring of the libido heard in the deep uncomplicated recesses of a child's mind. There is the tingling of flesh, the sensuous thrill of touch, when all the senses seem to be electrified by nature.

A Helena Rubenstein ad could not have put it better, or a plastic surgeon, or the director of a fat farm, or any other aspect of the culture that hates age and worships youth. Kiddie porno is only part of it, the nastier, less genteel part, but part of it nonetheless: the logical, ultimate fulfillment of the youth cult.

You wonder, after a while, what is going to happen. For the kids, it is easy to predict. The lucky ones end up talking to Lloyd Martin, "breaking down and crying," he says, "so relieved that it is finally over." They are the exceptions. Most are like Serena's friends, "dead," as she puts it, "burnt out on prostitution, drugs, or just life." It has happened already to the little girl who appeared in the film the cops watched that afternoon in New York. She is in a Catholic children's home now, where the authorities describe her as "very greatly disturbed." Such children will grow up, according to a Detroit police psychiatrist, "with no sense of modesty or privacy, no sense of the specialness of sex and the human body, basically, no moral sense at all." There was a kid like that whom the L.A. cops picked up recently. They asked him whether he had had sex with a pornographer. "No," he said. "I went down on him, and he went down on me, but we didn't have sex." The shrinks say that as an adult he will be subject to grotesque fears, and have difficulty experiencing normal sexual fulfillment. For others, there can be physical problems, too: among the very youngest, severe damage to the vagina and anus; in girls, an increased incidence of cervical cancer. Many will not be able to bear children. None will ever remember what it was like to be a child.

But what will happen to us, the adults? What has happened? Why does Lloyd Martin have to carry a picture around, a color shot of a very young boy, maybe seven, eyes wide with wonder and fear, having oral sex with a man in his forties? The boy is looking out to the person taking the picture, as if asking what to do. What are we telling him?

"I don't know who that guy is," Martin says of the adult in the picture. "But I am going to find him before I retire. I am going to get him." He pauses for a moment, as if trying to keep control. "Isn't this the pits?" he says finally.

No, Lloyd, this isn't the pits. This is the end of the fucking world.

—————————— **Chapter 21** ——————————

PREYING ON PLAYGROUNDS:
THE SEXPLOITATION OF CHILDREN
IN PORNOGRAPHY AND PROSTITUTION

C. David Baker

> But if anyone causes one of these little ones who believe in me to sin, it
> would be better for him to have a large millstone hung around his neck
> and to be drowned in the depths of the sea. Woe to the world because of
> the things that cause people to sin! Such things must come, but woe to
> the man through whom they come![1]

Seeking to implement this biblical injunction, legislators, law
enforcement officials, journalists, and the public in general
have sharply responded to a sudden flood of child pornography
and prostitution. Through the enactment of bold new laws,
increased enforcement, and severe public pressure, they have
gone about constructing large "millstones" as burdensome
deterrents to producers, distributors, and retailers of child
pornography in an attempt to curb the rapid growth of the
multimillion dollar child sexploitation[2] enterprise.

Unable to forecast the sudden appearance and rapid rise of
child sexploitation, scholars have been caught at a complete
surprise and legal literature has yet to touch upon the subject
fully. This comment will attempt to present an understanding of
this important concern by reviewing the prior legislative voids as
well as the problems confronting new legislation hastily drafted

---

1. Matthew 18:6,7 (New International Version of the New Testament).

2. The term *child sexploitation* refers to the sexual exploitation of minors for the
commercial profit of adults using children as prostitutes and as subjects in pornographic
materials, both obscene and non-obscene. Although the term is directed chiefly at adults
who exploit the children in sexual poses and acts for commercial benefit, it may also
include the acts of those who do so for their own gratification.

to prevent further spread of child sexploitation. Finally, after understanding how society has contracted this social disease, and the harm that it will ultimately produce, this comment will set forth a proposal designed to soothe the trauma of this new form of child abuse.

Understanding The Problem: A New Form Of Child Abuse

Emergence, Nature, and Scope of Child Pornography

Child pornography first began to cautiously appear in an "under-the-counter" fashion at adult bookstores in the late 1960s.[3] It consisted of little girls, eight to fourteen years old, posing nude in magazines called *Lollitots* and *Moppits*.[4] As the sexual appetite of pedophiles[5] increased, so did the demand for child pornography. By 1976, child pornography had become a featured item among obscenity dealers,[6] displaying in great volume and variety children aged three to sixteen in every conceivable sexual pose and act, heterosexual, and homosexual.[7] Such magazines graphically exhibit children as young as three

---

3. Up until 1968 much of the purported child pornography was mostly fakery, using young looking women who dressed in children's garments. They exposed themselves in suggestive poses and acts amongst playgrounds and toys and were referred to as "Young Lolitas." TIME. April 4, 1977 at 55.

4. G. Frank, *Child Pornography Industry Finds a Home in Los Angeles, L.A. Daily Journal*, Nov. 28, 1977, at 19, col. 1 (hereinafter cited as *Child Pornography in L.A.*).

5. Those adults whose sexual preference is for children.

6. Recognizing child pornography's feature billing the California Attorney General's Advisory Committee on Obscenity and Pornography noted in its REPORT TO THE ATTORNEY GENERAL ON CHILD PORNOGRAPHY IN CALIFORNIA (June 24, 1977) that recently, on a single page of the *San Francisco Ball*, an underground newspaper printed in Van Nuys, California, no less than thirty-four advertisements for sexual materials appeared of which eighteen offered child pornography and nine of those eighteen offered materials depicting bestiality. CAL. ATT'Y GEN. ON CHILD PORNOGRAPHY 5 (1977). (Hereinafter cited as CAL. ATT'Y GEN.)

7. *See* R. Lloyd, FOR MONEY OR LOVE: BOY PROSTITUTION IN AMERICA (1976) wherein the author documents the existence of at least 264 different magazines sold in adult bookstores across the country bearing names such as *Torid Tots, Night Boys, Lolita, Boys Who Love Boys, Lollitots* and *Children-Love* that depict children engaging in sexually explicit conduct.

years old "in couplings with their peers of the same and opposite sex, or with adult men and women. The activities featured range from lewd poses to intercourse, fellatio, cunnilingus, masturbation, rape, incest and sado-masochism."[8]

Because of its clandestine operation it is difficult to determine the exact extent of child pornography production, distribution, and sale. Until recently, it was always assumed that child pornography was produced, for the most part, in Europe and Scandanavia.[9] The public outcry, caused by recent publicity revealing the spread of child pornography, culminated in a series of Congressional Hearings[10] which revealed that police have uncovered major child pornography production centers in Los Angeles, New York, Chicago and several other large cities.[11]

The Sexually Exploited Child Unit of the Los Angeles Police Department estimates that 30,000 juveniles are sexually exploited annually in Los Angeles alone,[12] and of this number at least

---

8. SENATE COMM. ON THE JUDICIARY REPORT ON S. 1585, PROTECTION OF CHILDREN AGAINST SEXUAL EXPLOITATION ACT OF 1977, S. Rep. No. 95-438, 95th Cong., 1st Sess. 6 (1977), (hereinafter S. Rep. on 1585).

9. "Indeed, it is quite common for photographs or films made in the United States to be sent to foreign countries to be reproduced and then returned to this country in order to give the impression of foreign origin." S. Rep. on 1585, supra note 8, at 6. Accord: Child Pornography in L.A., supra note 3; J. Densen-Gerber & S. Hutchinson, Developing Federal and State Legislation to Combat the Exploitation of Children in the Production of Pornography, JLM/LEGAL ASPECTS OF MEDICAL PRACTICE 19 (Sept. 1977). (Hereinafter cited as Developing Legislation).

10. Proposed Amendments to the Child Abuse Protection and Treatment Act: Hearings on H.R. 6693 Before the House Education and Labor Subcommittee on Select Education, the House Judiciary Committee's Crime Subcommittee and the Senate Judiciary Subcommittee to Investigate Juvenile Delinquency, 95th Cong., 1st Sess. (1977). (Hereinafter cited as House Hearings on H.R. 6693).

11. However, child pornography is by no means limited to large urban centers. Pornographic photographs and films are generally taken in private homes, hotel rooms, or abandoned buildings and therefore may be produced in any small community. Indeed, the Senate Judiciary Committee noted the arrest of independent producers in such unlikely places as Port Huron, Michigan and Winchester, Tennessee. S. Rep. on 1585, supra note 8, at 6.

12. Testimony has also been offered that between January, 1976 and June, 1977 as many as 300,000 children have been subjected to sexual exploitation nationally. Child Pornography: Outrage Starts to Stir Some Action, U.S. NEWS. June 13, 1977, at 66 (Hereinafter cited as U.S. NEWS).

3,000 are under the age of fourteen.[13] Indeed, with its vast production facilities, film technicians, and printing houses, the "movie capital of the world" is the country's major center of the child pornography industry,[14] and Hollywood, once famous for its stars of the screen, has become the center for sexually exploited children.[15]

The child pornography boom has spawned an enterprise that grosses more than a half-billion dollars a year[16] and is still growing. Child pornographers cannot produce the material fast enough to meet the demand.[17]

Retail distribution of child pornography is an ideal investment that offers lucrative returns[18] while overhead is kept at a bare

---

13. CAL. ATT'Y GEN., *supra* note 6, at 16. *Accord:* L.A. Times, May 28, 1977, § 2 at 1, col. 4 (statement by Los Angeles Ass't Police Chief Daryl F. Gates at Congressional Hearings in Los Angeles.); *Developing Legislation, supra* note 9, at 19; J. Hurst, *Children—a Big Profit Item for the Smut Producer,* L.A. Times, May 26, 1977, § 2, at 1, col. 4 (Hereinafter cited as *Children—Big Profit*). It should be noted however that such estimates are speculative, and although no evidence can be found to confirm such figures, authorities are unable to refute it or show that it is in any way exaggerated. Nor can evidence be offered to show that the figures are not in actuality even higher for "a very high number of instances of this kind of sexual exploitation may go unreported, confounding any effort to arrive at an accurate estimate." CAL. ATT'Y GEN., *supra* note 6, at 17.

14. In October, 1977 Los Angeles Sheriff deputies arrested five adults and seized 500 films showing boys and girls in sexual acts. It was believed to be one of the largest child pornography distributorships in the nation. *Child Pornography in L.A., supra* note 4, at 19.

15. *See generally:* M. Wallace, *Kiddie Porn,* CBS 60 MINUTES. (produced by B. Lando, aired May 15, 1977). (Transcript of broadcast on file with the *Pepperdine Law Review.* Copyright © CBS Inc. 1977. All rights reserved). *See also: Children—Big Profit, supra* note 13, at 4.

16. U.S. NEWS *supra,* note 12, at 66; Los Angeles Police Investigator Lloyd Martin, an expert in the field of child sexploitation has stated that the industry may in fact be approaching a $1 billion-a-year business world wide. *Child Pornography in L.A., supra* note 4, at 19.

17. "Police and prosecutors have seized mailing lists that contain tens of thousands of actual and prospective child pornography customers." *Id.* Former L.A. Police Chief Ed Davis has stated that "The number of establishments dealing in porno material in the city of Los Angeles has increased from eighteen in 1969 to 143 in July of 1976—almost 800%." E. Davis, *Kid Porn: Is it "the Nadir of Man's Depravity"?,* L.A. Times, September 18, 1977, § 5, at 3, col. 1 (hereinafter cited as *Man's Depravity?*).

18. While producers and retailers also claim large benefits, as much as 70% of the profits accrue to the distributors who are the true beneficiaries of child sexploitation. Investigators point to evidence that some big distributors are placing their profits, as much as

minimum. Magazines that retail for $7.50 to $12.50 each can be produced for as little as thirty-five cents,[19] and a cheap home movie camera can be used for two hours in a private home or hotel to produce a one dollar film that will retail at $75.00 to $200.00 a copy.[20] The California Attorney General's Office concluded that, unless suppressed, the child pornography market will continue to increase:

> [I]n 1972, a poor-quality pamphlet was published in Hollywood, California entitled *Where the Young Ones Are*. The pamphlet listed 378 places in 59 cities of 34 states where ". . . the young can be found." Listed were such places as bowling alleys, beaches, arcades, parks and the like. The pamphlet reportedly sold 70,000 copies at $5.00 per copy. Moreover, at least two publications are presently being distributed on a nationwide basis which are apparently directed to child molesters.[21]

Child pornography is widely distributed through adult bookstores, on open display in some, while only in an "under-the-counter" fashion in others.[22] The primary means of distribution is by mail order catalogue[23] which permits a pedophile to

---

$650,000 at a time in one case, in foreign bank accounts. *Child Porn in L.A., supra* note 4, at 19.

19. Magazines are only one form of child pornography. Pedophiles can select ten to twelve minute film "loops," still photographs, slides, playing cards, video cassettes and a variety of other products. *S. Rep. on 1585, supra* note 8, at 6.

20. *Id. See also* Cal. Atty Gen., *supra* note 6, at 21.

One graphic example of the economics of child pornography was presented at the Committee's Chicago field hearing. A police officer testified how undercover officers of the Chicago Police Department were able to infiltrate a group that was using two fourteen year old boys to make a pornographic film for national distribution. The cost of producing this 200 foot film was $21 per copy and the retail selling price was to have been $100. At the time of their arrest, the producers of the film stated that they might have been able to sell as many as 10,000 copies of the film over a six-month period.

S. Rep. on 1585, supra note 8, at 6.

21. Cal. Atty Gen. *supra* note 6, at 21, 22. A child molester is one who makes indecent advances or sexually accosts minors of the opposite sex. *See, infra* note 48.

22. *S. Rep. on 1585, supra* note 8, at 6.

23. These distributors do their mail order business under many different company names, which they change regularly to avoid detection by law enforcement officials. The principal means by which the distributors advertise their pornographic wares are mailing lists that are purged every three months so as to reflect only those who purchase material,

order materials anonymously according to his or her own sexual preference[24] and to establish contacts with other pedophiles, or even child models.[25]

Authorities are split as to whether these high profits have attracted organized crime.[26] The New York State Select Legislative Committee on Crime recently found that the Mafia has begun to move back into prostitution, which it had largely abandoned in the 1930s, primarily because of the lucrative profits from child sexploitation.[27] Additionally, the Commission concluded that the Gambino Mafia family and other organized mobsters have extensive interests in child pornography enterprises.[28] The Commission's position was perhaps best stated by State Senator Ralph Morino, Chairman of the State Crime Commission, who said that, "Organized crime has no shame and will stoop to any outrage to make a buck."[29] In contrast, others, including California Attorney General Evelle J. Younger, believe that organized crime is holding back in fear of the public outrage at child pornography and enforcement crackdowns by police.[30]

Apart from organized crime few pornographers fit the stereo-

---

and to prevent unreceptive solicitees from complaining to the authorities. CAL. ATT'Y GEN., *supra* note 6, at 6,7.

24. Mail order material offers a wide selection of pornography from "hardcore" explicivity involving children in bizarre sexual activity with others (child or adult) to simple photographs of nude children, often in lewd poses. It is estimated that 80% of all child pornography is homosexual in nature. *Id.*

25. Indeed there appears to be an unofficial fraternity of thousands of pedophiles. In one recent San Francisco raid police confiscated among other things a mailing list containing 5,000 prospective child pornography customers. *See Child Pornography in L.A., supra* note 4, at 19. It should be noted however that all too often child pornographers have come to the attention of authorities merely because of inadvertence or mischance as a result of misdelivery of the mail or the breakdown of a film development computer. CAL. ATT'Y GEN., *supra* note 6, at 23.

26. Authorities have long known that organized crime is heavily involved in adult pornography. A California attorney general's report on organized crime said "80% of the production and distribution of adult pornography is mob controlled." *Child Pornography in L.A., supra* note 4, at 19.

27. TIME, *Youth for Sale on the Streets*, Nov. 28, 1977, at 23 (hereinafter cited as *Youth for Sale*).

28. *Id.*

29. N.Y. TIMES, June 1, 1977, § 1, at 7, col. 1.

30. *Child Pornography in L.A., supra* note 4, at 19.

type of "the grimy old man prowling juvenile hangouts."[31] In contrast, they are often wealthy, mobile, educated, and powerful pillars of the community getting rich off the exploitation of the powerless.[32] Regardless of the participant's societal status, however, it is clear that this new form of child abuse and obscenity has outraged the public. California's State Senator Newton Russell has articulated much of this growing opposition stating "[Child pornography] is a reflection of the societal and spiritual morality of this nation. If there is to be any reversal of the trend, the place to start is child porn."[33]

The Relationship Between Pornographic Material, Child Prostitution, and Child Molestation

Several authorities have found a close relationship between child pornography and the practice of child prostitution.[34] One is often a by-product of the other.[35] Children are invited to "parties" where they are encouraged to enter sexual acts so that photographs may be taken and circulated as advertisements for prostitution.[36] Frequently, the pictures are then reproduced and sold to distributors.[37]

Numerous examples are available of child sexploitation for adult profit.[38] A recent example of child prostitution involved a

---

31. U.S. NEWS, *supra* note 12, at 66 (report of Robert Leonard, president elect of the National District Attorneys' Association).

32. *Kiddie Porn, supra* note 15.

33. TIME, *Child's Garden of Perversity,* April 4, 1977 at 56 (hereinafter cited as *Garden of Perversity*).

34. *S. Rep. on 1585, supra* note 8, at 7.

35. *See generally Children—Big Profit, supra* note 13.

36. *See Garden of Perversity, supra* note 33, at 55.

37. *S. Rep. on 1585, supra* note 8, at 7, cites several examples and states that:
    One such case involved the Reverend Claudius (Bud) Vermilye, Jr. who operated a home for wayward boys in Winchester, Tenn. The Reverend Vermilye encouraged the young boys in his charge to engage in orgies and filmed the orgies with a hidden camera. He then sold the films to certain "sponsors" of the home and also arranged for some of the sponsors to come to the farm and have sex with the boys.

38. *Id.* An example noted by the Senate Committee was that of two men who founded a Boy Scout Troop of 40 boys in New Orleans. About ten boys were regularly selected to go

Chicago based operation known as the Delta Project.[39] Delta Project leaders devised a series of "Delta Dorms" located in large cities around the country. An adult pedophile known as the Delta Don and four or five young boys as Delta Cadets would operate each Delta Dorm. After being solicited through the mails and paying a fee as a Delta sponsor, adult pedophiles would be able to make appointments at the dorms or arrange to have a cadet sent home with him. While it appears that no Delta Dorm was ever founded before the Project was foiled by Chicago undercover investigators, several young cadets were found to be actively promoting the scheme through a multi-state publicity campaign in which they visited one potential sponsor after another.[40]

A few teenagers and young children live at home and "turn tricks" merely for pocket money.[41] Most, however, are runaways, "the products of broken homes and brutality, often inflicted by alcoholic or drug addicted parents."[42] Hungry for a meal and the slightest display of friendship they "take to the streets and use their body for survival and then, beaten by pimps and bereft of self esteem, live in fear of reprisal if they try to escape the racket."[43] New York City is the reputed center for juvenile prostitution with an estimated 20,000 runaways under age sixteen available for pecuniary sex[44] with roughly 800 pimps plying their services.[45]

---

on Scouting trips with a ring of adult males (including three millionaires) with whom they were strongly encouraged to engage in various homosexual acts while being filmed. At the time of the report's publication nineteen adult males had been charged in connection with the case and a scoutmaster had been sentenced to seventy-five years in prison. *See also* U.S. NEWS, *supra* note 12, at 66.

39. *S. Rep on 1585, supra* note 8, at 7,8.

40. Until recently, the shipment of boys across state lines for prostitution was not against any federal law as the Mann Act, 18 U.S.C. 2423 (1948), did not include males and pertained specifically only to prohibiting the interstate transportation of minor females for the purpose of prostitution. S. 1585 however, (passed by both houses of Congress January 24, 1977) amends 18 U.S.C. 2423 to prohibit the interstate transportation of *any minor* for the purposes of engaging in prostitution or prohibited sexual conduct.

41. *Youth for Sale, supra* note 27, at 23.

42. *Id.*

43. *Id..*

44. Pre-teen prostitutes only twelve years old regularly earn $200 a night in Chicago and in Los Angeles; police estimate that as many as 3,000 girls and boys under the age of fourteen are actively engaged in prostitution. *Id.*

45. *Youth for Sale, supra* note 27, at 23.

The vast amount of child pornography seized by police officers at the time of child molestation arrests has convinced many law enforcement agencies that "a direct relationship exists between pornographic literature of this kind and [the] molestation of young children."[46] Amazingly, in a Los Angeles Police Department investigation, where more than 100 victims and suspects were interviewed in over forty child molestation cases during a five month period,[47] pornographic literature, often exhibiting children, was found to be present in *every* case.[48]

Further, evidence indicates that in addition to personal gratification, child pornography is also employed by child molesters[49] "to arouse their victims[50] and to persuade very young children that such behavior is permissible."[51] The California Attorney General's Office noted the following example as illustrative:

> ... a 55 year old man was arrested for attempting to lure a five year old girl
> into his vehicle. In his possession was a brief case containing porno-
> graphic materials depicting children and adults. Because he was a

---

46. CAL. ATT'Y GEN., *supra* note 6, at 18.

47. October 1976 to March 1977.

48. CAL. ATT'Y GEN., *supra* note 6, at 20. "In interviews with a great many police officers the Committee was frequently told: 'I never arrested a child molester who did not have pornography in his possession.' Evidence obtained regarding recent arrests supports these statements." *Id.*

49. An adult heterosexual who is sexually aroused by young girls is normally referred to very broadly as a child molester but an adult homosexual who is sexually aroused by young boys is more specifically termed a *chicken hawk*. Young boys who serve as prostitutes for older men are commonly referred to as *chickens*.

50. CAL. ATT'Y GEN., *supra* note 6, at 19, lists the example of how "a 33 year old man showed pornographic films to his twelve year old victim. The films depicted nude males in homosexual activity and were intended to arouse the victim to commit homosexual acts with the suspect."

51. *Id.* at 19, 20 cites the example of:

> A 23 year old . . . man arrested for sexually molesting two little girls, aged eight
> and seven. At the time of his arrest he had in his possession a large quantity of
> pornographic material in which young girls were depicted. Also discovered
> were a number of nude photographs taken by the suspect of local children.
> Police also found a letter written by the suspect to the publisher of a magazine
> which depicts nude children and which is distributed by a mail order firm in
> Southern California. In the letter the suspect expresses the hope that his own
> little girls (ages two and three) will be able to appear in the publication "when
> they get a little older."

heterosexual, the emphasis of the publications was on young girls. Also in his briefcase was a supply of quality candy, lollipops, small dolls in factory wrappers, books containing pornographic stories, and a tube of petroleum jelly. A two dollar bill was clipped to the flap of the briefcase. This suspect had prepared a 'child molesting' kit which included a large supply of pornographic material.[52]

Thus, because of its apparent relation to child prostitution and molestation,[53] child pornography presents a greater danger than is at first apparent.[54]

Profile of a Sexually Exploited Child

From among the estimated 700,000 to one million children who run away from home each year[55] pedophiles can select thousands of dispossessed "stars" for their books, magazines, films, or prostitution rings.[56] The lonely and hungry runaways serve as a "ready pool of 'acting talent' . . . eager to pose for $5 or $10—or simply a meal and a friendly word."[57] Child sexploitaters

---

52. *Id.* at 19.

53. *Cf. Man's Depravity?, supra* note 17, at 3 (wherein the author attempts to show that an increase in sex-oriented establishments are accompanied by a comparable increase in the amount of crime for that area).

54. *Cf.* F. SCHAUER, THE LAW OF OBSCENITY (1976) wherein the author states:

> As to short-term effects there is fairly universal agreement among the studies done that exposure to erotica results in immediate sexual stimulation. . . . However, although there may very well be a cause-and-effect relationship (between pornography and sex offenders) the case histories do not present strong evidence of this. It may be just as well that the same mental or social aberrations which lead people to commit sex offenses also lead them to pornography . . .. While it seems clear that pornography cannot be shown to be the major cause of sexual antisocial acts, neither can it be completely excluded as a cause, at least among those who might otherwise be disposed. *Id.* at 60, 61.

See, e.g., REPORT OF THE COMMISSION ON OBSCENITY AND PORNOGRAPHY 640-654 (N.Y. Times, ed. 1970) (Minority Report of Charles H. Keating, Jr.). *See also* Hoover, *Combating Merchants of Filth: The Role of the F.B.I.,* 25 U. PITT L. REV. 469 (1964).

55. Recent findings of Senator Birch Bayh's Subcommittee on Juvenile Delinquency as noted in *Developing Legislation, supra* note 9, at 19. *See also, S. Rep on 1585, supra* note 8, at 8.

56. *See S. Rep. on 1585, supra* note 8, at 8.

57. *Garden of Perversity, supra* note 33, at 55.

recruit subjects at bus stations, hamburger stands, or amusement arcades offering gifts such as bicycles or drugs for sexual favors.[58] With small children, even candy or a trip to Disneyland may be sufficient consideration for sexual services.[59]

Lloyd Martin, head of the Los Angeles Police Department's Sexually Abused Child unit, has said, "Sometimes for the price of an ice-cream cone a kid of eight will pose for a producer. He usually trusts the guy because he's getting from him what he can't get from his parents—love."[60] Indeed, a Los Angeles Police Department investigation in September, 1976 revealed that:

> The victims contacted were found to be in need of supportive services. They expressed relief that their activities had been discovered. They often however, expressed some affection for their abusers, similar to that found among children abused by their parents. One victim told the officer, "He (the suspect) is my best friend."[61]

Not all sexually exploited children are runaways. Many come from broken homes.[62] Often parents and guardians are unaware of their children's sexual activity. In some of the most sordid cases, however, parents themselves have led or "sold" their children into pornography or prostitution.[63] Detective Martin has found "a constant rule seems to be that children under the age of nine are usually introduced to it (child pornography or prostitution) by their parents."[64] Often, parents involve their children because they themselves were once pornography stars or models,[65] or they may "sell" their children for money to support their

55. *S. Rep. on 1585, supra* note 8, at 8.

59. *Child Pornography in L.A., supra* note 4, at 19.

60. *Garden of Perversity, supra* note 33, at 55.

61. CAL. ATT'Y GEN., *supra* note 6, at 17.18.

62. They live apparently normal lives with their families and in school. *S. Rep. 1585, supra* note 8, at 8.

63. *Id.*

64. *Child Pornography in L.A., supra* note 4, at 19.

65. "Some children in child pornography are victims of incest. Parents will have intercourse with a son or daughter, then swap pictures with other incestuous parents or send the photos to a sex publisher. Sex periodicals, particularly on the West Coast, publish graphic letters on parents' sexual exploits with their own children." *Garden of Perversity, supra* note 33, at 55.

drug or alcoholic addictions.[66]

In a profile compiled by the Los Angeles Police Department from their investigations and interviews with pornographers,[67] the typical boy participant was described as:

1. Between the ages of 8 and 17;
2. An underachiever in school or at home;
3. Usually without previous homosexual experience;
4. From a home where the parents were absent either physically or psychologically;
5. Without any strong moral or religious affiliations;
6. Suffering from poor sociological development.[68]

The effect of child pornography and prostitution on its child participants is to produce psychological scarring and emotional distress for life.[69] New York psychoanalyst Herbert Freudenberger warns that "Children who pose for pictures begin to see themselves as objects to be sold. They cut off their feelings of affection, finally responding like objects rather than people."[70]

---

66. *See generally Children—Big Profit, supra* note 13, at 5, col. 1 (where a young woman states that she allowed her boy of nine and girl of eleven to be photographed in sexually suggestive poses for $150 because she had just finished school and needed money ". . . so the kids helped mom out.")

67. *S. Rep. on 1585, supra* note 8, at 8.

68. Such sociological factors prompted the Senate Judiciary Committee to remark:
   It should be emphasized that child pornography and prostitution are just individual aspects or symptoms of a larger context of social problems that confront the nation. Broken homes, alienated and runaway children, emotionally disturbed juveniles, alcohol and drug abuse among the very young, and wide spread child abuse are among the national problems that help create the milieus in which child pornography and prostitution can thrive. *S. Rep on 1585, supra* note 8, at 9.

The Committee concluded that:
   Against the backdrop of the breakdown of the family and the fundamental values of our society, questions must be asked regarding the adequacy of our educational system, the effectiveness of our social agencies, our ability to deal with poverty and unemployment, and the quality of our justice system. Child pornography and prostitution are deadly serious problems. But even more menacing is the fact that these are only tips of the iceberg. *Id.*

69. *Developing Legislation, supra* note 9, at 20.

70. *Garden of Perversity, supra* note 33, at 55. Many psychiatrists maintain that sexually exploited children are often unable to find sexual fulfillment as adults.

Further, authorities[71] generally agree that the deep psychological and humiliating impact of such sexual activity[72] perpetuates a vicious cycle whereby the degraded child joins other deviant populations: drug addicts, prostitutes, criminals, and pre-adult parents.[73] More tragic, however, is the fact that sexually exploited children tend to become sexual exploiters of children themselves as adults.[74]

Perhaps the affect on sexually exploited children is best summarized in the queries of Los Angeles Police Chief Davis, "Who could hold out any hope that children so abused in their formative years will ever make positive contributions to society? Child pornography has to be the nadir of man's depravity. What vice can possibly remain to be exploited?"[75]

---

71. *S. Rep. on 1585, supra* note 8, at 9. CAL. ATT'Y GEN., *supra* note 6, at 18, *Garden of Perversity, supra* note 33, at 55. *See generally* (authorities commenting on the harmful effect of disseminating pornographic materials to children) Dibble, *Obscenity: A State Quarantine to Protect Children,* 39 SO. CAL. L. REV. 345 (1966); Wall, *Obscenity and Youth: The Problem and a Possible Solution,* 1 CRIM. L. BULL. 8, 21 (1965); Note, 55 CAL. L. REV. 926, 934 (1967); Comment, 34 FORD L. REV. 692, 694 (1966); Green, *Obscenity, Censorship and Juvenile Delinquency,* 14 U. TORONTO L. REV. 229, 249 (1962); Lockhart and McClure, *Literature, The Law of Obscenity, and the Constitution,* 38 MINN. L. REV. 295, 373-385 (1954); Note, 52 KY. L.J. 429, 447 (1964). Especially *see* Dr. Gaylin of the Columbia University Psychoanalytic Clinic, reporting on the views of some psychiatrists in Gaylin, *The Prickly Problems of Pornography,* 77 YALE L.J. 579, 592-93 (1968) where he states:

> It is in the period of growth [youth] when these patterns of behavior are laid down, when environmental stimuli of all sorts must be integrated into a workable sense of self, when sensuality is being defined and fears elaborated, when pleasure confronts security and impulse encounters control—it is in this period, undramatically and with time, that legalized pornography may conceivably be damaging.

72. *But see* R. Currier, . . . *Or a Sign of Society's Continuing Blindness?* L.A. Times, § 5, at 3, col. 2 (wherein the author argues that child sexuality and eroticism with other children or adults is "natural, normal, healthy and good" and has in actuality been suppressed in our society as a result of the adult sexual revolution).

73. *Developing Legislation, supra* note 9, at 20.

74. *S. Rep. on 1585, supra* note 8, at 9.

75. *Man's Depravity?, supra* note 17, at 3. It is recognized that former Chief Davis is not a child psychology expert, but he is nonetheless very well acquainted with the problem as a respected authority on vice related crimes and founder of the Sexually Exploited Child Unit in Los Angeles.

Constructing An Effective And Proper Cure

The Ineffectiveness of Existing Applicable Law

The conclusion of the above overview is that child sexploitation is a new form of child abuse growing at an alarming rate whose effect is clearly damaging to the health of society as a whole, and the children so readily exploited. Strong, prosecutable, and effective law is urgently required to stall its spread and fill the void of existing state and federal legislation. Understandably, legislators could not have been expected to foresee child sexploitation's rapid rise.

Federal law presently prohibits the *distribution* of obscene materials. Four different agencies[76] are responsible for enforcing five federal obscenity laws which prohibit any mailing,[77] importation,[78] or interstate transportation of obscene materials,[79] broadcasts of obscenity,[80] as well as the interstate transportation of females under eighteen years of age for the purposes of prostitution.[81] Additionally, the public may request that there be no further delivery of unsolicited mailings or advertisements which are sexually offensive under the Anti-Pandering Act of 1968.[82]

These federal statutes are not "adequate weapons to combat child pornography and child prostitution."[83] No federal statute specifically regulates the distribution of sexual material *to* children, or the production, distribution, and sale of child pornography in interstate commerce.[84] Also, federal law prohibiting the interstate transportation of young females for

---

76. The Department of Justice, the Federal Bureau of Investigation, the Postal Service and the Customers Service.

77. 18 U.S.C. § 1461 (1948).

78. 18 U.S.C. § 1462 (1948).

79. 18 U.S.C. § 1465 (1955).

80. 18 U.S.C. § 1464 (1948).

81. 18 U.S.C. § 2423 (1948).

82. 39 U.S.C. § 3008 (1968).

83. *S. Rep. on 1585, supra* note 8, at 9.

84. *See Developing Legislation, supra* note 8, at 19.

purposes of prostitution[85] is silent as to such practice with young boys.[86] The gap is widened by the practice of federal authorities to initiate investigations only when large manufacturers or distributors, including organized crime, are involved.[87]

On the state level, forty-seven states and the District of Columbia have enacted statutes prohibiting the dissemination of obscene materials to minors.[88] However, only eight states have passed legislation to specifically prohibit the sexual exploitation of minors in pornographic materials or to regulate the distribution and sale of child pornography or child prostitution.[89]

---

85. 18 U.S.C. § 2423 (1948).

86. *Youth for Sale, supra* note 27, at 23.

87. *S. Rep. on 1585, supra* note 8, at 9, 10. Therefore most of the sources of child pornography and prostitution never came within the purview of the statute.

88. CAL. PENAL CODE § 311-312 (West 1966); COLO. REV. STAT. ANN. § 40-9-16 to 40-9-27 (1963); CONN. GEN. STAT. REV. § 53-243 to 53-245 (Supp. 1965); DEL. CODE ANN., Tit. 11, §§ 435, 711-713 (1953); FLA. STAT. ANN. § 847.0011-847.06 (1965 and Supp. 1968); GA. CODE ANN., § 26-6301 to 26-6309 a (Supp. 1967); HAWAII REV. LAWS § 267-8 (1955); IDAHO CODE ANN §§ 18-1506 to 18-1510 (Supp. 1967); ILL. ANN. STAT. C38 §§ 11-20 to 11-21 (Supp. 1967); IOWA CODE ANN. §§ 725.4-725.12 (1950); KY. REV. STAT. §§ 436.100-436.130, 436.540-436.580 (1963 and Supp. 1966); LA. REV. STAT. §§ 14:91.11, 14.92, 14.106 (Supp. 1967); ME. REV. STAT. ANN., Tit. 17, §§ 2901-2905 (1964); MD. ANN. CODE. Art. 27, §§ 417-425 (1957 and Supp. 1967); MASS. GEN. LAWS ANN., c. 272, §§ 28-33 (1959 and Supp. ... :8); MICH. STAT. ANN. §§ 28.575-28.579 (1954 and Supp. 1968); MO. ANN. STAT §§ 563.270-563.310 (1953 and Supp. 1967); MONT. REV. CODES ANN. §§ 94-3601 to 94-3606 (1947 and Supp. 1967); NEB. REV. STAT. §§ 28-926.09 to 28-926.10 (1965 Cum. Supp.); NEV. REV. STAT. §§ 201.250, 207.180 (1965); N.H. REV. STAT. ANN. §§ 571-A:1 to 571-A:5 (Supp. 1967); N.J. STAT. ANN. §§ 2A:115-1.1 to 2A:115-4 (Supp. 1967); N.C. GEN. STAT. §§ 14-189 (Supp. 1967); N.D. CENT. CODE §§ 12-21-07 to 12-21-09 (1960); OHIO REV. CODE ANN. §§ 2903.10-2903.11, 2905.34-2905.39 (1954 and Supp. 1966); OKLA. STAT. ANN. Tit. 21, §§ 1021-1024, 1032-1039 (1958 and Supp. 1967); PA. STAT. ANN. Tit. 18, §§ 3831-3833, 4524 (1963 and Supp. 1967); R.I. GEN. LAWS ANN. §§ 11-31-1 to 11-31-10 (1956 and Supp. 1967); S.C. CODE ANN. §§ 16-414.1 to 16-421 (1962 and Supp. 1967); TEX. PEN. CODE: ARTS 526, 5276 (1952 and Supp. 1967); UTAH CODE ANN. §§ 76-39-5, 76-39-17 (Supp. 1967); VT. STAT. ANN., Tit. 13, §§ 2801-2805 (1959); VA. CODE ANN. §§ 18.1-227 to 18.1-236.3 (1960 and Supp. 1966); W. VA. CODE ANN. §§ 61 and 8-11 (1966); WYO. STAT. ANN. §§ 6-103, 7-148 (1957).

89. CAL. LAB. CODE §§ 1309.5-1309.6 (West 1977) and CAL. PENAL CODE § 311.4 (West 1977); CONN. GEN. STAT. ANN. § 53-25 (1977); N.C. GEN. STAT. § 14-190.1, *et seq.*, (1971); N.D. CENT. CODE §§ 12.1-27, 1-03, (1975); N.Y. PENAL CODE § 263.05 (McKinney 1977) recently held unconstitutionally overbroad in St. Martin's Press Inc. v. Carey, 46 U.S. L.W. 2297 (Nov. 28, 1977); S.C. CODE ANN. § 16-414.1 *et seq.* (1977); TENN. CODE ANN. § 39-3013 (1975); TEX. CODE ANN. § 43.24 (1977) recently held unconstitutionally overbroad on its face in Graham v. Hill, No. A-77-CA-188 (W.D. Tex., filed Jan. 30. 1978).

State statutes covering sex crimes are generally of no avail because the physical acts involved in producing child pornography may fall short of the criminal criteria[90] or they may be worded so broadly as to discourage courts from applying them in terms of significant sanctions that are directly on point.[91] Another factor that makes it difficult to prosecute producers for sex abuse crimes is that while there may be ample evidence of such crimes in the pornographic material itself, the abused children are difficult to identify and rarely located.[92]

Child welfare provisions in state education laws often regulate the employment of children in sexual activities, and prohibit immoral acts, but generally are either not applicable when the child is working for a parent[93] (from which much pornography is derived[94]) or the penalties are so limited as to pose no real deterrent.[95]

Without any other effective alternatives available, most prosecution must be for contributing to the delinquency of a minor,[96] or under the state's general obscenity laws which make no distinction between children and adults as pornographic models.[97] Such offenses are almost always only misdemeanors and pose no real hazard to producers of child pornography, much less distributors and sellers, who accept the low risk of prosecution as a cost of doing business for such high profits.[98]

The ineffectiveness of existing laws becomes more evident when confronted with the difficult task of prosecution and conviction. Exploited children are rarely located to aid in prosecution. Producers insulate themselves by hiding behind a myriad of

---

90. *E.g.,* rape, sodomy, incest, etc. *Developing Legislation, supra* note 9, at 20.

91. *Id.*

92. *See Garden of Perversity, supra* note 33, at 55.

93. *E.g.,* MICH. ACT 157, PUBLIC ACTS of 1947 (as amended) § 409.14 (1967).

94. *See* text and material accompanying notes 62-66.

95. *E.g.,* N.Y. EDUC. LAW § 3231(a), (c) (1972).

96. And as discussed previously, finding the minor is no easy task. *See* text accompanying note 92.

97. *Garden of Perversity, supra* note 33, at 55. "One result: many lawyers believe that the genital pictures in *Lollitots,* however offensive, might be judged no more obscene under the law than similar photos of adult women in most men's magazines." *Id.*

98. As to profits, *see* text accompanying notes 16-21.

deceptive dummy corporations.[99] Perhaps more damaging is the fact that the courts themselves often discourage and frustrate the few criminal investigations that are successful. Such a case is that of Edward Mishkin, a leading wholesaler, who was arrested when New York City police, after a year's investigation, seized 1,200 pornographic films and magazines, many depicting children. Upon conviction he could have received up to a seven year prison sentence, but instead, was sentenced to weekends in jail for six months.[100]

More recently, Judge Margaret Taylor of the New York Family Court caused a public uproar when she dismissed prostitution charges against a fourteen year old girl, ruling that prostitution laws are unconstitutional because unmarried adults, including prostitutes and their customers, have a constitutional right to privacy in the pursuit of pleasure.[101] The judge stated in her decision that, "Sex for a fee is recreational . . . The arguments that prostitution harms the public health, safety or welfare do not withstand constitutional scrutiny."[102]

Due to the newness of the criminal offense, lack of applicable and effective legislation, and poor enforcement record, virtually no decisional law exists wherein the central issue was the sexual exploitation of children in pornography or prostitution. In *People v. Byrnes*[103] an eleven year old girl testified that her father had taken her to a photographer's home where he filmed her and her father engaging in various sexual acts. On appeal from his conviction for rape, sodomy, and incest, the father argued that he was convicted solely on the uncorroborated testimony of his daughter. The court, however, held that photos of the explicit acts had been properly admitted as evidence.

Similarly, in *State v. Kasold*,[104] the defendant was convicted on

---

99. *See Garden of Perversity, supra* note 33, at 55.

100. MacPherson, *Children: The Limits of Porn,* Washington Post, Jan. 30, 1977, § C, at 1.

101. L.A. Times, Jan. 26, 1978, § I, at 1, col. 5.

102. *Id.* at 17, col. 1.

103. 33 N.Y. 2d 343, 308 N.E. 2d 435, 352 N.Y.S. 2d 913 (1974).

104. 110 Ariz. 558, 521 P.2d 990 (1974).

evidence that included photos of himself exposing his genitals before a fully clothed little girl who had her back to the camera.[105]

A defendant had photographed a nude thirteen-year-old girl in *St. Paul V. Campbell*[106] and was convicted of disorderly conduct. On appeal the court declared that disorderly conduct was not the appropriate charge and reversed, pointing out that a conviction would certainly have been reasonable for contributing to the delinquency of a minor or employing a minor for immoral purposes.

Finally, in *People v. Burrows*[107] the California Court of Appeals affirmed Burrows' conviction for false imprisonment and using a minor in the preparation of obscene materials when an adult had bound his twenty year old victim[108] hand and foot, sexually abused him, and then photographed him in indecent positions.

In light of the above discussion, it is evident there are voids in existing state and federal legislation in the prevention of child sexploitation that must urgently be filled with new, effective, and constitutionally appropriate legislation.

Overcoming Constitutional and Practical Hurdles

Regulating child sexploitation is a difficult and complicated task. The area is emotionally charged and intellectually confusing. The chief problem confronting legislators is the blending of two distinct, but related problems: the abuse of children in producing the pornographic materials and its distribution and sale. Both areas must be approached separately before enforcement can effectively be applied and constitutional problems can be avoided.

Child pornography is in essence a hybrid industry composed

---

105. Concerning the employment of photos of a person's anatomy as criminal evidence in trial, *see* Annot., 9 A.L.R.2d 889, 923-26 (1950).

106. 287 Minn. 171, 177 N.W. 2d 304 (1970).

107. 260 Cal. App. 2d 228, 67 Cal. Rptr. 28 (1968).

108. At the time of the crime, the age of majority was twenty-one and therefore the twenty-year-old victim was still deemed a minor.

first of producers, who directly exploit the child physically to create a pornographic product, and secondly the close association of manufacturers, distributors, and retailers who cultivate and perpetuate the child pornography market.

Regulation of both aspects, the child abusing producer as well as the distribution and retail of the pornographic materials, must be dealt with individually and harmonized to provide the most powerful deterrent to the practice of child sexploitation. This would limit pornographic production and destroy the vast market upon which child sexploiters feed.

Penalizing producers alone would definitely not be enough to effectively deter child sexploitation or the child molestation encouraged by such pornographic material.[109] Legislation aimed solely at producers would only serve to drive them underground where they would continue their business. The already difficult problem of locating, prosecuting, and convicting child sexploiters would be even more difficult. Further, the common practice of film and magazine pirating will maintain retail supplies so that there will be no slack in the market. Distributors, who receive most of the profits, are the principal figures in the child pornography enterprise. Products can continually be reproduced to the point that child subjects could someday be seen by their own children.[110] Thus, for child pornography laws to be effective they must regulate not only production, but also the distribution and sale of the product as well.

Once the sexual exploitation is published in print or on film[111] it is then subject to first amendment scrutiny.[112] If it is considered legally obscene, it is not speech that is protectable by the first amendment. However, if not considered to be obscene[113] it is

---

109. *See* text and material accompanying notes 46-54 on the relationship of pornographic material to child molesting and abuse.

110. *See Child Pornography in L.A., supra* note 3, at 19.

111. Motion pictures are clearly protected by the first amendment as an expression of speech even if shown or sold for commercial purposes. *See* Joseph Burstyn Inc. v. Wilson, 343 U.S. 495 (1952).

112. U.S. CONST. amend. I provides in pertinent part: "Congress shall make no law . . . abridging the freedom of speech or of the press."

113. Simply because material is considered to be pornographic (the depiction of erotic

protectable expression which can*not* be infringed upon by the government.[114]

State and Federal legislators, responding to the urgent need, are proposing "a kind of end run around obscenity laws and the first amendment problems attendant thereto—a ban on sexually explicit pictures of children, whether legally obscene or not."[115] Proponents of the wide sweeping legislation maintain that it is directed at detering a specific type of *conduct*, child abuse, and is in no way seeking to impinge on free speech.[116] Child pornography is therefore perceived as a form of abuse rather than a form of obscenity.[117] An example of this type of law is H. R. 3913[118] which would make *any* proven involvement with the production and sale of explicit sex pictures of childs, *whether or not obscene*, a felony.[119] It therefore not only reaches *all* of the conduct sought to be deterred but also *all* of the parties involved in perpetuating it without ever coming under the purview of the first amendment. Attempting to regulate the conduct, child abuse law regulates non-obscene and obscene as well and therefore impinges on protected speech as well as unprotected.

---

behavior intending to cause sexual excitement) does not necessarily determine whether or not the material is obscene and unprotected speech.

114. Roth v. United States, 354 U.S. 476 (1957) (hereinafter cited as *Roth*) (wherein the Court stated for the first time its reason that obscenity was not protected because it was without redeeming social importance).

115. *Garden of Perversity, supra* note 33, at 55, 56. *See, e.g.,* N.Y. PENAL CODE § 263.05 (McKinney 1977); TEX. CODE ANN. § 43.24 (1977); Roth Amendment to S. 1585, Cong. Q. at 2205 (Oct. 15, 1977); H.R. 3913, 95th Cong., 1st Sess. (1977) (hereinafter cited as H.R. 3913).

116. *See* E. Goodman, *A Clear Case of Villainy,* L.A. Times, March 15, 1977, § 2, at 7, col. 1 where the author argues that:

> This is not a First Amendment issue. It is not a matter of legislating the sexual fantasies of adults. It's a matter protecting the real lives of young models. We can take kid porn out of the realms of sex and into the realm of power where it belongs. The children are victims, and kid porn is the exploitation of the powerless by the more powerful. That exploitation is as common to adult-child relationships as is protection.

117. *Garden of Perversity, supra* note 33, at 56.

118. H.R. 3913, *supra* note 115.

119. Thus, "salesmen in an adult bookstore could be prosecuted as an active participant in the crime of sexually exploiting the children pictured in the store's magazines." *Garden of Perversity, supra* note 33, at 56.

Opponents argue that since such legislation indiscriminately fails to discern between protected and unprotected obscene speech, it is void and unconstitutional for being overbroad.[120] *Roth v. United States*[121] stood for the principle that only non-obscene speech is protectable against infringement because obscenity was "utterly without redeeming social importance."[122]

The Supreme Court announced its most recent test for determining whether or not certain material is obscene in *Miller v. California*.[123] The Court said obscenity is determined[124] by testing whether the average person in the community would find the work *as a whole* appealing to the prurient interests[125] and lacking in serious social value.[126]

Still, despite the great reception accorded the test in *Miller*, and all the reams of print and legal scholarship accorded the subject,

---

120. For a good discussion on the doctrines of both overbreadth and vagueness *see* Grayned v. Rockford, 408 U.S. 104 (1972).

121. *Roth, supra* note 114.

122. Often referred to as the Roth-Memoirs test from the case of A Book Named John Cleland's Memoirs of a Woman of Pleasure v. Massachusetts, 383 U.S. 413 (1966) (hereinafter cited as *Memoirs*) wherein the Court held that the utter absence of redeeming social importance would not be presumed from the fact that material was "obscene," but rather it was an element which had to be proven in order to declare that the item was obscene.

123. Miller v. California, 413 U.S. 15 (1973) (hereinafter cited as *Miller*). After *Roth*, no majority would concur in a single substantive obscenity opinion until *Miller*.

124. The basic guidelines for the trier of fact must be: (a) whether the average person, applying contemporary community standards would find that the work taken as a whole, appeals to the prurient interest, (b) whether the work depicts or describes, in a patently offensive way, sexual conduct specifically defined by the applicable state law, and (c) whether the work, taken as a whole, lacks serious, literary, artistic, political, or scientific value. *Id.* at 74.

125. "Prurient interest" is said to refer to a morbid interest in sex, presumably as differentiated from a normal, healthy interest in the same subject. The normative and subjective aspects of this definition have been a source of continuing problems.

126. With respect to redeeming social value, the *Miller* Court said:
   We do not adopt as a constitutional standard the "utterly without redeeming social value" test of Memoirs; that concept has never commanded more than three Justices at one time. If a state law that regulates obscene material is thus limited, as written or construed, the First Amendment values applicable to the States (are) adequately protected by the ultimate power of appellate courts to conduct an independent review of constitutional claims when necessary. 413 U.S. at 24-25.

determining what is and what is not obscene is no easier a task than when the debate began.[127] Existing and proposed statutes that ban material depicting children engaged in or observing "*any* sexually explicit conduct"[128] prohibit the distribution and sale of protectable and socially valuable materials that may contain only brief portions of child nudity or sexual activity as part of a more meaningful overall purpose. Such a ban directed at actual conduct, as a form of child abuse, necessarily also regulates a form of free speech and therefore must comply with current obscenity standard as delineated in *Miller v. California;*[129] that "the average person applying contemporary community standards would find the work *taken as a whole,* appeals to the prurient interest . . . and whether the work, *taken as a whole,* lacks serious literary, artistic, political, scientific value."[130] (Emphasis added).

Such sweeping legislative prohibitions fall desparately short of *Miller* standards and are clearly overbroad.[131] Legislative critics and civil libertarians quickly point out that such highly acclaimed films as "The Exorcist," which contains a brief scene in

---

127. The difficulty is exemplified by the fact that such serious and critically acclaimed films as "Carnal Knowledge", and books like James Joyce's ULYSSES and D. H. Lawrence's LADY CHATTERLY'S LOVER have at one time or another been thought "obscene" by government censors. *See* DE GRAZIA, CENSORSHIP LANDMARKS (1968); B. Pines, *The Obscenity Quagmire,* 49 CAL. ST. B.J. 509 (1974); Jenkins v. Georgia, 418 U.S. 153 (1974); United States v. One Book Called "Ulysses", 5 F. Supp. 182 (S.D.N.Y. 1933), *aff'd,* 72 F.2d 705 (2d Cir. 1934), while such celebrated works of erotica as "Behind the Green Door", "Deep Throat", and "Devil in Miss Jones" have repeatedly been found not to be obscene. *See,* People v. Mitchell, No. 31458699 (Cal., L.A. Mun. Ct. 1974); People v. Gass, No. M, 106475 (Cal., Citrus Mun. Ct. 1974); City of East Detroit v. Adams, No. 0-6823 (Mich., E. Detroit Mun. Ct. 1974).

128. *See, e.g.,* H.R. 3913, *supra* note 115, N.Y. PENAL CODE § 263.05 (McKinney 1977); TEX. CODE ANN. § 43.24 (1977).

129. *Supra,* note 123.

130. 413 U.S. at 24.

131. Laws are unconstitutionally overbroad when they are susceptible of application to conduct protected by the first amendment. A statute which may be clear and precise as to the conduct proscribed nonetheless may be struck down as unconstitutionally overbroad where it sweeps within its ambit speech or conduct which is not subject to suppression. If so, it must be declared unconstitutional on its face, regardless of the fact that the conduct could be regulated by a more narrow statute. Grayned v. Rockford, 408 U.S. 104 (1972); Coates v. Cincinnati. 402 U.S. 611 (1971); Dandridge v. Williams, 397 U.S. 471 (1970).

which a minor simulates masturbation, and "Romeo and Juliet," where a minor appears briefly in the nude, would be prohibited under such legislation even though they are clearly not obscene.[132]

Likewise, even if new child pornography laws are not overbroad for prohibiting all materials depicting any and all child sexploitation, they may still be constitutionally void for vagueness because they often attempt to hedge beyond obscenity lines. Covering material containing "nudity,"[133] "sadism and masochism,"[134] "any other sexual activity,"[135] and other general terms without specifically limiting its regulation to obscene materials, such laws are too vague to be within the specificity required by *Miller*. These vagaries, like overbroad statutes, deter privileged

---

132. *See S. Rep. on S. 1585, supra* note 8, at 12-13. *Accord* H.R. Rep. No. 696, 95th Cong., 1st Sess. (1977) where the House Committee on the Judiciary concluded at 7:
> We agree that there is no First Amendment question in providing for prosecution of persons who abuse children. However, once those photos and films are reduced to magazines, movies, etc., numerous court decisions including Supreme Court decisions, make clear that they are permissible under the First Amendment guarantee of free speech unless they are proven to be obscene.
> Although H.R. 3913 purports to cover distributors and sellers as abusers, the fact is that they ordinarily are remotely removed from the actual abuse, and, in prosecuting them without showing any participation in the actual abuse, we are in fact prosecuting for the distribution or sale of the material.

133. *S. Rep. on 1585, supra* note 8, at 11 reviewing proposed legislation (S. 1011) which would prohibit the depiction of "Nudity, if such nudity is depicted for the purpose of sexual stimulation or gratification of any individual who may view such depiction" said:
> [The] language is so broad that it could conceivably prohibit such innocent scenes as "skinny dipping" or even nude snapshots of babies that were mailed to grandparents. This is particularly true since the proposed test for offensiveness is the sexual stimulation or gratification of *any* individual rather than using the standard of the *average* individual as required by the Supreme Court in Roth v. United States 354 U.S. 476 (1957) and Miller v. California 413 U.S. 445 (1973).

134. *See, e.g., id.* at 27, where the example is given that:
> "Sadism" and "masochism" are broad enough to cover activities which are not necessarily sexually oriented. They could include filmed episodes of physical mistreatment of orphans, child laborers or inmates of a juvenile detention facility or a child inflicting injury upon himself. Such portrayals would have no sexual appeal except, perhaps, to some tiny segment of society.

135. *Id.*, it was also noted that this phrase is so broad that it could conceivably prohibit such innocent conduct as hugging and kissing.

activity as well as obscene activity and therefore are unconstitutional.[136]

A recent case on first amendment overbreadth and vagueness is *Erznoznik v. City of Jacksonville*,[137] wherein the United States Supreme Court invalidated a local Florida ordinance which prohibited the showing, at certain locations, of motion pictures "in which the human male or female bare buttocks, human female bare breasts, or human bare pubic areas are shown . . ."

In striking down the ordinance, the Court noted that the restriction was broader than permissible. The Court stated that the ordinance:

> . . . sweepingly forbids display of all films containing any uncovered buttocks or breasts, irrespective or context or pervasiveness. Thus it would bar a film containing a picture of a baby's buttocks, the nude body of a war victim or scenes from a culture in which nudity is indigenous. The ordinance also might prohibit newsreel scenes of the opening of an art exhibit as well as shots of bathers on a beach. Clearly all nudity cannot be deemed obscene even as to minors.[138]

Child pornography statutes that reach protected expression as well as obscenity are therefore void on their face for overbreadth and may also be unconstitutional on grounds of vagueness.[139]

Recognizing it is inevitable that child pornography legislation

---

136. The United States Supreme Court has permitted broad standing to attack constitutionally overbroad statutes in order to prevent their existence from deterring others. For example, in Broadrick v. Oklahoma, 413 U.S. 601 (1973), the Court stated that the litigants would be permitted to challenge the statute not only because their own rights of free expression were violated but because the mere existence of the statute could cause others not before the court to refrain from engaging in constitutionally protected speech or expression. *See also* Gooding v. Wilson, 405 U.S. 518 (1972) and Lewis v. New Orleans, 415 U.S. 130 (1974). In Bigelow v. Virginia, 421 U.S. 809 (1975), the United States Supreme Court held that an actor had standing to challenge a statute as facially overbroad regardless of whether his own conduct could have been regulated by a more narrowly drawn statute. *See also* Doran v. Salem Inn, Inc., 422 U.S. 922 (1975) where the United States Supreme Court held that public bars had standing to raise a challenge, based on an alleged violation of the first and fourteenth amendments, to the overbreadth of a town ordinance prohibiting bust exposure.
137. 422 U.S. 205 (1975).
138. *Id.* at 213.
139. *Id. See also* Butler v. Michigan, 352 U.S. 380 (1957).

must subject itself to first amendment review,[140] some scholars argue that, as applied to children, the Supreme Court should broaden its present obscenity standards and create a new definition of obscenity.[141]

The Court has permitted certain justifiable infringements on the expression of free speech where as stated in *United States v. O'Brien*[142] regulation (1) is within the constitutional power of the government, (2) furthers an important or substantial governmental interest, unrelated to the suppression of free expression, and (3) imposes only an incidental restriction on an alleged first amendment right that is no greater than is essential to the furtherance of the interest.[143]

Child pornography laws legitimately seek to further the government's important interest in protecting its children from sexual exploitation.[144] It is within the government's power and is unrelated to free speech. Analogously, the U.S. Supreme Court in *Ginsberg v. New York*[145] upheld a New York statute which made it a crime to disseminate obscene materials to minors because the legislature could rationally conclude that the exposure of minors to obscene material is harmful to their "ethical and moral development."[146] The Court said states could properly seek to support the interests of parents in controlling their children's access to obscene material.[147] *Ginsberg's* great significance to child pornography laws, however, is that it promulgated double obsenity standards, one applicable to adults and the other, more expansive in nature, to children. *Ginsberg* cited with favor the opinion of the New York Court of Appeal in *Bookcase, Inc. v. Broderick*[148] that:

---

140. *Supra* note 129.
141. *See* CONG. Q., Nov. 12, 1977 at 2416.
142. 391 U.S. 367 (1968).
143. *Id.* at 377.
144. *See* Prince v. Massachusetts, 321 U.S. 138 (1944).
145. 390 U.S. 629 (1968).
146. *Id.* at 641.
147. *Id.* at 639.
148. 18 N.Y.2d 71, 218 N.E.2d 668 (1966).

Material which is protected for distribution to adults is not necessarily constitutionally protected from restriction upon its dissemination to children. In other words, the concept of obscenity or of unprotected matter may vary according to the group to whom the questionable material is directed or from whom it is quarantined. Because of the State's exigent interest in preventing distribution to children of objectionable material, it can exercise it power to protect the health, safety, welfare and morals of its community by barring the distribution to children of books recognized to be suitable for adults.[149]

Also in support of its expansive obscenity definition for children the Court repeated the concurring opinion of Chief Judge Fuld in *People v. Kahan*[150] where he stated:

While the supervision of children's reading may best be left to their parents, the knowledge that parental control or guidance cannot always be provided and society's transcendent interest in protecting the welfare of children justify reasonable regulation of the sale of material to them. It is, therefore, altogether fitting and proper for a state to include in a statute designed to regulate the sale of pornography to children special standards, broader than those embodied in legislation aimed at controlling dissemination of such material to adults.[151]

It has been argued that the logic of *Ginsberg* should be applied to the abuse of minors in the production of obscene material to justify the recognized infringement that child pornography laws may impose on free expression.[152] If the state can constitutionally protect a minor's welfare by restricting materials available to him or her, it follows that the state possesses authority to prohibit publication of sexually explicit materials which use minors as subjects.

In face of the strong constitutional protection accorded non-obscene material,[153] it cannot be concluded, with any certainty, that this rationale for the regulation of child pornography will

---

149. *Id.* at 75, 218 N.E. 2d at 671.

150. 15 N.Y.2d 311, 206 N.E.2d 333 (1965).

151. *Id.* at 312, 206 N.E. 2d at 334.

152. *Developing Legislation, supra* note 9, at 23.

153. *See* Erznoznik v. City of Jacksonville, 422 U.S. 205 (1975); Butler v. Michigan, 352 U.S. 380 (1957).

withstand constitutional attack.[154] It should be noted that whereas *Ginsberg* dealt with the dissemination of obscenity *to* children, thus restricting the seller's right to distribute to children and the children's right to buy, child pornography laws concern the *production* and distribution of pornographic materials in which children are subjects, and denies access by anyone, child or adult, to such material. The Senate Judiciary Committee reported in its review of proposed federal legislation prohibiting the sexual exploitation of children:

> It was the opinion of the experts who testified before the Committee that virtually all of the materials that are normally considered child pornography are obscene under the current standards. Thus they can be prohibited under the existing federal obscenity statutes. Indeed as was noted earlier, federal authorities have already begun an extensive crack down on child pornography. In comparison with this blatant pornography, non-obscene materials that depict children are very few and very inconsequential. Thus it would be extremely unwise to jeopardize the effectiveness of any federal effort to combat hard core child pornography by also attempting to prohibit the sale and distribution of such non-obscene and relatively innocent materials as "The Exorcist" and "Romeo and Juliet".[155]

Therefore, little would be lost by isolating the two areas of production and distribution and sale of child pornography, and handling them separately. The child abuse inherent in pornography production can be entirely prohibited by broad legislation unrelated to first amendment rights. At the same time increased penalties and extensive crackdowns on distributors and retailers will greatly enhance the deterrent effectiveness of present obscenity statutes while still staying safely within the bounds of first amendment confines.

Such a delicate balance appears to weigh in the favor of first amendment rights over any justifiable infringement, but this balancing decision is undoubtedly one that will ultimately be decided by the U.S. Supreme Court. Until then, it appears that initial confrontations have been decided in favor of free speech

---

154. *Accord, S. Rep. on 1585, supra* note 8, at 27.
155. *S. Rep. on S. 1585, supra* note 8, at 13.

rights narrowly limiting child pornography legislation pertaining to publishers, promoters, distributors, and sellers. In *St. Paul's Press, Inc. v. Carey*,[156] a Federal District Court in New York granted a preliminary injunction preventing enforcement of a New York statute making it a felony to produce or promote any performance that includes sexual conduct by a child. In so deciding the court concluded that:

> The New York legislature may have decided that it is too difficult if not impossible to stop this exploitation of children by going after only those who produce the photographs and movies, and that the most expeditious if not the only practical method of law enforcement is to dry up the market for this material by imposing severe criminal penalties on those promoting, distributing, advertising and selling the product. If so, the court believes there is a serious question whether the state, in choosing to punish publishers, distributors, advertisers and booksellers for their activities with respect to a non-obscene book, has chosen the least drastic means of accomplishing its goal consistent with preserving first amendment rights.[157]

Similarly, in *Graham v. Hill*,[158] the Federal District Court for the Western District of Texas declared a hurriedly enacted Texas child pornography statute[159] unconstitutionally overbroad. The court recognized the important state interest in deterring the sexual exploitation of minors,[160] but nonetheless stated "In this area, (free speech) the Court must be vigilant to safeguard

---

156. 46 U.S. L.W. 2297 (Nov. 28, 1977).

157. *Id.*

158. No. A-77-CA-188 (W.D. Tex., filed Jan. 30, 1978).

159. TEX. PENAL CODE § 43.25 (1977) provides as follows:

(a) A person commits an offense if, knowing the content of the material, he sells, commercially distributes, commercially exhibits, or possesses for sale, commercial distribution, or commercial exhibition any motion picture or photograph showing a person younger than 17 years of age observing or [sic] engaging in sexual conduct.

(b) It is an affirmative defense to prosecution under this section that the obscene material was possessed by a person having scientific, educational, governmental, or other similar justification.

(c) An offense under this section is a felony of the third degree.

160. Graham v. Hill, *supra* at 5:

The Court's task is made even more difficult in a case such as this, where the

legitimate first amendment rights, even if to do so may in some cases be a distasteful task."[161]

Because the Texas statute failed to require that the work be found obscene, the *Graham* court pointed out that "the statute would permit the suppression of a motion picture, and the imprisonment of a theatre manager or owner, regardless of whether or not, taken as a whole, the work is obscene."[162] Further, unwilling to expand its definition of obscenity as to children[163] it was stated that:

> The Court does not believe, either, that § 43.25 could pass constitutional muster as written on the justification that it is a measure to protect the safety and welfare of minors, or to prevent their exploitation and abuse. If the statute were limited to prohibiting the depiction of minors actually engaging in sexual conduct, or even if the statute merely prohibited the observance of actual sexual conduct by minors, the Court would likely have no hesitation in declaring its constitutionality. *See Ginsberg v. New York*, 390 U.S. 629 (1968). But the blanket prohibition in § 43.25 against exhibiting motion pictures just because they contain a scene in which a young person is shown observing sexual conduct, without any prerequisite that the film be obscene or that the minor's part in the film in any way involves sexual exploitation, renders the statute overbroad. In light of the total failure to require that the material proscribed by § 43.25 be obscene, the Court cannot avoid the conclusion that the statute clearly is overbroad, and that its deterrent effect on protected conduct is both real and substantial, especially considering the severe sanctions for violation of the statute.[164]

Thus, overbroad state child pornography statutes have not faired well initially, but undoubtedly more confrontations between child abuse laws and first amendment rights have yet to

---

state through its criminal laws seeks to control what it views as a serious problem created by the exploitation of minors in the making of pornographic photographs and films. This is an important matter; accordingly, the Court must and does give strong consideration to the state's interest in enforcing the policy expressed in the statute, and the Court by no means depreciates the state's concern for minors or its attempt to protect them.

161. *Id.* at 6.
162. *Id.* at 7.
163. *See* textual material accompanying notes 137-152.
164. Graham v. Hill, *supra* at 10.

take place.

Another important issue presented by child pornography laws is the imposition of criminal responsibility on parents who participate in the sexual exploitation of their children.[165] Legislators could rationally conclude that children are unable to make a free and understanding decision to participate in prohibited acts.[166] Further, parents who allow their children to participate in sexually explicit activities are central figures in the child pornography process.[167] It has been argued that children have a right of privacy with respect to the dignity of their bodies,[168] however, since a child's constitutional rights are subject to the control of its parents (at least until adolescence)[169] it is unclear what right a child possesses independent from his parent.[170] It is clear, however, that a parent's control does not include the right to engage in an unlimited variety of sexual activities in the home[171] nor is there a right of privacy in family sexual affairs if photographs are taken with parental approval.[172]

Still another requirement that must be met if child pornography laws are ever to pass constitutional muster concerns the "knowledge" of the defendant. In *Smith v. California*[173] the court struck down, on free expression grounds, a Los Angeles city ordinance that imposed strict liability without requiring any element of knowledge.[174] The court articulated principles appli-

---

165. *See Developing Legislation, supra* note 9, at 21.

166. Ginsberg v. New York 390 U.S. 629 (1968).

167. *See* United States v. Perry, 389 F.2d 103 (4th Cir. 1968); Call v. United States, 265 F.2d 167 (4th Cir. 1959), wherein suppliers of sugar and containers to illicit distillers were convicted under 26 U.S.C. § 5686(a) (1958), which forbids possession of property with intent to violate the internal revenue laws.

168. *Recent Decisions*, 12 DUQUESNE L. REV. 645 (1974).

169. *See* Note, *Torture Toys, Parental Rights and the First Amendment*, 465 S. CAL. L. REV. 184, 188-201 (1972).

170. *See* Note, *Parental Consent Requirements and the Privacy Rights of Minors: The Contraceptive Controversy*, 88 HARV. L. REV. 1001, 1008-09 (1975).

171. *See* Cheesebrough v. State, 255 So. 2d 675 (Fla. 1971), *cert. denied*, 406 U.S. 976 (1972).

172. *Cf.* Lovisi v. Slayton, 363 F. Supp. 620 (E. D. Val. 1973), *aff'd on other grounds*, 539 F.2d 249 (4th Cir. 1976).

173. 361 U.S. 147 (1959).

174. *See also* Near v. Minnesota, 283 U.S. 697 (1931).

cable here: in order to be constitutionally sound, any law restricting possession or distribution must require that the producer, possessor, or distributor know *both* that the material is obscene *and* that a minor under the stated age is depicted therein.[175]

In light of the clandestine fashion in which child pornography is produced, the prosecution will not always be able to sustain such a burden of proof. It will often be difficult to prove the minority of the actor unless he or she is identified and produced in court or other competent evidence of the actor's age is available.[176] It is not necessary, however, to show the defendant knew specifically the minor's age but only that he or she was in fact a minor.[177]

A final caution pertaining to the drafting of realistic penalties and sanctions for violating child pornography statutes is in order. In the wake of public outrage accompanying the disclosure of the nature and extent of child exploitation, several proposed bills provided for extremely harsh penalties.[178] Prosecutors find

---

175. *Smith* would also appear to prevent a state from requiring a bookseller or publisher from inspecting or reading every publication that he or she wishes to sell in that this would restrict the material that is available to the public to that which the seller is able to review. Such a requirement would severely limit the public's access to non-obscene material and therefore is impermissible. The exact mental element required is still in debate:

> We need not and most definitely do not pass today on what sort of mental element is requisite to a constitutionally permissible prosecution of a bookseller for carrying an obscene book in stock; whether honest mistake as to whether its contents in fact constituted obscenity need be an excuse; whether there might be circumstances under which the State constitutionally might require that a bookseller investigate further, or might put on him the burden of explaining why he did not, and what such circumstances might be. Doubtless any form of criminal obscenity statue applicable to a bookseller will induce some tendency to self-censorship and have some inhibitory effect on the dissemination of material not obscene, but we consider today only one which goes to the extent of eliminating all mental elements from the crime.

361 U.S. at 154.

176. S. *Rep on 1585, supra* note 7, at 28.

177. *See* United States v. Hamilton, 456 F. 2d 171 (3d Cir. 1972) stating that the Mann Act, 18 U.S.C. § 2423 (1948) does not require that the Government prove the girl's age in transporting her interstate for immoral purposes.

178. *See, e.g.,* H.R. 6693, 95th Cong., 1st Sess. (1977) (as introduced) which as originally

juries very reluctant to convict defendants in cases where there is even the slightest doubt if it means subjecting them to severe penalties.[179] For this reason penalties must be severe enough to act as a formidable deterrent to both small and large scale child exploiters and still be reasonable enough so as not to present an impediment to attaining convictions.

Therefore, strong and effective child pornography laws should approach the hybrid problem separately, deal with the producer as a child abuser but distributors and retailers as sexual exploiters subject to first amendment obscenity standards. Parents too, who actively participate in the sexual exploitation, must be subjected to criminal liability if they fail in their parental responsibilities. Violators must know that the material is obscene and that a minor is depicted therein and the penalties which they are subject to must be strong deterrents but still reasonable in light of the offense.

Proposed Legislation

Suddenly aware of child pornography and prostitution's rapid growth a shocked public has demanded immediate legislative action. Former Mayor of New York Abraham D. Beame voiced commonly shared fears before the New York State Crime Commission saying "We have not yet sunk to the level of savage animals, but if we don't draw the line against pornography today, and specifically against child pornography, we can kiss good-bye to civilization as we know it and cherish it."[180]

ON THE STATE LEVEL

Under pressure to deal with such sentiments, lawmakers have

---

drafted provided for penalties of up to twenty years imprisonment and fines of up to $50,000 or both. *See also,* Cal. A. B. 1597 (1977) (as introduced) which provided for punishment of up to $100,000 a year and imprisonment of up to eleven years or both (which are longer than the five, six or seven year terms that California provides for attempted or second degree murder).

179. *See* B. Pines, *The Obscenity Quagmire,* 49 CAL. ST. B.J. 509, 514 (1974).

180. N.Y. Times, June 1, 1977, § I, at 7, col. 1.

hastily responded with a flood of new laws. The House Committee on the Judiciary in surveying all enacted, pending, and expected state laws which prescribe sexual child abuse and the production of child pornography noted that:

> Prior to the 1977 legislative sessions, very few states had laws prohibiting the use of children in obscene materials or performances and those that did exist were generally written in broad language without adequate powers for prosecution. During this past year, however, 24 states considered legislation to outlaw this exploitation of children. Of these 24 states, the unusually high number of 15 states enacted strong, comprehensive laws and final approval is expected before the year's end in an additional 6 states. In addition to these 21 states with new statutes, the states of West Virginia and North Dakota had previously enacted laws in 1974 and 1975 respectively.
>
> Legislative action will without a doubt be even more complete by the time legislatures adjourn in 1978. A number of the states indicated that legislation will be introduced in their upcoming sessions, and in many cases, bills have already been introduced. The 3 states that did not approve the bills last year will resume their consideration, and an additional 11 states will be considering legislation. In all these states, I can assure you the interest in passing legislation is very strong. It is very likely therefore that in 1978, 37 states will have adopted thorough prohibitions against using children sexually for preparing pornographic materials. I know of no other issue where state lawmakers have been able to react so quickly and completely to a problem confronting their states, as in curbing the sexual exploitation of children.[181]

As previously noted, at present there are only eight states with laws specifically pertaining to child pornography,[182] prior to 1977 there were only four,[183] the expected total by mid-1978 is thirty-seven.

Recent legislation designed to effect a quick and stern remedy for such child abuse may raise serious constitutional problems[184] but has also spawned varied and innovated responses that offer

---

181. H. Rep. No. 696, 95th Cong., 1st Sess. at 9 (1977). Testimony of California Assemblyman Kenneth Maddy presenting the results of the study to the Subcommittee.

182. *Supra*, note 88.

183. North Carolina (1971), West Virginia (1974), North Dakota (1975), and Tennessee (1975).

184. *See* notes 152-155 and accompanying text.

great promise towards the goal of eradicating from society the sexual exploitation of children in pornographic materials and prostitution.

Many states, like New York and Texas,[185] approach the issue broadly and treat producers, distributors, and retailers as child abusers without regard to the first amendment. As has already been discussed, such laws have definite difficulties in passing constitutional muster.[186] Several states[187] presently attempt to reach only the producers and thereafter make no distinction between the distribution and sale of obscene material that depicts children in sexually explicit conduct and that which does not. Other states, including California,[188] contemplate double-barrelled legislative attack which treats producers as child abusers

---

185. N.Y. PENAL CODE § 263.05 (McKinney 1977); TEX. CODE ANN. § 43.24 (1977); both held unconstitutionally broad. See textual material accompanying notes 153 *et seq.*

186. *See* notes 152-155 and accompanying text.

187. *E.g.*, N.C. GEN. STAT. § 14-190.1, *et seq.* (1971); TENN. CODE ANN. § 39-3013 (1975).

188. *See* CAL. LAB. CODE §§ 1309.5-1309.6 (West 1977) and CAL. PENAL CODE § 311.4 (West 1977) covering production of child pornography.

Labor Code § 1309.5 provides:

(a) Every person who, with knowledge that a person is a minor under 16 years of age, or who, while in possession of such facts that he should reasonably know that such person is a minor under 16 years of age, knowingly sells or distributes for resale films, photographs, slides, or magazines which depict a minor under 16 years of age engaged in sexual conduct as defined in Section 311.4 of the Penal Code, shall determine the names and addresses of persons from whom such material is obtained, and shall keep a record of such names and addresses. Such records shall be kept for a period of three years after such material is obtained, and shall be kept confidential except that they shall be available to law enforcement officers as described in Section 830.1 of the Penal Code upon request.

(b) Every retailer who knows or reasonably should know that such films, photographs, slides, or magazines depict a minor under the age of 16 years engaged in sexual conduct as defined in Section 311.4 of the Penal Code, shall keep a record of the names and addresses of persons from whom such material is acquired. Such records shall be kept for a period of three years after such material is acquired, and shall be kept confidential except that they shall be available to law enforcement officers as described in Section 830.1 of the Penal Code upon request.

(c) The failure to keep and maintain the records described in subdivisions (a) and (b) for a period of three years after the obtaining or acquisition of such material is a misdemeanor. Disclosure of such records by law enforcement officers, except in the performance of their duties, is a misdemeanor.

Labor Code § 1309.6 provides:

(a) Any person who violates any provision of Section 1309.5 shall be liable for a civil penalty not to exceed five thousand dollars ($5,000) for each violation, which shall be assessed and recovered in a civil action brought in the name of the people of the State of California by the Attorney General or by any district attorney, county council, or city attorney in any court of competent jurisdiction.

(b) If the action is brought by the Attorney General, one-half of the penalty collected shall be paid to the treasurer of the county in which the judgment was entered, and one-half to the State Treasurer. If brought by a district attorney or county counsel, the entire amount of penalty collected shall be paid to the treasurer of the county in which the judgment was entered. If brought by a city attorney or city prosecutor, one-half of the penalty shall be paid to the treasurer of the county and one-half to the city.

Penal Code § 311.4 provides:

(a) Every person who, with knowledge that a person is a minor, or who, while in possession of such facts that he should reasonably know that such person is a minor, hires, employs or uses such minor to do or assist in doing any of the acts described in Section 311.2, is guilty of a misdemeanor.

(b) Every person who, with knowledge that a person is a minor under the age of 16 years, or who, while in possession of such facts that he should reasonably know that such person is a minor under the age of 16 years, knowingly promotes, employs, uses, persuades, induces, or coerces a minor under the age of 16 years, or any parent or guardian of a minor under the age of 16 years under his or her control who knowingly permits such minor, to engage in or assist others to engage in either posing or modeling alone or with others for purposes of preparing a film, photograph, negative, slide, or live performance involving sexual conduct by a minor under the age of 16 years alone or with other persons or animals, for commercial purposes, is guilty of a felony and shall be punished by imprisonment in the state prison for three, four, or five years.

(c) As used in subdivision (b), "sexual conduct" means any of the following, whether actual or simulated: sexual intercourse, oral copulation, anal intercourse, anal oral copulation, masturbation, bestiality, sexual sadism, sexual masochism, any lewd or lascivious sexual activity, or excretory functions performed in a lewd or lascivious manner, whether or not any of the above conduct is performed alone or between members of the same or opposite sex or between humans and animals. An act is simulated when it gives the appearance of being sexual conduct.

SEC.4. (a) If any provisions of this act or the application thereof to any person or circumstances is held invalid, such invalidity shall not affect other provisions or applications of the act which can be given effect without the invalid provision or application, and to this end the provisions of this act are severable.

SEC.5. Notwithstanding Section 2231 of the Revenue and Taxation Code, there shall be no reimbursement pursuant to that section nor shall there be any appropriation made by this act because the Legislature recognizes that during any legislative session a variety of changes to laws relating to crimes and infractions may cause both increased and decreased costs to local government entities and school districts which, in the aggregate, do not result in significant identifiable cost changes.

whether or not the material is obscene, and deals with distributors
and retailers of "obscene"[189] materials depicting minors under
first amendment analysis.[190]

SEC.6. This act is an urgency statute necessary for the immediate preservation of the public peace, health, or safety within the meaning of Article IV of the
Constitution and shall go into immediate effect. The facts constituting such
necessity are:

Recent findings have indicated the use of children in pornographic materials
is increasing at an alarming rate. Los Angeles County alone estimates that
30,000 cases of child and teenage molestation, including cases of child
pornography, will occur in 1977. Due to the seriousness of this problem, the
Legislature declares that laws prohibiting the use of children in pornography
must take effect immediately.

189. California and several other states still maintain as their definition of obscenity the
test declared in *Roth, supra* note 113, that the material be "utterly without redeeming
social importance." The Roth Test places an onerous burden of proof on the prosecution.
See Man's Depravity?, supra note 17, at 3. In contrast however, the Supreme Court's most
recent test in *Miller, supra* note 122, requires that it need only be shown that the material
"lacks serious literary, artistic, political, or scientific value," a difficult but still much
easier task. Cal. A.B. No. 1820 (April 25, 1977) which would call for abandoning the Roth
Test in favor of the Miller Test is presently being considered.

190. *See* CAL. PENAL CODE § § 311.2, 311.9 (West 1977) dealing with the manufacture,
distribution, and retail of obscene material depicting children in sexually explicit
conduct.

Penal Code § 311.2 provides:

(a) Every person who knowingly sends or causes to be sent, or brings or
causes to be brought, into this state for sale or distribution, or in this state
possesses, prepares, publishes, or prints, with intent to distribute or to exhibit to
others, or who offers to distribute, distributes, or exhibits to others, any obscene
matter is guilty of a misdemeanor.

(b) Every person who knowingly sends or causes to be sent, or brings or
causes to be brought, into this state for sale or distribution, or in this state
possesses, prepares, publishes, or prints, with intent to distribute or to exhibit to
others for commercial consideration, or who offers to distribute, distributes, or
exhibits to others for commercial consideration, any obscene matter, knowing
that such matter depicts a person under the age of 18 years personally engaging
in or personally simulating sexual intercourse, masturbation, sodomy, bestiality, or oral copulation is guilty of a felony and shall be punished by
imprisonment in state prison for two, three, or four years, or by a fine not
exceeding fifty thousand dollars ($50,000), in the absence of a finding that the
defendant would be incapable of paying such a fine, or by both such fine and
imprisonment.

(c) The provisions of this section with respect to the exhibition of, or the
possession with intent to exhibit, any obscene matter shall not apply to a
motion picture operator or projectionist who is employed by a person licensed
by any city or county and who is acting within the scope of his employment,

The effect of such state laws is generally to make activities
which are misdemeanors under general obscenity statutes felon-

---

provided that such operator or projectionist has no financial interest in the
place wherein he is so employed.

(d) Except as otherwise provided in subdivision (c), the provisions of
subdivision (a) or (b) with respect to the exhibition of, or the possession with
intent to exhibit, any obscene matter shall not apply to any person who is
employed by a person licensed by any city or county and who is acting within
the scope of his employment, provided that such employed person has no
financial interest in the place wherein he is so employed and has no control,
directly or indirectly, over the exhibition of the obscene matter.

Penal Code § 311.9 provides:

(a) Every person who violates Section 311.2 or 311.5, except subdivision (b) of
Section 311.2, is punishable by fine of not more than one thousand dollars
($1,000) plus five dollars ($5) for each additional unit of material coming within
the provisions of this chapter, which is involved in the offense, not to exceed ten
thousand dollars ($10,000), or by imprisonment in the county jail for not more
than six months plus one day for each additional unit of material coming
within the provisions of this chapter, and which is involved in the offense, such
basic maximum and additional days not to exceed 360 days in the county jail, or
by both such fine and imprisonment. If such person has previously been
convicted of any offense in this chapter, or of a violation of Section 313.1, a
violation of Section 311.2 or 311.5, except subdivision (b) of Section 311.2, is
punishable as a felony.

(b) Every person who violates Section 311.4 is punishable by fine of not more
than two thousand dollars ($2,000) or by imprisonment in the county jail for
not more than one year, or by both such fine and such imprisonment. If such
person has been previously convicted of a violation of former Section 311.3 or
Section 311.4, he is punishable by imprisonment in the state prison.

(c) Every person who violates Section 311.7 is punishable by fine of not more
than one thousand dollars ($1,000) or by imprisonment in the county jail for not
more than six months, or by both such fine and imprisonment. For a second and
subsequent offense he shall be punished by a fine of not more than two
thousand dollars ($2,000), or by imprisonment in the county jail for not more
than one year, or by both such fine and imprisonment. If such person has been
twice convicted of a violation of this chapter, a violation of Section 311.7 is
punishable as a felony.

SEC. 3. If any provision of this act or the application thereof to any person or
circumstances is held invalid, such invalidity shall not affect other provisions or
applications of the act which can be given effect without the invalid provision
or application, and to this end the provisions of this act are severable.

SEC. 4. This act is an urgency statute necessary for the immediate preservation of the public peace, health or safety within the meaning of Article IV of the
Constitution and shall go into immediate effect. The facts constituting such
necessity are:

The proliferation of child pornography and the use of minors as subjects in

ies when children are sexually depicted therein.[191] Some states are contemplating enhanced penalties that become more severe as the age of the child depicted in the sexually explicit matter becomes younger. California provides variable penalties for distributors and retailers which increase with the amount of material confiscated; the statute provides effective deterrence and appropriate punishment for distributors and retailers whether they operate on a small or large scale.[192]

Such legislation generally also provides criminal liability for those parents who knowingly allow or cause their children to be involved in such sexually explicit conduct. Another innovative device employed by California is requiring all distributors[193] and retailers[194] who knowingly deal with child pornography to keep a record of all names and addresses of persons from whom such material is acquired for a period of three years. Violation subjects the distributor or retailer to a civil penalty of up to a $5,000 fine.[195]

States, through numerous innovations and remedies, are sure to develop strong, effective, and prosecutable laws to govern child pornography.

ON THE FEDERAL LEVEL

From its constitutional right to regulate commerce[196] Congress derives its legislative power to bar any article it may deem

---

child pornography pose a serious threat to the health and welfare of a large
number of minors in California which necessitates immediate redress.

191. *Compare* CAL. PENAL CODE § 311.2(a) (West 1977) providing misdemeanor punishment for manufacture and distribution of adult obscenity, with § 311.2(b) providing felony punishment of two, three, or four years and/or a fine of up to $50,000 for the same activity but with material depicting children in any sexually explicit manner.

192. *See* CAL. PENAL CODE § 311.9 (West 1977) providing a penalty for distribution of not more than $1,000 plus five dollars for each additional unit confiscated and imprisonment for not more than six months plus one day for each additional unit.

193. *See* CAL. LAB. CODE § 1309.5(1)(a) (West 1977).

194. *See* CAL. LAB. CODE § 1309.5(1)(b) (West 1977).

195. Such a record keeping requirement is of tremendous aid to law enforcement officers in combating the largely clandestine child pornography enterprise, but it also raises serious constitutional fifth amendment issues by the state requiring defendants to, in essence, testify against themselves. It is not within the scope of this comment to address the constitutional problem created by registration.

196. U.S. CONST. art. I, § 8, cl. 3.

undesirable from interstate or foreign commerce of the mails,[197] and to prohibit the manufacture of an article within a state if it will affect interstate or foreign commerce.[198] Congress may also punish conduct which has only a potential affect on interstate commerce and therefore can prohibit any child pornography as long as the producer knows, has reason to know, or intends that the materials will move in and affect interstate or foreign commerce.[199]

In the midst of the growing public concern over the welfare of sexually exploited children, in the first months of the 95th Congress, four bills[200] dealing with the sexual exploitation of children were introduced in the Senate and a series of bills,[201] one with 124 co-sponsors, was introduced into the House of Representatives. Ultimately each developed and passed its own legislation. The House bill[202] was broad and sweeping and made no distinction between obscene and non-obscene. The Senate bill[203]

---

197. *See, e.g.*, United States v. Orito, 413 U.S. 139 (1973); United States v. Darby, 312 U.S. 100 (1941); and Periara v. United States, 347 U.S. 1 (1954).

198. *See, e.g.*, United States v. Darby, *supra* at note 197; Wickard v. Filburn, 317 U.S. 111 (1942); and United States v. Wrightwood Dairy Co., 315 U.S. 110 (1942).

199. *See, e.g.*, United States v. Addonizio, 451 F. 2d 49 (3d Cir. 1971); and United States v. Prano, 385 F. 2d 287 (7th Cir. 1967).

200. S. 1011, S. 1499, S. 1585, and S. 1040.

201. H.R. 3913, 3914, 4571, 5326, 5474, 5499, 5522, 6351, 6734, 6747, 7254, 7468, 7522, 7834, 7895, 8059.

202. H.R. 8059, 95th Cong., 1st Sess. (1977).

203. S. 1585; 95th Cong., 1st Sess. (1977). *See S. Rep. on 1585, supra* at note 8 at 17, 18 where the Senate Judiciary Committee stated:

> The Committee has carefully considered the suggestion that the Federal laws be extended to make illegal the sale and distribution of materials whose production involved the use of minors in sexually explicit conduct as defined in Section 2251. The Committee recognizes, however, that the sale and distribution of such material cannot be approached in the same manner as its production. Attempts to prohibit the sale and distribution of such material necessarily involve an evaluation of the content of materials in question. Consequently, the Supreme Court in Miller v. California, 413 U.S. 15 (1973) has held that in determining whether material is obscene and loses its First Amendment protection, the material must be judged in its entirety. Therefore, the Committee is of the view that an attempt to make illegal the sale and distribution of material regardless of whether such material when taken as a whole is obscene, would run counter to present Federal constitutional law as ennunciated by the Supreme Court in Miller.

was more defined and limited to production of pornographic materials involving children under sixteen and was designed to avoid any confrontation with the first amendment. However, when the Senate bill went to the floor, an emotional floor battle led many senators to agree with the statement of Senator Hatch that "If we want to rid this country of child pornography, we must go after distributors of this filth with tough standards, not the watered-down obscenity standards for adults."[204] Further, it was hoped that the Court would use more stringent obscenity standards than those for adults.[205] Ultimately, the Senate adopted Senator Roth's amendment to the bill providing for criminal penalties for knowingly distributing or selling child pornography whether or not it was obscene.

Finally, in deference to the first amendment, the Senate and House Conference Committee added the word "obscene" to the Roth amendment before the bill was passed by both houses and became law. It thus decided to be safe within the first amendment and adopted the hybrid approach by punishing producers of child pornography as child abusers on one hand and sellers and distributors of *obscene* material depicting children in sexually explicit conduct on the other.[206] In analyzing the effectiveness of the finished law, Senator Kildee, author of the House bill, stated that:

> the term "obscene" would weaken the bill as a strictly child abuse measure but it should still cover virtually all child pornography. Since this law will make sellers and distributors of child pornography accessories to child abuse, its existence will discourage sales and will give

---

In considering the possibility that the Court would apply a broader obscenity standard in cases of child sexploitation the Committee concluded that:

> While the Court has indicated that different standards may apply to the dissemination of allegedly obscene material to juveniles, it has not intimated that different standards should apply to the dissemination of materials which portray juveniles in sexually explicit conduct, and the Committee believes that such an approach would not pass constitutional muster.

Id., at 18.

204. Cong. Q., Oct. 15, 1977, at 2131.
205. *See* textual material accompanying notes 138-153.
206. *See* Cong. Q., Nov. 12. 1977, at 2416.

convictions not possible under present law. Also, since we did not define "obscene" in the bill, we hope it may lead the court to adopt our definition of sexually explicit conduct as a separate definition for obscenity where children are concerned.[207]

The new federal law[208] prohibits producers from using any child under sixteen to engage or assist in any sexually explicit conduct in the production of any visual or print medium.[209] Parents, too, are equally liable if they knowingly permit such conduct.[210] However, such parent or legal guardian must have control over the actions of the child when permitting the child to engage in sexually explicit conduct.[211]

Distribution and sale, however, of obscene materials under federal obscenity statutes was already a felony.[212] Therefore Congress *doubled* the penalties whenever the materials depicted children in sexually explicit conduct.[213]

The new law also updates the Mann Act[214] to prohibit the interstate transportation of young boys under eighteen, as with young girls, to engage in prohibited sexual conduct.

Other Factors of Influence

Strong and effective legislation alone cannot solve the problem of child pornography and prostitution and this comment would be remiss if it did not briefly observe other important factors that can control the spread of child pornography. The deterioration of the family and the fundamental values of our society, poverty and unemployment, inadequate education and social agencies, and a general lack of caring in an impersonal society provides the

---

207. *Id. See also* text accompanying notes 108-155.
208. 18 U.S.C. § § 2251-2253 (1977).
209. 18 U.S.C. § 2251 (a) (1977).
210. 18 U.S.C. § 2251 (b) (1977).
211. CONF. REP. No. 601, 95th Cong., 1st Sess., at 6 (1977).
212. *Supra*, notes 77-82.
213. 18 U.S.C. § 2252(b) (1977) providing for up to $10,000 or imprisonment up to 10 years, or both, for a first time offender; $15,000 and 15 years, or both, for a second time offender.
214. 18 U.S.C. § 2253 (1977).

perfect environment in which child sexploitation can fester and grow.

In April, 1977, the Los Angeles Police Department credited a substantial decline in the amount of books, magazines, and films depicting children in sexually explicit acts to "vigorous law enforcement and public pressure, including considerable publicity about the subject."[215]

Even the broadest law under the most expansive definition of obscenity requires effective enforcement. Enforcement agencies should be well trained and acquainted with the child pornography industry and wherever possible special child sexploitation units, like that of the Los Angeles Police Department, should be set up to concentrate specifically on the overlapping problems of child pornography, child prostitution, runaways, and child molestation.[216] Prosecutors should be specially trained in order to insure convictions. Further, all state agencies should be well acquainted with the nature and extent of child sexploitation and prepared to deal harmoniously with each other. Enforcement should be swift and begin intensively against the most offensive material and continue down to the imposition of civil penalties and injunctions for certain parties where the imposition of criminal liability would be inappropriate.[217]

Public pressure may well be the strongest deterrent to the child pornography and prostitution markets.[218] Educational programs can be presented to organizations that deal with children to recruit public involvement in the battle by being able to recognize early symptoms of a sexually exploited child or reporting observations of child exploitation. Public awareness reduces the

---

215. CAL. ATT'Y GEN., *supra* note 6, at 4.

216. *Id.* at 30.

217. *E.g.*, such as against photographic laboratories which process films depicting children engaged in sexual conduct, which have been found to be "untouched links" in the process from production to ultimate retail sale of child pornography. CAL. ATT'Y GEN., *supra* note 6, at 25.

218. During the April, 1977 child pornography decline, as a result of public pressure, it was reported that Reuben Sturman, the primary national distributor of pornography, notified his 800 distributors and his 100 retail stores that he would not provide defense money for anyone in his employ who is arrested for selling or distributing child pornography. CAL. ATT'Y GEN., *supra* note 6, at 4.

amount of child pornography and prostitution available, encourages support of police enforcement efforts, and encourages a change in the "community attitudes" used to determine whether or not material is obscene in the *Miller*[219] test.

Conclusion

The sexual exploitation of children for profit in pornography and prostitution is growing at an alarming rate. Child pornography affects not only the child subjects but is also connected with other forms of child abuse and molestation. Thousands of children are involved in a business that has grown into a multimillion dollar industry.

Child pornography is a hybrid problem comprised of child abuse both in the product's creation and the distribution and sale that creates the market. The problem *cannot* be remedied unless both areas are properly approached. Statutes that attempt in a sweeping fashion to legislate both protected as well as unprotected speech are overbroad and cannot pass constitutional muster. Therefore production of child pornography must be controlled through strong child abuse laws and the market must be discouraged through effective first amendment legislation that offers harsh penalties for materials depicting children in any sexually explicit manner.

"Such things must come, but woe to the man through whom they come!"[220]

---

219. *Supra* note 122.
220. Matthew 18:7 (New International Version of the New Testament).

Chapter 22

THE PEDERASTS*

PARKER ROSSMAN

In the early 1960s I stumbled onto a problem which seems to be largely ignored by society and where scientific research is very deficient—especially considering its deep impact on the lives of those involved. In the course of counseling some deeply troubled men, I was led to explore the world of the pederast, eventually getting acquainted with over 1,000 men who were erotically attracted to young boys. I also interviewed more than 300 boys involved with such men.

On Studying the Sexual Underground

I began the study in an effort to help some men, fathers of families, responsible citizens in their communities, who were being blackmailed, having fallen into the hands of a pimp who suggested they might like to try a new sort of sexual experience. The first of these I met was a professional man from the Midwest who had come to New York City to attend a study conference and to visit the World's Fair. He had observed and participated in two "orgies," where he had gotten acquainted with several other men who were victims of the pimp. Through these men I became acquainted with several more, scattered across the country, and I was distressed to find that large numbers of children, particularly 12-, 13- and 14-year-olds, were being prostituted.

Although my first reaction was to draft proposals for better guidance and supervision of children, it occurred to me that the more important question was, who are the customers? I found

*From *Society, 10(3)*:29-35, April 1973. Courtesy of *Trans* Action Inc., Rutgers—The State University, New Brunswick, New Jersey.

myself heavily engaged in counseling in an area where I knew little, attempting to deal with the problems of pederasts—not merely those being blackmailed, but those struggling with temptation and guilt. One glimpse of this anguish is well portrayed in the recent film, *Death in Venice*, where the film-maker stresses the dismay of a man who discovers that he is erotically attracted to a young boy (somewhat of a misreading of the Thomas Mann novel from which the film was made).

The pederasts I met desperately needed to talk to someone they could trust. They required help and support to stay out of trouble. So in an effort to help, I surveyed the vast literature on pederasty: legal cases, medical, analytic, psychiatric, and psychological case studies; historical, anthropological and biographical material. As will be suggested in a forthcoming bibliographical article on pederasty in the *Journal of Sex Research*, some of the thinly disguised autobiographical novels may provide accurate data needed to counterbalance the existing inadequate, incomplete and subjective research on pederasty.

Without intending it and without legitimated qualifications, I was propelled into an extended research project, more comprehensive than anyone has yet attempted, the only exception being Dr. Ettore Mariotti of Naples, whose medical research was banned and burned earlier in this century. He died a broken man, and I, too, have found that research into pederasty may endanger one's career and may even endanger one's life when it leads to an exploration of child prostitution.

Because of the caution, fear and secrecy of pederasts, I do not believe anyone else has had such an opportunity. Certainly, no one else has written a report on such extensive interview data. This article is not intended as a preliminary report of findings, but rather as a statement of some hypotheses for further research and as a proposal for the creation of an interdisciplinary research team which would undertake a study of pederasty and pedophilia. New insights into homosexuality also might be produced by more adequate research into the sexual experience of children and of children with adults. It is clear to me that no one discipline, no one scholar is adequately equipped to deal with the complexities which my research has uncovered.

How and where does one find pederasts? Unlike homosexuals, there are no pederast associations in the United States. Yet, each pederast knows another; and across a decade one can therefore be led from person to person. If one is trusted he can in time become acquainted with the secret pederasts who never reveal themselves unless they get into trouble or go to a psychiatrist. One can begin to speak now of a "homosexual community," but pederasts are isolated from one another by fear and suspicion of each other. As G. W. Henry suggests in his book, *All the Sexes,* the number of pederasts is much larger than is commonly known or supposed.

There are mailing lists of persons who order pederast books, photographs and other materials. Before it became illegal to send unsolicited advertisements of pornography, a number of European firms sent mailings to discover potential customers. There are now (in Europe) coded mailing lists of as many as 50,000 Americans who have purchased such materials. I have sorted through a number of such lists and I found one dealer who had in his files 1,800 returned questionnaires from American pederasts who reported their activities and interests to suggest the sorts of printed materials they would be interested in buying. The majority of these were professional men: teachers, doctors, social workers—with university professors heading the list. And the questionnaires suggested that most of them ordered books and pictures as fantasy substitutes for criminal sexual activity. Those 1,800 questionnaires further indicated that such persons often went overseas, or at least far from home, if they engaged in pederast sexual acts. These questionnaires seemed to confirm what I had learned from my counseling interviews—that these pederasts tended to have sex without love with young prostitutes when away from home; and at the same time these men had affectionate, non-sexual relationships with boys at home.

This provisional answer to the question of *who* led to yet another question: why? And the pederasts I was counseling also wanted to know how unique their experience was. One of them offered to pay for sending out a questionnaire asking for autobiographical information: when did these pederasts first become aware of their temptations and desires? What was the nature of their fantasies and experience? Selecting initially 1,000 names from a commercial list, I wrote 500 persons, on five continents, to ask if they could supply me with data or bibliography on child prostitution—since it was assumed no one would admit he was a pederast. I received an astonishing volume of replies, with newspaper clippings, articles and personal experiences. Most of the persons who wrote said that they loved children and would do anything they could to stamp out abuses and exploitation of children.

I wrote again, personally typed letters on an MTST tape typewriter, to the second 500 names as well as to those who had replied to the first letter, asking for the names of persons who might be able and willing to supply data about pederasty, especially asking who would be willing to fill out an anonymous questionnaire or be interviewed. The replies were disappointing. Not many were willing to fill out even the most confidential or anonymous questionnaire. Those who finally did fill out a questionnaire were not truthful. Later, in personal interviews, many admitted that the truth was exactly the opposite of what they had written.

It should be noted that whereas an increasing number of homosexuals believe they have a battle to fight for law reform and some public acceptance, pederasts have no such illusion. Most of them are deeply fearful and resentful of any publicity, research or public notice. Some persons even threatened my life if I should pursue such a study or publish results. Many others, however, replied that they would be interested in talking to me confidentially, often adding an appeal for help. Some were very dismayed at having once engaged in a criminal act and intended never to do so again. Others were so fearful of their pederast fantasies and temptations that they would hardly shake hands with a boy. Some had felt they could not afford therapy, and others had found therapy unhelpful.

At this point I had what turned out to be a foolish notion—that one might experiment with a sort of Alcoholics Anonymous group for pederasts who needed and wanted the help and support of others to keep from yielding to temptation. So partly as a device for gathering more data into the "why," I tried convening some discussion meetings, which were useful only in revealing the overwhelming difficulties of group conversation. So, on the suggestion of several persons, I initiated a series of round-robin letters, in which pederasts wrote anonymously of their sexual fantasies, dreams and experiences. This project continued across five years, involving several hundred persons.

I began by asking the questions I had developed for a questionnaire, and essay replies were mailed to other participants for comment. In addition to personal experience and autobiographical statements, the round-robin newsletters included information on pederast books, films, articles—the equivalent finally of nearly 5,000 double-spaced typewritten pages, which drew together nearly all of the available data on pederasty from all sources, for extensive comments from pederasts themselves. Those who received and commented on this material included pediatricians (one who read and discussed it all with his wife), psychiatrists, social scientists, politicians, policemen, parole officers, clergy—including a bishop—social workers, scholars of various disciplines. Many of these persons, of course, were not pederasts, but were sex researchers and scholars of other disciplines. The plan had been to deposit all this material at the Institute of Sex Research at Indiana University.

The most substantial aspect of the research consisted of in-depth interviews, which were possible only after a basis of trust was established—even then some would talk to me only anonymously, and one man only in the dark. I would like to express public appreciation here to the many men, some distinguished in their fields of work, who not only were willing to reveal to me things they had never dared to tell anyone before, but who in many cases traveled great distances at their own expense to meet me when I was in Paris, Beirut, Tangiers, Sydney, Toronto as well as many American cities.

What Is A Pederast?

The one contribution I should perhaps be expected to make on the basis of such extensive research would be a definition of pederasty, but the more one knows about such a subject the more difficult it becomes to establish adequate definitions, for one has learned a thousand exceptions for a thousand qualifications and complications. One cannot define pederasty without stating controversial hypotheses.

André Gide in his *Journal* wrote: "A pederast is a lover of young boys and I am one." Note that this does not necessarily define pederasty in terms of an erotic attraction to boys, nor is the pederast thus defined as one who engages in sexual acts with boys, although Gide does report such sexual activity in his autobiography, *If It Die*. Rather the pederast sees himself as one who loves boys in all the meanings of the word love.

Our difficulty with the word *pederast* is that it covers many types, some as widely different as virgin and rapist. Can one word be used to include them all? I am especially not willing to limit the word *pederast* to those who are engaging in illegal sex acts, but insist on including a large majority who have never had a first homosexual experience. Who then is a pederast? As with homosexuals, I am content to let them define themselves. A pederast is someone who accepts the label and identifies himself as such, chaste or promiscuous.

It is generally assumed that pederasty is a subdivision of homosexuality, pederasts being those homosexuals who prefer "chicken" (young boys). In my judgment such homosexuals are only one type of pederast. If one defines a homosexual as a person who engages in homosexual acts, then many pederasts are homosexuals. The only kind of sex act a man can have with a boy is a homosexual act. However, most homosexuals are eager to disassociate themselves from pederasty, being honestly horrified at the thought of homosexual relations with a child. Some further feel that, to accomplish legal reform to their advantage, restrictions on homosexual activity among consenting adults must be removed at the price of stricter laws against sex acts with children. Never mind the psychological damage done to children by dragging them to court on matters that should be handled medically and psychiatrically. Many homosexuals find it convenient to forget their own childhood emotions and experiences. And questioning the relationship between homosexuality and pederasty, one faces the question: who is a consenting adult? If the age of consent is 18 or 21, then many homosexuals are in fact pederasts. On the other hand, if the age of consent is puberty or age 14 as in some countries, then much pederasty becomes homosexuality, for many of the children we are discussing would then be considered adults.

More important, however, is the fact that a large percentage of pederasts are not exclusively attracted to males and are not homosexual if one uses the common sense definition: a homosexual is a man who is erotically attracted to an adult male. Some pederasts are admittedly homosexual; some consider themselves bisexual and should be more accurately called pedophiliacs— being equally attracted to young girls. Many pederasts relate sexually to women very well, and as researchers on homosexuality have amply shown, are married, and have children. Many of the accepted psychoanalytic theories of pederasty simply do not seem to apply to them at all. Also many pederasts have a deadly fear of "homosexual boys," for homosexual youngsters tend to panic at emotions they are unable to manage, or they become insanely jealous and demanding. Our understanding of pederasty must therefore be enlarged to include a much greater variety of experience, as indicated by our interviews.

Five Types of Pederasty

Adequate definitions of pederasty must take account of at least five types of pederasty:

First, the smallest category is the "temporary or substitute" pederast who sleeps with a boy when women are not available. Usually he does so only infrequently, is quite cautious, and does not really consider himself to be a pederast. This type was in the past commonly found at sea; for example see Jean Bosq's *Le Vice Marin,* which helped remove young boys from French ships because of its evidence that the ship captain was accurate when he remarked that "after six weeks at sea the sodomy laws no longer apply." But ship crews no longer include young boys and most voyages are relatively short in duration. Steps have also been taken to eliminate pederasty in other traditional breeding grounds —young boys are generally not jailed in adult prisons, and women are much more available to the army.

I would also include in this category those individuals who are essentially heterosexuals who in search of new sexual kicks become the customers for young male prostitutes at home and abroad. For example, there is the tourist who patronizes the boys brothel in Bangkok and tells his friends that for a different kick they should try young boys that are available in many tourist cities. And there is a great deal of pederasty among Americans in Vietnam, as there was among the French before them for the same reasons—not because of a lack of women.

Second is the category of "criminal or exploitative pederasts," including pimps of young boys, gangsters who run pederast hangouts, blackmailers and others on the fringes of society where many are engaged extensively with women. Some of these pederasts limit their sexual activity almost exclusively to young boys and do consider themselves to be pederasts. There is often a great deal of legal and personal risk involved in this type of activity. It is important to note that many of these people have passionate affection for boys, and they may be the most authentic survivals of the substitute type. Many of them had their definitive sexual experiences in reformatories. Across their formative teenage years and sometimes into their twenties, they had regular sexual intercourse and even passionate affairs with younger inmates. They not only developed a taste for sex with young boys, they became very skilled at seduction and learned to give and receive pleasure of a radically different kind than they have with women.

Third, some of these men who became addicted to boys in reformatories become the "promiscuous pederast" type. This category includes those men who cruise cheap motion pictures and regularly pick up the hustlers available in most cities. Many of these are lower-class men. Those I interviewed included bakers, clerks in hotels and stores, bus drivers, milk routemen, policemen.

Most men in this category are exclusively pederasts and consider themselves as such. Some have already been arrested and can no longer get good jobs. Others are careless and cynical because of fatalism. Taking risks is a part of the game. Some make sexual propositions to every boy they meet, to see which will respond. They are not likely to use drugs, alcohol or force, as some in the previous category, but many are frankly exploitative. Some are callous, others are mentally ill. There is, indeed, such variety in this category that it ought to be a dozen categories. It should be noted that the criminal and cautious types are the only ones considered in most of the theories of cause and cure.

Fourth are the "careful pederasts." These men generally do not limit themselves solely to young boys but are quite aware of their inclination toward pederasty. They generally have a good deal of money and they avoid sexual contact with boys except in carefully protected situations, thereby minimizing legal and personal risks. Some, for example, would never touch a boy in the United States, but make special trips to other countries. One man has sexual relations only with the children of call girls he befriends and baby-sits for. Another pays a sizeable monthly income to a widow whose son he is educating. I learned of two "father-son sports clubs" where fathers traded their own sons on camping trips. There have been a number of arrests in relation to one of these groups in the Los Angeles area. I found a town of 8,000 people in the Midwest where a group of men have paid for the college education of a series of boys across 20 years, in exchange for sexual favors when the boys were younger. Because of the care with which they protect themselves, these men do not usually fall into the hands of the law—unless they make careless mistakes or violate their own rules for some reason. One basic rule of the careful pederast, for example, is never to mix business with pleasure.

Responsible Pederasts

Fifth, "responsible pederasts" are those men, often wealthy and of good education and position, who avoid any kind of sexual contact or involvement with children. Aware of their problem and temptations, they bend over backwards to protect themselves, some refusing to have anything to do with organizations where young boys will be present. Many of these men in their first interviews with me swore that they have never had any kind of sexual contact with a boy—at least not since they were young teenagers themselves. Later, however, many of them admitted that "some years ago" they had slipped once or twice, and they live in mortal fear that it will be discovered even yet. There are certain common factors in causing them to slip. Frequently they are not prepared to handle a seductive and seducing child, particularly one with previous sexual experience. Further the irresistible child was one who not only was aroused and demanding, but also revealed a very touching sexual hunger: "I was so fond of that child I simply could not refuse him." The third typical factor, however, is the development of strong resistance, having succumbed in this way. Being repentant, angry that he was naive and unprepared, the responsible pederast is determined to make sure that he never succumbs again.

I detected that many of them have moods that go up and down and that from time to time they do have weak moments when their resistance is low—such as some evening when in a distant and anonymous city they meet a young hustler. This is the most neglected group in pederast research and therapy. Mostly they report that analysts and psychiatrists do not take them seriously, if they report some temptations which they seem to have pretty well under control.

Finally, within each of the above categories, what we actually find is a continuum of attitudes and experiences, and many of the thousand persons who have provided data do not fit exactly into any of the above categories.

While it is useful to know how many pederasts there are, how they make contacts with boys, and the extent and type of sexual activity, there are, however, more crucial questions, revolving around the nature of the sexual experience upon life, personality, morals, values, attitudes and emotions of those who have the experience. Further, to speak of "sexual experience" points to the fact that we are concerned with more than sex acts, that is, with the meanings and interpretations given to such acts and to the emotions surrounding unfulfilled desires. For while the literature for the most part emphasizes the types and frequency of unusual sexual acts, the sexual activity of pederasts is for the most part extremely limited. Many, in fact, except for the promiscuous category, have experienced a sexual act with a boy only once or twice in a lifetime, often years ago. A high percentage of the promiscuous category are sexually active only when they are away on vacations or overseas.

Pederast Morality

At one of my early meetings with pederasts, those present pointed out that every one of them would draw a line at some point, in terms of his own moral standards:

- Some would never touch a boy, certainly not sexually.
- Others thought it was all right to hug and caress a boy, but not kiss.
- Others thought it was acceptable to kiss and to masturbate the boy.
- Others would fellate a boy, but considered anal intercourse a crime.
- The large majority would make the above decisions in accordance with the wishes of the boy. They would do what he desired and no more.
- None would touch a child not yet pubescent, because that boy would not be interested or aroused.
- Some would never touch a child unless there was mutual affection.
- Others, however, considered it a game or sport to seduce a young adolescent, especially one who wanted to play the game.
- Others would never seduce a boy, but would indulge in sexual acts with an experienced boy prostitute—especially away from home.

As I extended my interviews, this list grew longer and longer, suggesting an almost infinite variety of attitudes and experiences. In his ideal world, where he lives most of the time and for most of the years of his life, the pederast—except for certain criminal and promiscuous types—loves and protects boys.

What does he enjoy in sexual relations with a boy? The pederast enjoys giving the boy pleasure, perhaps in the sense of "enjoying the pleasure of the other," which Sartre in *Saint Genet* uses to interpret the writings of that French author. They do not kiss boys, usually, because boys do not want to be kissed, so the pederast contents himself with the teasing and wrestling which a boy enjoys. Because a pederast truly wants a boy's affection, he follows the boy's sexual lead rather passively, becoming sexually active only as affection grows and as the boy wishes. Most said: "You never really have to seduce a boy. Give him time and he will seduce you." They generally agreed that those who fall into the hands of the police are the ones who have forgotten that rule.

The Consenting Boys

What do boys enjoy sexually? While I did get the chance to talk, in limited ways, to the young lovers of some pederasts—and more meaningfully and constructively with older boys and young men who had been such lovers in the past—I could not interview a truly representative sample of children. Most of my data on the attitudes and experience of boys is from interviews with boy prostitutes. In any event, some clear impressions emerge from hearing men and boys describe their experiences.

It was generally agreed that boys respond to men's overtures, or even seek men out, for four main reasons or combinations of them: (1) some boys are hungry for affection, (2) some mainly want money and gifts (and not always because of poverty), (3) some want adventure, new experiences, kicks other than sexual ones. Some at a rather young age see "playing the queers" as an exciting game to play until they are old enough for girls, (4) mostly, however much they may hide behind other reasons, boys indulge in sexual activity with men because they greatly enjoy being fellated. They are highly aroused by a sexually stimulating culture, and they want sex education and sexual kicks.

Lower-class delinquent boys are more likely to have been seduced than other youngsters. In nearly all cases the boys were first seduced by youngsters of their own age or slightly older. While this is more characteristic of the boy prostitutes (and therefore of those I interviewed), the adult pederasts I interviewed verified that this was indeed typical of most of their lovers. The sexually experienced boy is not only more available and more tempting to the pederast, but he often takes initiative in proposing sexual relations, especially in a situation of mutual trust and affection.

In most cases, the actual sexual intercourse of man with boy is much more like a game than like love-making with a woman. Indeed, a large number of boys in America, and also in England, use the term "fun and games" to talk about such activity. The boy who would react angrily to any suggestion that he had ever indulged in homosexual activity, or in sexual perversions, or love-making with males, would often admit to "fun and games." I do not know how extensive it is for adolescents to view sexual activity as a sport, but it seems to be very typical of those boys who are involved with pederasts, and seems to characterize the adolescent memories and fantasies of a high percentage of pederasts of all categories.

Therefore, instead of discussing the extent to which pederasts and boys are indulging in oral intercourse, anal intercourse or masturbation—for the first two are perhaps much more rare than commonly supposed—it might make much more sense to study the types of sexual games that are played, in which oral or anal intercourse are sometimes the penalty for the loser or the reward for the victor. There are gambling games, sporty games related to boxing and wrestling, sexual competitions and contests. There is the "hunt and chase," and there are other courtship games. One might well speak of "healthy" games and "sick" games, for some—especially as developed in juvenile penal institutions—come to involve teasing, sadistic spanking, psychological torture, prostitution, mock marriages, and even rape. There are sporty games which involve very little emotion and fantasy, and there are highly charged emotional experiences in which fantasy is a major dimension of the game.

It is often pointed out that how adults react and what adults say to interpret sexual acts may be much more influential, much more crucial in the emotional development of the child than the actual sexual act in which he may have been involved. Perhaps it is even more crucial how the child interprets and fantasizes over his own sexual experience. There is an emotional point at which a homosexual affirms his identity: "All right I am a homosexual. Now I understand myself," and where the pederast says to himself: "I am a pederast. I didn't ask to be a pederast. How did it happen?" Most pederasts, if they have an opinion at all, think that it happened to them at puberty, in relation to fantasies and solitary pleasures long before they had any sexual contact with another person of either sex.

Erotic Attraction

Many pederasts reported that they were conscious of a strong erotic attraction to boys before they had any idea of the type of sexual contact they would desire. This is not true of those who actively participated in sexual games during their own adolescence. Those who did tend to desire the types of sexual contact which they came to enjoy during adolescent sex games. The actual nature of the games was less important than the fantasies which accompanied and interpreted the sex play, adding a pleasurable emotional dimension to the games. Interestingly enough, when one questions pederasts about the nature of those fantasies, especially the ones they remember or still repeat because of their emotional or pleasurable significance, they most often mention four types:

- inventing new games or elaborating upon habitual games as they might be played in the future
- reliving an adolescent sexual experience or elaborating an imaginary adolescent experience which was meaningful at that time
- fantasizing an encounter with the "ideal boy," a "love story"
- refantasizing an adolescent masochistic game or dream

The aim of the fantasy is genital pleasure and the accentuation of genital pleasure, and the successful fantasy is one which provides either the stimulus to masturbation or the "warm emotional glow" or sexual pleasure without masturbation. The most successful fantasies are generally a reliving of experiences of early adolescence, which grow deeper and more routine each time they are relived.

It is my hypothesis that pederasty's origin lies in the experience and interpretation of intense and exciting personal pleasure in sexual experiences at puberty and following. Wendell Pomeroy warns, in *Boys and Sex*, that adolescent homosexual play "may become so pleasurable" that a boy "will not give himself an opportunity to develop a heterosexual life." For many pederasts it may well be that the adolescent sex games were so pleasurable that he continues them alongside other types of sexual experience in later life. It seems to me that a neglected aspect of research into homosexuality and pederasty is the study of pleasure. This becomes more crucial in a time when "sex as fun" and "fun culture" take deeper root in the attitudes of the younger generation. The emphasis on the study of clinical and neurotic aspects of homosexuality, for example, as sickness, has simply understressed the role of pleasure in determining what people will do sexually.

What role do daydreams and masturbation fantasies play in the pederast's sexual pleasure, in his temptations and desires, in his self-concept of pederast and justification of his behavior? What is the difference between "man-boy love affairs" and sex games which take place in a non-love situation? How do these different experiences affect the sexual socialization and sexual behavior of various individuals? There are no clearcut answers to these questions. Indeed, some adolescents appear to engage in a great deal of sex play with little emotional impact, while the lives of others are deeply colored by one isolated sexual experience. Research is needed into the nature of sexual pleasure, especially when not in the context of a loving relationship, and into the sexual fantasies of children and young adolescents as related to the development of pederast and homosexual tendencies. We have only scratched the surface—our answers have suggested new questions. Research into pederasty has been inadequate because we haven't even known what questions to ask.

Chapter 23

POLICY RECOMMENDATIONS
ON CHILD PORNOGRAPHY CONTROL

LeRoy G. Schultz

1. Policy aimed at control and prevention must be based on sound data, informed intelligence, and rationality. Such resources are lacking at present. There is a marked need for objective data based upon research, and such research should be supported by the Office of Child Development, D.H.E.W., as they now have the necessary staff and other resource potential including a national focus.

2. Since some introductory evidence indicates runaway minors are recruited by the "porno trade," each community and state should begin to strengthen its social services for such youth, with reasonable funding from both tax-supported and United Way support. (See J. Gordon and J. Houghton: *Final Report, N.I.M.H. Runaway Youth Program* Center for Studies of Child and Family Mental Health, Jan. 31, 1977.)

3. Since persons involved in protective and authority roles, such as teachers, scout masters, adoptive and foster parents, staff of children's institutions, etc., may be recruitment agents of the sex-industry, reasonable screening and surveillance of such persons is recommended within the current framework of law.

4. At present there is a dissatisfaction, by concerned groups, with the amount of time, resources, and staff of law enforcement and social welfare agencies devoted to problem control, particularly in large urban areas. A national inte-

grated effort by all related law enforcement agencies is required.

5. The generalization that all minors are psychologically traumatized is unwarranted at this time, pending further research. It creates a credibility gap and negative self-fulfilling aspect to make such assumptions. If the problem is one of morals rather than trauma, this should be honestly acknowledged.

6. Each state must, after deliberations, establish a realistic "age of consent" for voluntary sexual behavior. Society owes each minor (14-18 years) the right to choose his own sexual welfare, unless conditions contra-indicate, with the minor sharing in decisions of the "conditions" (See Chapter 25).

7. There is a marked need to come to grips with the issue of sex education, including answering the questions of why, when, how, and to what end. Minors should be given reasonable power to influence choice of subject matter in the public school system. The sin of parental sexual ignorance should not be visited upon helpless children, if the result is sexual abuse.

8. Policy makers, legislators, and city councilmen and women should be alerted to the strong possibility that a liberal policy on pornography reduces the incidence of child molestation (Kutchensky, 1973).

9. Some of the new laws prohibiting child pornography, simply overlap existing laws which have been in force for many years. Films and photos can be staged, filmed, and packaged quickly, with frequent change in locale so that detecting at this stage is nearly impossible. Transportation and distribution of the film may prove more likely of police intervention. A recent Pittsburgh court case indicates that film studios are recruiting minors over the age of consent, but who have the body and face of a child.

10. Penalities on conviction of child pornography laws should provide deterrent sentences in terms of fines and imprisonment. Fines should reflect the profits the crime pays.

11. New legislation should in no way interfere with legitimate research by bonafide research agencies dealing with solutions to the problem, or relevant related defensible research interests. Such projects should be cleared through the local police department or prosecutor's office.

12. Hysteria and anxiety-mongering by the news media should in no way affect policy makers or enforcers with enacting premature laws. Carefully drafted laws, with reasonable time for deliberation, stand the best chance of avoiding first amendment objections.

Section VI

SEXUAL EMANCIPATION

"The judges of normality are present everywhere. We are in the society of the teacher-judge, the doctor-judge, the educator-judge, the social worker-judge: It is on them that the universal reign of the normative is based, and each individual, wherever he may find himself, subjects to it his body, his gestures, his behavior, his aptitudes, his achievements."

M. Foucalt: *Discipline and Punishment*
New York, Pantheon, 1977, p. 304.

Chapter 24

SEXUAL EMANCIPATION — AN INTRODUCTION

LeRoy G. Schultz

It may be difficult for the reader to think of the "other side of the coin" of sexual abuse, after the previous series of readings. Society, the school, juvenile court, and the family are likewise child-molestors through the crime of omission. We willfully and maliciously withhold sexual information. We do not teach children how to make decisions regarding sexuality, and we deny them the learning experience and experiment of the real thing. Healthy sexual integration is made most difficult through a total social system oppression of normal sexuality. No balanced evaluation of the issue of child and minor sexual abuse is possible if we continue to deny that children and minors have sexual interests and drives. A look at contemporary age of consent laws (see appendix in Chapter 25) shows that we are a long way from being guided solely by the utilitarian aim of preventing demonstrable harm to victims. Our laws consist of a wierd medley of prohibited behaviors, couched in quaint Victorian language, originating in different historical periods of providing penalties that are unrelated to the presumed harmfulness or prevalence of the behaviors in question. As the next chapter indicates, social workers, judges, and mental health workers seem to have gathered all available data and arranged them to fit previously established theses, a kind of adolescent vulnerability as middle-class dogma. Our social control agencies continue to go after minors who simply refuse to slip through adolescence gracefully.

Setting a universal age of consent is almost impossible, considering the normal conflict in values and differential access of power to influence policy. The consumers of "protection" have never been asked to participate, to decide. While both sides fight it out, the important value of freedom of choice goes to the adult victors. While the determination of age of sexual consent is a matter for the legislature, it may be the courts that must push a legislature filled with re-election anxiety. The court may be the minors' only ombudsman and protector against antisexual parents and other social institutions (1).

REFERENCES

(1) Comment: Do children have the right to be incorrigible? *Brigham Young University Law Review*, Vol. 1976, 1976, pp. 659-691.

Chapter 25

THE AGE OF SEXUAL CONSENT: FAULT, FRICTION, FREEDOM

LeRoy G. Schultz

Western civilzation has never been capable of rationally nor humanely accommodating sexual expression in combination with the changing emancipation of minors. The history of changing definitions of the "legal age of consent" is one of suffering at the hands of adults, who always were presumed to have the "best interest of the child" uppermost or operating from a "for their own good" ideology. Sexual expression and childhood have traditionally been viewed as areas of social life that could pose threats to the social order unless held in check. Vigorous efforts to control both were characterized by fear, brutality, and superstition.[1,2]

Children and minors have historically been viewed as rightless, immature, incapable of sound decisions, harbingers of evil or total innocents, id-dominated animals in need of punishment, and property of parents. Such concepts of children and minors influenced the legal doctrine that shaped the definition of the age of consent, in the early period of history.[3,4] The struggle for "children's rights" the past 200 years suggest a slow incremental series of steps, sometimes forward, as we tiptoe towards a new concept of childhood and adolescence and perhaps even a "Bill of Rights" for youth. This chapter will deal with the evolution of the legal doctrine of "age of consent" in relation to youthful sexual expression and in turn relate both to present patterns of sexual behaviors. Since our common law heritage springs predominantly from England and our social customs from England and the mainland of Europe, historical data from both will be cited. The values and definitions of childhood and adolescence change over time and up until very recently these changes have resulted in *increasing* the age of consent for a wide variety of reasons, not all of which appear defensible today.

357

The literature on the "age of consent" is sparse and full of time gaps, so that making generalizations is hazardous and intellectual synthesis is difficult and the reader is cautioned.

Consent and History

The "age of consent" or the "age of minority" shifted over time to accommodate changing values, technology, and concepts of the science of childhood and adolescence. People in each historical period had to determine for themselves the "age of consent."

"Age of consent" in earliest times referred to a minor's rights and duties, in general, on reaching adulthood: at a later historical period, it specifically became identified with the age at which sexual consent could be freely given. As early as 585 A.D. males of the upper class or nobility were considered "of age" at seventeen years,[5] this being the general age at which boys were strong enough to carry armour and weapons. Barbaric tribes throughout Europe set the "age of consent" at fifteen years, apparently due to the lightweight armour common.[5] However, in early Rome, the issue of "age of consent" centered on the child's capacity to understand property laws, i.e. not to be taken advantage of in inheritance, and was set at age fourteen years. Thus, very early, both physical maturity and cognitive elements were popular criteria in "age of consent" determination.

In England by the time of the Magna Carta, the age of consent was moved to age twenty-one years.[5] Increasing the age was attributed to the introduction of extra-heavy armour (the mail shirt), the need for expert horsemanship, and warfare training.[5] France, mean-while, set the age of consent at seventeen years, claiming that boys (girls did not matter as yet) were physically and mentally capable of transacting business and cultivating land at such an age.[5]

Regarding girls, the law was quick to take a protective position. Under early English common law, it was not a crime for men to engage in consensual sexual intercourse with a female of any age, but by the latter half of the thirteenth century, legislation was enacted making it a crime to ravish a "damsel" under the age of twelve years, her consent being immaterial.[6] By the 16th century, the age of consent was reduced to ten years of age[7] and it was this law that was transported to the American colonies.[8]

Exception to the general "age of consent" usually occurred when the couple involved opted for marriage. In Rome, Justinian fixed the minimum age for marriage at fourteen years, providing the couple had parental consent to marry.[5] Under the Statute of Philip and Mary, fathers were given control over marriage of their daughters if she were to marry before age sixteen years.[1] Children, during this period of history were viewed as a means of improving the parent's estate, by choosing her husband for her. Sexual activity was restricted to the marital state only. In some instances, children as young as seven years were "pre-married" to other persons, sometimes adults, chosen by the parents, with a legal marriage to follow at the girl's age of sixteen years, thus assuring a good property arrangement.[5] In the event that the children who were "pre-married" had sexual intercourse and pregnancy resulted before the female reached age sixteen years, the couple was considered legally married by the community. The then current folklore, codified into law, held that girls menstruate at age fourteen years, i.e. become sexually mature, and boys of this age were sexually impotent and sterile.

Justice, or a concept of children's rights, by even rudimentary standards were simply irrelevant to children up to as late as 1850. Children were not legally protectable persons. Their value lay in their potential to advance family fortune. They were protected as a means to an end, not the end itself. Early marriage and pregnancy were essential to survival, since life was short by today's standards and infant mortality was high. By the seventeenth century, the ecclesiastical court of England ruled that boys of fourteen years and girls of twelve years could marry with their father's consent,[1] and most did marry at an early age. The result was a large child and public welfare problem. Couples could not support themselves or their children, and many became public charges, straining community budgets. The seriousness of the problem of caring for hundreds of welfare infants in each village can be gauged by efforts of control. In 1583, the Englishman, Stubbes, sensing the approaching bankruptcy of his town over child welfare costs, proposed that the age of consent be moved to age twenty-one years, with capital punishment for violators.[9,10] Stubbes' proposal may be the first recorded instance of "age of consent" criteria being of an economic character in terms of social welfare. A girl's sex organs, her reproductive potential, was of considerable economic value, a "treasure" that she lacked sufficient judgment to use or give away unless she was past a certain age.[11]

In England, for generations, the church had policed the sexual activities of minors through the Arch Deacon Court's meetings held weekly.[1] If the church discovered pregnancy among unmarried minors, both the minors and their parents were punished, thus setting a precedent of parental responsibility for children's acts. The Arch Deacon Courts appeared more concerned with the welfare costs of sexual activity than with sexual activity *per se*. Since girls were the ones who became pregnant and who posed a threat to family stability, it was they who were viewed as a community threat, with subsequent legislation supporting what is known today as the sexual double standard. This standard suggests girls be held to a higher standard of morality than boys, a heritage that colors so-called "status offenses" today.

Up to 1880, English courts held that if a child gave voluntary consent to sexual intercourse, a charge of sexual assault could not be made, no matter what her age.[12,13] In 1885, the Criminal Law Amendment was passed, setting age thirteen years as the limit on a consent defense and age sixteen years as the age at which she could legally consent to sexual intercourse.[14] Raising the age of consent in 1885 to 16 years was due, in part, to the campaign and social action of reformist Josephine Butler, in her efforts to rid England of child prostitutes.[15,16] During the period 1840 to 1885, large numbers of girls were entering houses of prostitution to escape the hardships of farm life and the suffering and poor wages of the "sweat shops" of the city, or simply, unemployment. Butler and her social action groups tried to rehabilitate the prostitutes on a voluntary basis, coupled with a strong dose of religion. This attempt met with failure as the prostitutes either were not interested in "being saved" or had no access to the rehabilitation program. The income received from prostitution could not be matched by conventional women's employment. Responding to this failure, Butler was successful in having passed a new law, which was to be of great impact on minors' sexual freedom. The newly passed law, the Criminal Law Amendment Act of 1885, gave Butler and her group the power to use police in removing young prostitutes from the streets even *against their will* up to the age of sixteen years. The spirit of this new law contended that the sexual freedom of minor girls was second to society's duty to protect her *from herself.* Girls who resisted being rescued or rehabilitated were to be arrested; thus, the young girl moved from being a victim to being a criminal or delinquent. The extent of this spirit can be learned from court rulings. One such ruling claimed to end "animal lust and the moral degradation of man and the destruction of womanhood"[17] and to protect "society, family and infants."[18] The state's role as sex moral supremist was further entrenched by decisions holding that "a boy or man must resist a voluptuous, abandoned woman who solicits him" or suffer the penalty for statutory rape[19] and that "even if the girl is older than the boy, and more aggressive than him, or the real seducer or a common prostitute seducing a fifteen year old boy, the boy will be guilty and the girl innocent."[20] The legislature and the court simply echoed the prevalent values of those in power, one being that a woman or girl under age eighteen does not possess sufficient knowledge of the factors needed to decide on engaging in sexual behavior,[21] nor would society teach such knowledge. The girl finds herself in a double bind. Without knowledge there could be no lawful consent, since consent requires freedom to excise the powers of choice and awareness of the implications of that choice.[22]

Since there were no ecclesiastical courts in the United States, their role was filled by state legislators and judges who echoed the moralistic constraints of the time. Age of sexual consent for girls ranged from a low of seven years in Delaware to a high of eighteen years in Massachusetts, with many states choosing age sixteen years.[23] All states, however, had to make one exception to statutory rape for the boy or man, and "incorrigibility" for the girl, and this occurred if the sexually active couple decided to marry. To put it another way, a married girl of fourteen years of age could make excellent choices regarding sexual activities, while her seventeen-year-old single sister could not.

The legal notion of age of consent has tried to shift with the times, but its historical substance was based on feudal and nineteenth century values, some of which were transported to America. The premises were—

1. the physical strength of minors
2. the cognitive power of minors
3. the child as parental property
4. the social need to control illegitmacy
5. the moral need to control child prostitution
6. the social need to control "sexually acting out" girls

These aspects were seized upon by reformers, "child savers," and feminists working to protect minor girls from themselves.

Giving Consent Too Soon

Shortly after the establishment of the juvenile court in America (1899), its focus broadened to include not just the neglected and abused child, but a whole range of preventive services for youngsters needing "protection" and "control." By the 1890s, minors in need of control were no longer diagnosed by court and social science professionals as "precocious" but were put under the new label "immature."

The originator of the concept of adolescence, G. Stanley Hall, warned of the adolescents' "perversion, crime and secret vice."[24] The acceptance of such characterizations, along with other social forces, resulted in a deluge of protective legislation. Juvenile delinquency became a social focus only after the concept of adolescence became popular. The model of the good adolescent was the opposite of the new stigma "delinquent," i.e. precocious and independent of authority. Expanding on Hall's work, other social scientists described adolescence as a period of dangerous instability, vulnerability, and narcissism.[30] Activities for adolescents were to be constructed differently than those of adults, with separation of the sexes, thus assuring the isolation of youth from "adult" pleasures and premature discovery, of the sexual life. Youth were to be protected not only from other's property, but from themselves and from a wide range of so-called status offenses, by legislatures and their implementing arm, the social control agencies. By the turn of the century, the sharp distinction between children and minors who were abused and neglected and those who were delinquent eroded away, and the state completed its power over minors. Laws written to protect minors began referring to them as "depraved, wicked and evil." In the absence of a strong family or church, the creation of the reformatory was essential. The "proper" adolescent was to be shaped by social science, social workers, and physicians. This shaping process was not more humane than what preceded it. The early treatment of sexual expression in minors, now labeled delinquency or incorrigibility, constitutes a dark chapter in history.[25,27]

TABLE 25-I. NEW YORK FAMILY COURTS SEXUAL INCORRIGIBILITY DISPOSITIONS IN PERCENTAGES*

Charge	Court Referral	Detained	Adjudicated	Probation
Undesirable Boyfriend	64	43	57	40
Sexual Misbehavior	67	33	33	33
Promiscuity	80	50	50	50
Staying out overnight	56	47	42	18
Undesirable companion	44	55	27	11
Prostitution	100	0	0	0
Cohabitation	100	0	0	0
Spent night with male	100	0	0	0

*From *Yale Law Review* Vol. 83, 1974, pp. 1383-84.

The social reformer, Josephine Lowell, agitated the legislature and it passed a bill creating the first institution for "... erratic ... women who are easily yielding to lust" in Newark, N.Y. in 1878.[28] All women regardless of age were viewed as sexually vulnerable and childlike in defenselessness, and any budding sexual activity in minor girls was viewed as a sign of mental retardation or illness.[29,30] In an age in which sexual feelings and pleasures were restricted to men, females engaging in sexual activity voluntarily were presumed to be automatically "unwilling," even if legally married.[31] Rosenheim summarizes: "The dominant theme of the new [juvenile court establishment] has been child protection. It presupposes passivity of children as its ideal. It permits the possibility that the passive can become corrupted or misguided. Child protection thus encompasses the tasks of both salvation and re-education. These are the underlying purposes of social legislation for children. Together with the older laws of parent and child laid down over seven centuries, they form the modern framework for the definition and implementation of permissible standards of behavior by and towards youth."[32]

Adolescence was now itself the cause of delinquency. While in Dicken's time (1840s) juvenile crime was attributed to the evil influence of adults, by 1890 it was the child's conduct that was the determinant of later adult crime. While in 1850 crime was considered a moral disease, by 1900 this had been reversed: immoral behavior should be treated as a crime. These new social changes in attitudes towards minors broadened the jurisdiction of the juvenile court, and the social control agencies it supports, and could now include normal behavior thus criminalizing behavior once left to private discretion.

Between 1880 and 1960 the *parens patriae* doctrine, including the criminalization of normal traditions of youth, went essentially unchallenged. For example, in 1944 the United States Supreme Court held that "The power of the state to control the conduct of children reaches beyond the scope of its authority over adults."[33] However, the 1960s and 1970s were to witness a veritable revolution in the rights of minors throughout much of society and its institutions, and subsequently due process protections were extended to minors. While due process protection left intact current illegal behaviors as defined by the juvenile court law, questions and challenges were beginning to be raised as to the meaning of vague behaviors such as "incorrigible," "beyond control," and "endangering his own welfare," and the psychiatric diagnosis (actually a social condemnation) of "sexually acting out." Despite vagueness, 50% of all minors incarcerated in one state were there because the court had ruled them "ungovernable," which in the case of girls meant giving sexual consent too soon.[34] In a last ditch stand, the state of New York attempted to defend the current age of consent law by denying sexually active minors the right to control pregnancy by denying them access to contraceptive technology. The court ruled that the state's right to control sexual behavior of minors "cannot be justified."[35] Justice Stevens, concurring, added that sex control laws have a "symbolic effect" and constitute a form of "propaganda" and Justice Rehnquist, concurring, stated ". . . (The State) may not use its police power to legislate in the interests of its concept of the public morality as it pertains to minors."[35] Such opinions, along with other social data, may foretell of expected changes in our concept of the age of consent.

Reality Today

There is no longer any justification for the juvenile laws' support of a neo-Victorian attitude towards sexual consent. Most of the rationale offered to support consent standards, certain statutory rape provisions, and some female status offenses are no longer acceptable to large segments of America, if they ever were. In short, they may be viewed as victimless crimes, or more realistically, a reflection of adolescent preference. A reappraisal of their negative affects is timely.

While children and adolescents may have always been sexually active in the past,[36] it is doubtful that the level of sexual activity has ever been higher than today. Several recent reliable national studies of minors' sexual behavior reveal that—

- at age 15 years, 18 percent of American white girls have had sexual intercourse; at age 16, 25.5 percent have had sexual intercourse; female blacks were 38 percent sexually active by age 15[37]
- at age 7 years many black girls have had or witnessed sexual intercourse, if they live in the ghettos[38]
- by age 12 years, 13 percent of females have had intercourse; and by age 15 years, 56 percent of females are sexually active[39, 40]

- the average age of first intercourse was 12.8 years, with 14 percent of girls reporting first intercourse below age 9 years[41]

How courts relate to these research findings can be learned from studying the intake patterns of one large juvenile court in terms of sexual behavior charges (Table 25-I). The names of the behaviors usually disguise their sexual nature.

Sexual charges bring more serious court attention than crimes for girls; 62 percent of all "ungovernability" cases at intake are girls, with 44 percent over the age of fifteen years.[42] The sexually active girl has been made the little vixen of *parens patriae*. At no level of society does minority status make sexual activity inaccessible, whatever the official norms may be. Yet, it is the poor, minority girl who ends up in juvenile court or the

TABLE 25-II. JUVENILE COURT INTAKE FOR THREE MONTH PERIOD*.

Sexual Allegation	Number of Girls Charged
General Sexual Misbehavior	6
Spent Night With Male	3
Cohabitation	1
Promiscuity	5
Prostitution	1
Disapproved Boyfriend	25
Disorderly Conduct	7
Runaway	96
Keeping Overnight Hours	25
Keeping Late Hours	46

*From Note, *Ungovernability: The Unjustified Jurisdiction*, 83 YALE LAW J. 1408 (1974).

correctional institution. Her middle-class peer with the same "problem" has options beyond the court for solution. Both the court and the legislature ultimately must come to grips with the fact that the basic intellectual capacities are present very young and that complex moral and political reasoning can take place at least by age twelve or fourteen years.[43, 44] *Parens patriae* has become an insecure, over-protective father who, reminiscing upon his own sexual past, resists the natural sexual emancipation of his daughter, continuing to stick his head in a Victorian sand trap.

No group in our society possesses a more ambiguous legal position than the youth. Their status as a "person" under our constitution is subject to doubt. The law, despite its cherished protection of individual freedom, justifies this strict control by its own overriding concern for the child's best interests. Unlike adults, a child and, in some instances, an adolescent have almost no say in self-determination because of immaturity. The parent and the state (both poor surrogate lobbies) speak for the child from his/her very conception, often engaging in open warfare. Even after puberty and during adolescence, the child's voice is unheard and unheeded. The best interests of an individual must remain uncertain because of underlying philosophical dilemma and differing viewpoints of the three parties. Special rules laid down by parents and the state[45, 47] are likely to be contradictory and burdensome when they unnecessarily obstruct a child's understanding of an experimentation with accepted adult behavior patterns.

Several recent trends suggest a "breaking of the ice" on consent law somewhat more in keeping with the real world of adolescence. One trend is to lower the age of sexual consent. For example, New York dropped from 18 to 17 years in 1967, Hawaii from 16 to 14 years, Illinois and Wyoming from 18 to 16 years, Pennsylvania from 16 to 14 years in 1976, and South Dakota from 16 to 15 years in 1977[45] (see chapter appendix).

Another positive trend is for states to do away with the "sex of the actor" requirement, so that females can be charged with sex crimes against children. For example, Maryland defines the crime as "any female over 18 to carnally know a male under 14."[45]

Another trend is to reduce the penalty for statutory rape if the actor is but a few years older than his partner. For example, Colorado requires that the male actor be at least two years older than his partner to sustain the charge of statutory rape. While such trends appear to be mere nibbles at the edges of a big problem, they constitute promising changes in an area not historically noted for changing at all. Some five states have created "free zones" in their sex laws, so that voluntary sexual intercourse for those between fourteen and eighteen years is not the law's concern if they do so with each other only.[45] It would appear that age fourteen years should be the age of sexual consent.

Another proposed legal change having impact on the sexual behavior of youth is one that calls for removal of all status offenses from the jurisdiction of the juvenile court,[48] although the intent of the change can be subverted by those of a different persuasion.[49] Even if the ABA recommendations were to gain acceptance, or if "free zones" were created for youth's sexual experimentation, there is still a snag. States can still place charges of "fornication," "lewd behavior," "carnal knowledge," "corrupting morals," etc., against those it chooses to go after, or those who because of income cannot fight with the legal weapons of the middle class, or those who are simply defenseless against an oppressive society by virtue of their age. They want participation, not protection. The sexually emancipated minor is here now.

APPENDIX

Statutory Rape in the United States*

ALABAMA	Age of consent for female is 12; May be capital offense to have intercourse with female under 12; Lesser offense to have carnal knowledge of female over 12 and under 16, but not applicable to boys under 16.
ALASKA	No one 16 or older may have carnal knowledge of a female under 16.
ARIZONA	Age of consent for female is 18.
ARKANSAS	Class C felony if anyone 18 or older has intercourse with anyone under 14; Class A Misdemeanor if anyone 20 or older has intercourse with anyone under 16; Class B misdemeanor if anyone has intercourse with anyone under 16.
CALI- FORNIA	Age of consent for female is 18. Physical ability of male under 14 to accomplish penetration must be proved.
COLORADO	Age of consent for female is 16, but for male to be guilty he must be at least two years older than female.
CONNECTI- CUT	Class B felony if male has intercourse with female under 14; Class C felony if male is 18 or older and has intercourse with female under 16.
DELAWARE	Class B felony if male has intercourse with female or male under 12; Class E felony if male has intercourse with female under 16 and male is at least four years older than female.
DISTRICT OF COLUMBIA	Age of consent for females is 16.

---

*American Civil Liberties Union, 1978.

FLORIDA   Capital offense if actor is over 18 and victim 11 or younger; Life felony if actor under 18 and victim 11 or younger; 1st degree felony if victim is 11 through 17 and actor in a position of familial, custodial or official authority over victim and uses authority to coerce victim's submission; 2nd degree felony for any person to have intercourse with another person under 18, of previous chaste character (no defense that victim was of previous unchaste character when lack of chastity caused solely by intercourse between victim and defendant).

GEORGIA   Age of consent for female is 14.

GUAM   Age of consent for female is 16.

HAWAII   Age of consent for female is 14.

IDAHO   Age of consent for female is 18.

ILLINOIS   No one over 17 may have intercourse with anyone under 16; Affirmative defense that actor reasonably believed victim was 16 or older.

INDIANA   Age of consent for female is 16; Greater punishment if female is under 12.

IOWA   Age of consent for female is 16, but it is also illegal for anyone over 21 to have sexual intercourse with a female under 17.

KANSAS   Age of consent is 16.

KENTUCKY   Class A felony if anyone has intercourse with another person under 12; Class C felony if actor 18 or over has intercourse with another person under 14; Class D felony if actor 21 or older has intercourse with another person under 16.

LOUISIANA   Capital offense if anyone has intercourse with female under 12 (lack of knowledge of female's age no defense); Lesser crime if anyone over 17 has carnal knowledge of female 12 through 16 when when age difference between actor and victim is more than 2 years.

MAINE   Illegal for anyone to have carnal knowledge of female under 14; Lesser crime for anyone 18 or older to have carnal knowledge of female 14 and 15.

MARYLAND Illegal for anyone to have carnal knowledge of any woman under 14; Lesser crime for anyone 18 or older to carnally know any female between 14 and 16; Illegal for any female over 18 to carnally know any male under 14.

MASSA-CHUSETTS   Age of consent for female is 16.

MICHIGAN Age of consent for female is 16.

MINNESOTA Anyone who carnally knows female under age of 10 subject to life imprisonment; When female 10 through 13, actor subject to imprisonment from 7 to 30 years; When female is 14 through 17, actor subject to imprisonment from 0 to 7 years.

MISSIS-SIPPI   Capital offense if person 18 or older has intercourse with female under 12 (Lesser penalty if actor 13 through 17); Lesser crime for any male to have carnal knowledge of female of previously chaste character, over 12 and under 18 who is younger than himself.

MISSOURI Capital offense if any person carnally knows female under 16. (Effective in 1979: Class A felony for any person to have intercourse with another person under 14; Class B felony for any person to have intercourse with another person 14 or 15; Class D felony for any person 17 or older to have intercourse with another person who is 16; Reasonable belief that victim is over age is a defense.

MONTANA   Age of consent for female is 16; More serious crime if actor is more than 3 years older than victim; Defense that actor reasonably believed victim to be over 16 (no defense of reasonable belief if victim was under 14).

NEBRASKA Illegal for anyone over 18 to have intercourse with another person under 16.

NEVADA Illegal for anyone 18 or older to have intercourse with another person under 16; more serious crime if actor 21 or older.

NEW HAMP-SHIRE Age of consent is 13; Also illegal for actor to have intercourse with victim 13 through 15 when actor is related, a member of same household or in position of authority over victim and uses authority to coerce victim's submission.

NEW JERSEY Illegal for anyone over 16 to have intercourse with woman-child under 12; Less serious crime for anyone over 16 to have intercourse with woman-child 12 through 15.

NEW MEXICO Illegal for anyone to have intercourse with child under 13; Less serious crime if actor is in a position of authority over child age 13 to 16 and actor uses authority to coerce victim's submission.

NEW YORK Class B felony when man has intercourse with female under 11; Class D felony when male, 18 or older, has intercourse with female under 14; Class E felony when male, 21 or older, has intercourse with female under 17.

NORTH CAROLINA Illegal for anyone to have intercourse with female under 12 (capital offense if actor over 16 and victim a virtuous female child under 12) (Lesser penalty if actor 16 or under); Felony if male has intercourse with female 12 through 15 who has never before had intercourse with anyone; Misdemeanor if female has intercourse with male under 16.

NORTH DAKOTA Felony when one person engages in a sexual act with another under 15; Misdemeanor when one person 18 or older engages in a sexual act with another age 15 through 17.

OHIO First degree felony for anyone to have intercourse

with another person under 13 (whether or not actor knows the age of the victim); Third degree felony for person 18 or older to have intercourse with another person when actor knows the other person is 13, 14 or 15 (but if actor is less than 4 years older than victim, crime is a misdemeanor).

OKLA-HOMA Illegal for male to have intercourse with female under 16 (may be capital offense if male over 18 and female under 14); Lesser crime if female 16 or 17 and of previous chaste and virtuous character; No conviction of male can be had for either offense if female over 14 and male 18 or under; Physical ability of male under 14 to accomplish penetration must be proved in all cases.

OREGON Class A felony when any person has intercourse with a female under 12; Class B felony when any person has intercourse with a female under 14; Class C felony when any person has intercourse with a female under 16 (no defense that actor did not know age of victim or that he believed her age was over 16).

PENN-SYLVANIA Illegal for any person 18 or older to have intercourse with any other person under 14; No defense that actor did not know age of victim or that he believed child was over 14.

RHODE ISLAND Age of consent for female is 16.

SOUTH CAROLINA First degree criminal sexual conduct for anyone to have intercourse with another person under 11 if actor is at least 3 years older than victim; Second degree for anyone to have intercourse with another person 11 through 14 if actor is at least 3 years older than victim; Second degree for anyone in a position of familial, custodial or official authority over victim age 14 or 15 and uses authority to coerce victim's submission.

SOUTH   Age of consent is 15.
DAKOTA

TENNESSEE Illegal for anyone to have intercourse with female
            under 12; Equally illegal for anyone to have inter-
            course with female 12 through 17 (but for this
            offense, no conviction may be had based on un-
            supported testimony of victim, and when victim
            is over 14, evidence of a female's reputation for
            want of chastity admissible on behalf of actor);
            Nothing shall authorize conviction of actor when
            female victim over 12 is a bawd, lewd or kept fe-
            male.

TEXAS   Age of consent for female is 17; Defense that fe-
            male 14 or older engaged in prior promiscuous
            sexual intercourse; Affirmative defense that actor
            was not 2 years older than victim.

VERMONT   Age of consent for female is 16.

VIRGINIA   Illegal for anyone to have intercourse with female
            under 13; Fourth class felony for anyone to have
            intercourse with female 13 or 14; Sixth class
            felony if actor is a minor and victim 3 years or
            more his junior; Fornication if actor is a minor
            and victim less than 3 years his junior; In all cases,
            if victim is 14 or older and of bad moral repute
            and lewd female, actor may be found guilty only
            of contributing to delinquency of a minor or
            fornication.

WASHING-   First degree statutory rape for anyone over 13 to
TON   have intercourse with another person under 11;
            Second degree for anyone over 16 to have inter-
            course with another person 11 through 13; Third
            degree for anyone over 18 to have intercourse with
            another person 14 or 15.

WEST   Age of consent is 16. First degree sexual assault if
VIRGINIA   anyone 14 or older has intercourse with another
            person under 11: Third degree if anyone 16 or

older has intercourse with another person under 16 and at least 4 years younger than actor; Affirmative defense that actor did not know victim's age unless he was reckless in his failure to know.

WISCONSIN Illegal for anyone to have intercourse with another person 12 or under; Lesser crime for anyone to have intercourse with another person over 12 and under 18 (Person under 15 cannot give consent; Person 15 to 17 presumed incapable of consent but presumption can be rebutted).

WYOMING Illegal to have intercourse with anyone under 12 if actor at least 4 years older than victim; Lesser crime if victim under 16 and actor at least 4 years older than victim; Affirmative defense that actor reasonably believed victim to be 16 or older (no defense if victim under 12).

REFERENCES

1. I. Pinchbeck and M. Hewitt: *Children in English Society*, Vol. 1 and 2. Toronto, University of Toronto Press, 1969.
2. J. Kett: Adolescence and youth in 19th century America. *Journal of Interdisciplinary History*, 2:283-298, 1971.
3. S. Schlossman and S. Wallach: The crime of precocious sexuality: Female juvenile delinquency in the progressive era. *Harvard Educational Review*, *48(1)*:65-94, 1978.
4. A. Platt: *The Child Savers.* Chicago, University of Chicago Press, 1977.
5. T. James: The age of majority. *American Journal of Legal History*, *4*:22, 1969.
6. Statute of Westminister I, 3 Edward I c. 34 (1275).
7. The Common Informer's Act, 18 Elizabeth c. 7 (1576).
8. Nider v. Commonwealth, 140 Ky. 684, 689, 131 S.W. 1024 (1910).
9. P. Stubbes: *The Anatomie of Abuses.* 1897, p. 97.
10. E. Shorter: Illegitimacy, sexual revolution and social change in Europe. *Journal of Interdisciplinary History*, 2:237-272, 1971.
11. Note: Forcible and statutory rape: An exploration of the operation and objectives of the consent standards. *Yale Law Review*, *62*:75-95, 1952.
12. H. Foster and A. Freed: Offenses against the family. *University of Missouri at Kansas City Law Review*, *32*:35, 1964.
13. Reg. v. Webb, 2 Carr and K, 937 (1848).
14. Criminal Law Amendment Act 1885, 48, 49, Vet. c. 69.

15. A. Butler: *Portrait of Josephine Butler*. London, Faber and Faber, 1954, pp. 131-141.
16. D. Pivar: *Purity Crusade*. Westport, Cn., Green Wood, 1973.
17. *Arena*, Vol. 3. 1891, p. 382.
18. People v. Ratz, 115 Cal. 132, 46, Pac. 915 (1896).
19. People v. Cureale, 137 Cal. 534, 538, 70, Pac. 468, 470 (1902).
20. 138 Cal. 467, 71. Pac. 564 (1903).
21. People v. Gordon, 70 Cal. 467, 468, 11, Pac. 762, 763 (1886).
22. People v. Nerdegreen, 106 Cal. 211, 214, 39, Pac. 607, 608, 46 Am. St. Rep. 234, 236, (1895).
23. L. Kanowitz: Law and the single girl. *St. Louis University Law Journal, 11*:300-319, 1967.
24. J. Gillis: *Youth and History*. New York, Academic Press, 1974, pp. 133-184.
25. G. Baker-Benfield: *The Horrors of the Half Known Life*. New York, Harper and Row, 1976.
26. A. Comfort: *The Anxiety Makers*. London, Nelson, 1967, pp. 69-113.
27. J. Money and H. Musaph: *Handbook of Sexology*. New York, Elsevier, 1977, pp. 269-281.
28. R. Mennel: *Thorns and Thistles: Juvenile Delinquency in the U.S., 1825-1940*. Hanover, N.H., University Press of New England, 1974, p. 71.
29. D. Taylor: Denied the power to do the good. *Journal of Social History*, 480, 1977.
30. I. Ray: The insanity of women caused by seduction *American Journal of Insanity, 23*:270, 1866.
31. M. Pearson: *The 5-Pound Virgins*. New York, Saturday Review Press, 1972, p. 20.
32. M. Rosenheim: The child and the law. In E. Grotberg: *200 Years of Children*. Washington, D.C. U.S. DHEW., 1976. p. 438.
33. Prince v. Mass., 321 U.S. 158, 170 (1944).
34. A. Conway and C. Bagdan: Sexual delinquency: Persistence of the double standard. *Crime and Delinquency*, 133, April, 1977.
35. G.P.O. Slip Opinion (1977), Cary, Gov. of N.Y., *et al*. v. Popula. Services International *et al.*, *Appeal from* U.S. Dist. Ct. Southern Dist. of N.Y. No. 75-443, *Argued* 1-10-77, *Decided* 6-9-77.
36. P. Cutright: The teenage sexual revolution and the myth of an abstinent past. *Family Planning Perspectives, 4(1)*:24-31, 1972.
37. M. Zelnik and J. Kantner: Sexual and contraceptive experience of young unmarried women in the U.S., 1976 and 1971. *Family Planning Perspectives, 9(2)*:55-73, 1977.
38. J. Ladner and B. Hammond: *Socialization into Sexual Behavior*. New York, Society for the Study of Sexual Problems, 1967.
39. R. Sorenson: *Adolescent Sexuality in Contemporary America*, New York, World, 1973, p. 214.
40. K. Schoof-Tams: Differentiation of sexual morality between 11 and 16 years *Archives of Sexual Behavior, 5(5)*:353-370, 1976.

41. M. Finkel and D. Finkel: Sexual and contraceptive knowledge, attitudes and behavior of male adolescents. *Family Planning Perspectives, 7(6):* 256-259,1975.
42. Note: Ungovernability: The unjustified jurisdiction, *Yale Law Journal, 83:*1408, 1974.
43. Governor's Special Commission on the Age of Majority, *Summary,* 1971, at 2, State of Michigan.
44. E. Boulding: Children's rights, *Society, 15(1):*40, 1977.
45. The strange world of statutory rape, *Children's Rights Report, 2(6):*March 1978.
46. S. Prevost: Statutory rape: A growing liberalization. *South Carolina Law Review, 18:*254-266, 1966.
47. A. Grey: Civilizing our sex laws. *Journal of Society of Teachers of Law, 13:* 106-112, 1975.
48. Institute of Judical Administration and ABA Joint Commission on Juvenile Justice Standards, Part I (1977) Non-Criminal Misbehavior.
49. D. Gilman: How to retain jurisdiction over status offenses: Change without reform in Florida. *Crime and Delinquency, 22:*48-51, 1976.

BIBLIOGRAPHY

SEXUALITY AND SEXUAL ABUSE THROUGH TIME

Acton, L.: *The Function of the Reproductive Organs in Childhood, Etc.* London, 1857.

Are low wages responsible for women's immorality? *Current Opinion, 54*:402-408, 1913.

Aries, P.: *Centuries of Childhood.* New York, Vintage, 1962, pp. 100-128.

Barber, R.: The Criminal Law Amendment Act of 1891 and the age of consent. *Australian and New Zealand Journal of Criminology, 10*:95-113, 1977.

Brushfield, L.: Sex and insanity. *Journal of Mental Science, 18*: 231-32, 1873.

Bullough, V.: *Sexual Variance in Society and History.* New York, Wiley, 1976, Chp. 16-20.

Clarke, E.: *Sex In Education: A Fair Chance for Girls.* Boston, Osgood, 1874.

Colby, C.: Mechanical restraints of masturbation in young girl. *New York Medical Record, 52*:206-209, 1897.

Cutright, P.: Teenage sexual revolution and the myth of an abstinent past. *Family Planning Perspectives, 4*:24-31, 1972.

DeLima, A.: *Our Enemy the Child.* New York, New Republic Press, 1923.

DeMause, L.: *The History of Childhood.* New York, Psychohistory Press, 1974, pp. 44-50.

DePauw, J.: Illicit sexual activity and society in 18th century Nantes. In R. Forster and O. Ranum: *Family and Society.* Baltimore, Johns Hopkins University Press, 1976, pp. 145-191.

Douglass, A.: *The Feminization of American Culture.* New York, Knopf, 1977.

Engelhardt, H.: The disease of masturbation: Values and concepts, *Bulletin of the History of Medicine, 48*:234-248, 1974.

Eyer, A.: Clitoridectomy for the cure of masturbation in young girls. *International Medical Magazine, 3*:259-262, 1895.

Fee, E.: Psychology, sexuality and social control in victorian England. *Social Science Quarterly, 58*:632-646, 1978.

Flandrin, J.: Repression·and change in the sexual life of young people. *Journal of Family History, 2*:196-210, 1977.

Foster, R. and Ranum, O.: *Deviants and the Abandoned in French Society.* Baltimore, Johns Hopkins University Press, 1978, pp. 6-8.

Gerson, J.: *De Confessioni Mollicei.* 1706.

Gilbert, A.: Doctor, patient and onanist disease in the 19th century. *Journal of History of Medicine,* July, 1975.

Goldberg, J. and Goldberg, R.: *Girls on city streets: A study of 1400 cases of rape.* New York, American Social Hygiene Association, 1935, pp. 155-183.

Haeberle, E.: Historical roots of sexual oppression. In H. and J. Gochros: *The Sexually Oppressed.* New York, Association Press, 1977, pp. 3-37.

Haller, J. and R.: *The Physician and Sexuality in Victorian America.* Urbana, University of Illinois Press, 1974.

Hardy, J.: *The Unnatural History of the Nanny.* New York, Dial, 1973, Chp. 8.

Harrison, F.: *The Dark Angel.* New York, Universe Books, 1978.

Hunt, D.: *Parents and Children in History.* New York, Basic Books, 1970, Chp. 8.

Jacobi, A.: On masturbation and hysteria in young children. *American Journal of Obstetrics, 8*:595-96, 1876.

James, T.: The age of majority. *American Journal of Legal History, 4*:21-33, 1960.

Kelly, C.: On some changes in the legal status of the child since Blackstone. *International Review, 13*:83-99, 1882.

Kennedy, D.: *Birth Control in America.* New Haven, Yale University Press, 1970.

Kett, J.: *Rites of Passage: Adolescence in America, 1790 to the Present.* New York, Basic Books, 1977.

Lerman, P.: Delinquency and social policy: A historical perspective. *Crime and Delinquency,* 383-393, Oct. 1977.

Levine, M. and A.: The more things change: A case history of child guidance clinics. *Journal of Social Issues, 26*:19-34, 1970.

Levy, S.: Interaction of institution and policy group: The origin of sex crimes legislation. *The Lawyer and Law Notes, 5*:3-12, 1971.

Lind, M.: The sexualization of female crime. *Psychology Today,* 43-46, Aug. 1974.

Litin, A. et al.: Parental influence in unusual sexual behavior. *Psychoanalytic Quarterly, 37*:36-45, 1956.

Mawby, R.: Social action and crime theory: Josephine Butler. *Howard Journal of Penology, 14*:30-42, 1975.

May, G.: *Social Control of Sex Expression.* London, 1930.

May, M.: Innocence and experience: The evolution of the concept of juvenile delinquency in mid-nineteenth century. *Victorian Studies, 17*:7-29, 1973.

McDougall, J.: Primal scene and sex perversion. *International Journal of Psychoanalysis, 53*:371-384, 1972.

Moll, A.: *The Sexual Life of the Child.* New York, Emerson, 1912.

Newman, R.: Masturbation, madness and modern concepts of childhood and adolescence. *Journal of Social History, 8*:1-18, 1975.

Ordahl, L and G.: A study of delinquent and dependent girls. *Journal of Delinquency, 3*:55-63, 1918.

Pearce, F. and Roberts, A.: The social regulation of sexual behavior and the development of industrial capitalism in Britain. In R. Bailey and J. Young: *Contemporary Social Problems in Britain.* Lexington. Ma, Heath, 1973, pp. 51-72.

Peto, A.: The etiological significance of primal scene. *Psychoanalytic Quarterly, 44*:177-190, 1975.

Pfohl, S.: The discovery of child abuse. *Social Problems, 24*: 310-23, 1977.

Pivar, D.: *Purity Crusade: Sexual Morality and Social Control 1868-1900.* Westport, Cn, Greenwood Press, 1973.

Platt, A.: *The Child Savers: The Invention of Delinquency.* Chicago, University of Chicago Press, 1969.

Plumb, J.: The new world of children in 18th century England. *Past and Present, 67*:64-95, 1975.

Quaife, G.: The consenting spinster in peasant society. *Journal of Social History*, *11*:228-241, 1977.

Ray, I.: Insanity of women produced by desertion or seduction. *American Journal of Insanity*. *23*:272-280, 1866.

Rose, V.: Rape as a social problem: A by-product of the feminist movement. *Social Problems*, *25*:75-89, 1977.

Rosenberg, A. and E.: The legacy of the stubborn and rebellious son. *Michigan Law Review*, *74*:1097-1165, 1976.

Rosenberg, C.: Sexuality, class, and role in 19th century America. *American Quarterly*, *25*:131-153, 1973.

Rothman, D.: The state as parent. In W. Gaylin et al.: *Doing Good: The Limits of Benevolence*. New York, Pantheon, 1978, pp. 69-96.

Ruggiero, G.: Sexual criminality in early Renaissance. *Journal of Social History*, *8*:18-37, 1975.

Saffady, W.: Fears of sexual license in the English reformation. *History of Childhood Quarterly*, *8*:18-37, 1975.

Schlossman, S. and Wallach, S.: The crime of precocious sexuality: Female juvenile delinquency in the progressive era. *Harvard Educational Review*, *48(1)*:65-94, 1978.

Shade, W.: A mental passion: Female sexuality in Victorian America. *International Journal of Women Studies*, *1*:13-29, 1978.

Shorter, W.: On writing the history of rape. *Signs*, *3(2)*:471-82, 1977.

Sinbaldi, G.: *Geneanthropeia*. 1642.

Smart, C.: *Women, Crime and Criminology*. Boston, Routledge, Kegan, Paul, 1976.

Stone, L.: *The Family, Sex and Marriage in England: 1500-1800*. New York, Harper and Row, 1977, Pt.5.

Strong, B.: Sex and incest in the 19th century family. *Journal of Marriage and the Family*, *35*:457-460, 1973.

Symposium: The shame of America: Age of consent laws in the U.S. *Arena*, *9*:192-215, 1895.

Tarnowski, B.: *Anthropological, Legal, and Medical Studies on Pederasty in Europe*. New York, Falstaff, 1933.

Tomes, N.: A Torrent of Abuse. *Journal of Social History*, 328-345, Spring 1978.

Trudgitt, E.: *Madonnas and Magdolens: The Origins and Development of Victorian Sex Attitudes.* New York, Holmes and Meier, 1975.

Tylor, P.: Denied the power to choose the good: Sex and Mental defect in American medical practice, 1850-1920, *Journal of Social History,* 472-489, 1977.

Universal Pictures: *Traffic in Souls.* 16 mm., 65 min., 1913 (Rockefeller White Slavery Commission).

Walowitz, J. and D.: We are not beasts of the field: Prostitution and the poor in Plymouth. In M. Hartman and L. Banner: *Clio's Consciousness Raised.* New York, Harper, 1974, pp. 192-225.

Worthington, G. and Topping, R.: *Specialized Courts Dealing With Sex Delinquency.* New York, Hitchcock Press, 1925.

SEXUAL DEVELOPMENT

Adams, J.: *Sex and the Single Parent.* New York, Coward, McCann, Geoghegan, 1978.

Adilman, P.: Mary and her mother. *Adolescence, 9:*199-200, 1974.

Ball, J. and Logan, N.: Early sexual behavior of lower class delinquent girls. *Journal of Criminal Law, Criminology and Police Science, 51:*209-214, 1960.

Beigal, H.: Children who seduce adults. *Sexology, 40(7):*30-34, 1974.

Bennett, W. and Delattre, E.: Moral education in the schools. *The Public Interest,* 81-98, Winter 1978.

Broderick, C.: Children's romances. *Sexual Behavior, 2(5):*16-21, 1972.

Broderick, C.: Sexual behavior of pre-adolescents. *Journal of Social Issues, 22:*6-21, 1966.

Bryt, A.: Adolescent sex crises. *Medical Aspects of Human Sexuality,* 8-40, Oct. 1976.

Campbell, A.: What makes a girl turn to crime? *New Society, 39:*172-173, 1977.

Char, W. and McDermott, J.: Children's exposure to homosexuals. *Medical Aspects of Human Sexuality,* 81-90, August 1977.

Cohen, K.: Children's sexual preoccupation as a reaction to difficult family relationship and parents anxieties about sex. *Journal of Child Psychiatry, 2*:205-220, 1951.

Cohen, M. and Friedman, S.: Nonsexual motivation of adolescent sex behavior. *Medical Aspects of Human Sexuality,* 8-39, September 1975.

Conway, A.: Sexual Delinquency. *Crime and Delinquency,* 39-40, April 1977.

D'Augelli, J. and D'Augelli, A.: Moral reasoning and premarital sexual behavior. *Journal of Social Issues, 33(2)*:46-66, 1977.

Dreifus, C.: Pre-adolescent sexuality. *Women, 3(1)*:2-6, N.D.

Fleming, A.: *For The First Time.* Berkeley, Medallion, 1976.

Furstenberg, F.: *Unplanned Parenthood.* New York, Free Press, 1976, Chapter 3.

Gadpaille, W.: A consideration of two concepts of normality as applied to adolescent sexuality. *Journal of the American Academy of Child Psychiatry, 15*:679-692, 1976.

Gagnon, J.: Sexuality and learning in the child. *Psychiatry, 28*: 212-228, 1965.

Gispert, M. et al.: Sex experimentation and pregnancy in black adolescents. *American Journal of Obstetrics and Gynecology, 26*:459-466, 1976.

Greene, N. and Esselstyn, T.: The beyond control girl. *Juvenile Justice, 23*:79-99, 1972.

Heagarly, M.: Sex and the pre-school child. *American Journal of Nursing, 74*:1479-1482, 1974.

Hopkins, J.: Sexual behavior in adolescence. *Journal of Social Issues, 33(2)*:67-85, 1977.

Jackson, M.: The motives of children who yield to temptation to steal. *Australian and New Zealand Journal of Criminology, 3*:231-237, 1970.

James, J.: Early sexual experience and prostitution. *American Journal of Psychiatry, 134*:1381-1385, 1977.

Kanter, J. and Zelnick, M.: Sexual experience of young single women in U.S. *Family Planning Perspectives, 4*:9-18, 1972.

Kaplan, H.: Can you ruin your daughter's sex life? *Harpers Bazaar, 109*:119-120, October 1976.

Konapka, G.: *Young Girls: A Portrait of Adolescence.* Englewood Cliffs, N.J., Prentice Hall, 1975.

Ladner, J. and Hammond, B.: Socialization into sexual behavior. *Society for the Study of Sexual Problems*, 1967.

Lester, E.: On the psychosexual development of the female child. *Journal of the American Academy of Psychoanalysis*, *4*: 515-528, 1976.

Lister, L.: Adolescents. In H. and J. Gochros: *The Sexually Oppressed*. New York, Association Press, 1977, pp. 41-53.

Lovko, K. and Wagner, P.: Signs of sexual difficulties in adolescents. *Medical Aspects of Human Sexuality*, *10(7)*:104-118, 1976.

Martin, N. et al.: Genetical, environmental and personality factors influencing the age of first sexual intercourse in twins. *Journal of Biosocial Science*, *9*:91-97, 1977.

Martinson, F.: Eroticism in infancy and childhood. *Journal of Sex Research*, *12*:251-262, 1976.

Messer, A.: The phaedra complex. *Archives of General Psychiatry*, *21*:213-218, 1969.

Miller, P. and Simon, W.: Adolescent sexual behavior: Context and change. *Social Problems*, *22*:58-76, 1974.

Mitchell, J.: Moral growth during adolescence. *Adolescence*, *10*:221-226, 1975.

Oaks, W. et al.: *Sex and the Life Cycle*. New York, Grune and Stratton, 1976, pp. 19-66.

Parcel, G.: Sex and the pre-schooler. *Texas Medicine*, *73*:37-41, 1977.

Reenshaw, D.: Sexuality in children. *Medical Aspects of Human Sexuality*, *5*:62-74, 1971.

Reevy, W.: Child sexuality. In A. Ellis and A. Aborband: *The Encyclopedia of Sexual Behavior*. New York, Hawthorne, 1967, pp. 258-267.

Rubenstein, J.: Young adolescents sexual interests. *Adolescence*, *9*:487-496, 1976.

Satterfield, S.: Common sex problems of children and adolescents. *Pediatric Clinics of North America*, *22*:643-654, 1975.

Schofield, M.:*The Sexual Behavior of Young People*. Boston, Little-Brown, 1967.

Schmidt, G. and Siqush, V.: Change in sexual behavior in young males and females between 1960—1970. *Archives of Sexual Behavior,* 2:27-45, 1972.

Scrignar, C.: Sex and the underage girl. *Medical Aspects of Human Sexuality,* 2:34-39, 1968.

Sorenson, R.: *Adolescent Sexuality in Contemporary America.* New York, World Books, 1972.

Tams, K. et al.: Differentiation of sexual morality between 11 and 16 Years. *Archives of Sexual Behavior,* 5:353-370, 1976.

Trainer, E.: *The Lolita Complex.* New York, Paperback Library, 1966.

Turner, E.: Attitudes of parents of deficient children toward sex behavior. *Journal of School Health,* 548-550, December 1970.

Weiss, B.: Earlier menstruation, longer adolescence. *Psychology Today,* 8(6):59, 1974.

Zelnick, M. and Kanter, J.: Sexuality and contraceptive experiences of young unmarried women in the U.S., 1976 and 1971. *Family Planning Perspectives,* 9: 55-73, 1977.

MEDICAL/PSYCHIATRIC ASPECTS

Bourg, R.: Clinical and therapeutic study on rape. *Obstetric-Gynocological Survey,* 17:566-567, 1962.

Braen, G.: *Rape Examination.* 16 m.m., 20 min., 1976, Abbot Motion Picture Library, Chicago, Illinois.

Breen, J. et al.: The molested young female. *Pediatric Clinics of North America,* 19:717-725, 1972.

Camps, F.: *Legal Medicine.* Baltimore, Williams and Wilkins, 1968, pp. 424-431.

Eaton, A. and Vastbinder, E.: The sexually molested child. *Clinical Pediatrics,* 8:438-441, 1969.

Elmer, E.: Follow-up study of traumatized children. *Child Abuse and Neglect: The International Journal,* 1(1):105-109, 1977.

Emerson, J.: Behavior in private places: Realities of the gynecological examination. In H. Dreitzed: *Recent Sociology, No. 2.* New York, McMillan, 1970, pp. 74-97.

Feigan, G.: Morbidity caused by anal intercourse. *Medical Aspects of Human Sexuality,* 177-186, June, 1974.

Folland, D. et al.: Gonorrhea in pre-adolescent children: An inquiry into source of infection and mode of transmission. *Pediatrics, 60*:153-156, 1977.

Furst, S.: *Psychic Trauma.* New York, Basic Books, 1967.

Gundlack, R.: Sexual molestation and rape reported by homosexual and heterosexual women. *Journal of Homosexuality,* 2:367-372, 1977.

Herjanic, B.: Sexual abuse of children: Detection and management. *Journal of the American Medical Association, 239*: 331-333, 1978.

Henslin, J. and Biggs, M.: The sociology of the vaginal examination. In J. Henslin: *Studies in the Sociology of Sex.* New York, Appleton-Century-Crofts, 1971, pp. 243-272.

Jaffe, A.: Sexual abuse and herpetic infection in children. *Journal of Pediatrics, 89*:338, 1976.

National Audiovisual Center: *Sexual Abuse, Part 5: Medical Indicators of Child Abuse and Neglect.* Filmstrip, 1977, GSA, Washington, D.C.

National Center on Child Abuse and Neglect: *Sexual Abuse: The Family.* 16 m.m., 30 min., 1977, OHD, POB 1182, DHEW Washington D.C. 20013

Paul, D.: The medical examination in sexual offenses. *Medicine, Science and Law,15*:154-162, 1975.

Paul, D.: Medical examination of a live rape victim and the accused. *Legal Medicine Annual, 137*:137-153, 1977.

Paul, D.: The medical examination in sex offenses against children. *Medicine, Science and the Law, 17*:251-258, 1977.

Peters, J.: Child rape: Defusing the time bomb. *Hospital Physician, 9*:46-47, 1973.

Potterat, J. et al.: Prepubertal infections with Neisseria gonorrhoeae. *Journal of the American Venereal Disease Association, 5*:1-3, 1978.

Power, D.: Paedophilia. *Practitioner, 218*:805-811, 1977.

Rengrose, C.: Pelvic reflexes in rape complainents. *Canadian Journal of Public Health, 68*:31, 1977.

Robinson, G. et al.: Review of child molestation and alleged rape cases. *American Journal of Obstetric Gynecology,110*: 405-406, 1971.

Roth, E.: Emergency treatment of raped children. *Medical Aspects of Sexual Behavior*, 88-91, August, 1972.

Rothbard, M. and Greenberg, H.: Gynecological health problems: Sexually abused adolescent females. *New York State Journal of Medicine*, 76:1483-1484, 1976.

Schmidt, B. and Kemp, C.: The pediatrician's role in child abuse. *Current Problems in Pediatrics, 5(5):*1-6, 1975.

Seiden, A. and Grassman, M.: Proposed additional guidelines for hospital care, child victims. In *Recommendations and Report of the Citizens Advisory Council on Rape.* Ill., Cook County, 1975.

Sgroi, S.: Comprehensive examination for child sexual assault. In Burgess, A. et al.: *Sexual Assault of Children and Adolescents.* Lexington, Ma., Lexington Books, 1978, pp. 143-158.

Sgroi, S.: Kids with clap: Gonorrhea as an indicator of child sexual assault. *Victimology*, 2:236-250, 1977.

Skolnick, A.: The myth of the vulnerable child. *Psychology Today, 11(9):*56-60, 65, 1978.

Swerdlow, H.: Trauma caused by anal intercourse. *Medical Aspects of Human Sexuality*, 93-98, July 1976.

tenBensel, R.: *Trauma: Clinical and Biological Aspects.* New York, Plenum Medical Book Co., 1975, pp. 249-272.

Terrell, M: Identifying the sexual abused child in the medical setting. *Health and Social Work*, 2:112-130, 1977.

Underhill, R. and Dewhurst, J.: The doctor cannot always tell. *Lancet, 8060(1):* 375-376, 1977.

Weinberger, J. and Kantor, M.: Possible sequelae of trauma and somatic disorder in early life. *International Journal of Psychiatry in Medicine, 7(4):*337-350, 1976/77.

INTERVIEWING/INTERROGATING SEX ABUSED YOUTH

Admissability of deposition of child of tender years. *American Law Review, 30:* 2d., 771.

Andrews, J.: The evidence of children. *Criminal Law Review*, 769-777, 1964.

Brown, W.: Police-victim relationships in sex crime investigation, *The Police Chief, 37:*20-24, 1969.

Burgess, A. and Holmstrom, L.: Interviewing victims. In A. Burgess et al.: *Sexual Assault of Children and Adolescents.* Lexington, Ma, Lexington Books, 1978, pp. 171-180.

Burgess, A. and Holmstrom, L.: The child and family during the court process. In A. Burgess et al.: *Sexual Assault of Children and Adolescents.* Lexington, Ma, Lexington Books, 1978, pp. 205-230.

Burgess, A. and Laszlo, A.: Court use of hospital records in sex assault cases. *American Journal of Nursing, 77*:64-81, 1977.

Burgess, A. and Laszlo, A.: When the prosecutrix is a child: The victim consultant in cases of sexual assault. In E. Viano (Ed.): *Victims and Society.* Washington, Visage, 1976, pp. 382-390.

Carstens, C.: The rural community and prostitution. *Journal of Social Hygiene, 1*:539-544, 1915.

Chicago Police Department: *Interviewing the Juvenile Sex Victim and Offender.* Training Bulletin 25, Vol. 5, 1964.

Competency of children as witnesses. *American Jurisprudence* (lst. ed. 129 et.seg.).

Expert evidence in cases involving children. *Western Australia Law Review, 12*:139-152, 1975.

Flammang, C.: Interviewing child victims of sex offenders. In L. Schultz: *Rape Victimology.* Springfield, Ill., Charles C Thomas, 1975, Chap. 15.

Freud, A.: The child as a person in his own right. *Psychoanalytic Study of the Child, 27*:621-625, 1972.

Freud, A.: On difficulties of communicating with children: The lesser children in chambers. In J. Goldstein and J. Katz: *The Family and the Law.* New York, Free Press, 1965.

Gelles, R.: Methods of studying sensitive family topics. *American Journal of Orthopsychiatry, 48*:408-424, 1978.

Gibbens, T. and Prince, J.: *Child Victims of Sex Offences.* London, Nell, 1963.

Herren, R.: Evidence of children and adolescents concerning sex offenders. *International Criminal Police Review, 96*: 385-390, 1956.

International Association of Chiefs of Police: *Interviewing the Child Sex Victim.* Gathersburg, MD., IACP, Training Key No.224, 1975.

Juvenile justice. *Newsweek,* 22, June 27, 1977.

Keefe, M.: Police investigation in child sex assault. In A. Burgess et. al.: *Sexual Assault of Children and Adolescents.* Lexington, Ma., Lexington Books, 1978, pp. 159-170.

Lawder, L.: Notes on questioning children. *Law and Order, 20*: 50-53, 1972.

Libai, D.: The protection of the child victim of a sexual offense in the criminal justice system. In L. Schultz: *Rape Victimology.* Springfield, Il., Charles C Thomas, 1975, Chap. 17.

McBarnet, D.: Victim in the witness box: Confronting the stereotype. Center for Socio-legal Studies, Wolfson College, Oxford, Great Britain, 1976 mimeo.

Mehrabian, A. *Non-Verbal Communication.* Chicago: Aldine, 1972, Chp. 9 "Children's Communication."

People vs. Oyola, 6 NY 2d. 259, 189 NYs 2d., 203, 160 NE 2d. 494. "Testimony is easily implanted in minds of children by interested persons."

Perils of doing your duty. *Time, 109*:13-14, June 6, 1977.

Prahm, H.: Psycho-social aspects of sexual offenses against children. *Abstracts of Criminology and Peneology, 15*:706, 1975.

Qualifying an infant witness to testify. *American Jurisprudence Proof of Facts, 6*:333-338.

Reifen, D.: Protection of children involved in sexual offenses. *Journal of Criminal Law, Criminology and Police Science, 49*:222-229, 1958.

Richette, L.: *The Throwaway Children.* New York, Dell, 1973, pp. 212-233.

Roznoy, M.: The young adult: Taking a sexual history. *American Journal of Nursing, 76*:1279-1282, 1976.

Saperstein, A.: Child rape victims and their families. In L. Schultz: *Rape Victimology.* Springfield, IL., Charles C Thomas, 1975, Chap. 16.

Schultz, L.: Interviewing the sex offenders victim. *Journal of Criminology, Criminal Law, and Police Science, 50*:448-452, 1960.

Scutt, J.: Fraud and consent in rape. *Criminal Law Quarterly*, *18*:312-324, 1975.

Sebba, L. and Cahan, S.: Sex offenses: Genuine and doubted victims. In I. Drapkin and E. Viano: *Victimology*, Vol. 5, Lexington, Ma, Heath, 1975, Chap. 2.

Stevens, D. and Berliner, L.: Special techniques for child witnesses. Washington, D.C., Center for Womens Policy Studies, 1976.

Sgroi, S.: Child sexual assault: Some guidelines for investigation and assessment. *Response to Intrafamily Violence and Sexual Assault, 1(5)*:2-3, Oct. 1977.

Towne, A.: A community program for protective work with girls. *Journal of Social Hygiene, 6*:57-71, 1920.

Trankell, A.: *Reliability of Evidence*. Stockholm, Sweden, Bechman, 1972.

Trankell, A.: Was Lars sexually assualted? *Journal of Abnormal and Social Psychology, 56*: 1958.

Yarrow, L.: Interviewing children. In P. Mussen: *Handbook of Research Methods in Child Development*. New York, Wiley, 1960.

TREATMENT

ACI Films: *Child Molesters: Facts and Fiction*, 1977, 16mm., 30 minutes. Box 1895, 12 Jules Lane, New Brunswick, N.J., 08902.

American Film Advertising: *Sexual Abuse: Identification, Management and Treatment*, audio-tape, Part 1 and 2. Six 11th Street N.E., Atlanta, Ga., 30309, 1978.

Anant, R.: Verbal aversion therapy with a promiscuous girl, *Psychological Reports, 22*:796-799, 1968.

Anthony, J.: The syndrome of the psychological invulnerable child. In J. Anthony and C. Kaupernik: *The Child and His Family*. New York, Wiley, 1974.

Bellack, A. et al.: Social skills training for non-assertive children: A multiple baseline analysis. *Journal of Applied Behavioral Analysis, 10*:183-195, 1977.

Bender, L. and Grugett, A.: Follow-up on report on children

who have atypical sexual experiences. *American Journal of Orthopsychiatry, 22*:825-837, 1952.

Berger, E.: The compleat advocate. *Policy Sciences, 8*:69-78, 1977.

Berman, L. and Jensen, D.: Father-daughter interaction and the sexual development of adopted girls. *Psychotherapy, 10*: 253-255, 1973.

Binder, J. and Krohn, A.: Sexual acting out as mourning process in female adolescent in-patients. *Psychiatric Quarterly, 48*: 193-208, 1974.

Blanchard, E. and Able, G.: Case study of biofeedback treatment of rape induced cardiovascular disorder. *Behavior Therapy,* 7:113-119, 1976.

Breen, J. et al.: The molested young females.*Pediatric Clinics of North America, 19*:717-725, 1972.

Burgess, A. et al.: Counseling the child rape victim. *Issues in Comprehensive Pediatric Nursing,* 45-57, November 1976.

Capraro, V.: Sexual assault of female children. *Annals of the New York Academy of Sciences, 142*:170-185, 1967.

Chaneles, S. and Brieland, D.: *Sexual Abuse of Children: Casework Implications.* Denver, Co., American Humane Association, 1967.

Chiatz, T.: Handling promiscuous teenage girls in court clinics. *International Journal of Offender Therapy, 17*:110-111, 1972.

Clarke, A. and Clarke, A.: *Early Experience: Myth and Evidence.* Riverside, N.Y., Free Press, 1976.

Cornthwailti, S.: Oral and rectal coitus among female gonorrhea contacts. *British Journal of Clinical Practice, 28*:305-306, 1974.

Crum, R.: Counseling rape victims. *Journal of Pastorial Care, 28*:112-121, 1974.

Davis, L.: Touch, sexuality and power in residential settings. *British Journal of Social Work, 5*:397-411, 1976.

DeFrancis, V.: *Protecting the Child Victim of Sex Crimes Committed by Adults.* Denver, Co., American Humane Association, 1969.

Doermer, W. et al.: Correspondence between crime victims needs and public services. *Social Service Review, 50*:482-490, 1976.

Easson, W.: Special sexual problems of the adopted adolescent. *Medical Aspects of Human Sexuality,* 7:92-103, 1973.

Eaton, A. and Vastibinder, E.: The sexually molested child. *Clinical Pediatrics,* 8:438-441, 1969.

Eist, H. and Mandell, A.: Family treatment of ongoing incest. *Family Press,* 7:216-232, 1968.

Faust, E. et al.: A Survey of Services Given Sexual Abuse Cases, with a Training Design for Protective Service Workers. MSW thesis, College of Social Work, University of South Carolina, 1976.

Feigan, G.: Morbidity caused by anal intercourse. *Medical Aspects of Human Sexuality,* 117-186, June 1974.

Finch, S.: Sexual activity of children with other children and adults. *Clinical Pediatrics,* 6:1-12, 1967.

Finkel, N.: Stress, traumas, and trauma resolution. *American Journal of Community Psychology,* 3:173-178, 1975.

Finlayson, A.: Social network as coping resources. *Society, Science and Medicine,* 10:97-103, 1976.

Freiberg, P. and Bridwell, M.: A therapy intervention model for rape and pregnancy. *The Counseling Psychologist,* 6:15-24, 1976.

Freidman, A.: *Therapy of Sexually Acting Out Girls,* Palo Alto, Ca., Behavior Science Books, 1970.

Furst, S.: *Psychic Trauma.* New York, Basic Books, 1967.

Gagnon, J. and Simon, W.: The child molester. *Redbook,* 54-60, February 1969.

Gorham, C.: Not only the stranger. *Journal of School Health,* 36:341-344, 1966.

Gerson, A.: Promiscuity as function of father-daughter relationships. *Psychological Reports,* 34:1013, 1014, 1974.

Gianturco, D.: The promiscuous teenager. *Southern Medical Journal,* 67:415-418, 1974.

Goodman, J.: The behavior of hypersexual girls. *American Journal of Psychiatry,* 133:662-668, 1976.

Hardgrove, G.: An interagency network to meet the needs of rape victims. *Social Casework,* 245-253, April 1976.

Harris, E.: Safe on the streets. *PTA Magazine,* 65:34-35, April 1971.

Hayman, C. et al.: A public health program for sexually assaulted females. In H. Gochros and L. Schultz: *Human Sexuality and Social Work*, New York, Association Press, 1972, pp. 321-333.

Help for the family coping with incest. *Practice Digest, 1(2)*: 19-22, 1978.

Hogen, W.: Brief guide for office counseling: The raped child. *Medical Aspects of Human Sexuality, 8(11)*:129-130, 1974.

Kiefer, R.: Brief guide to office counseling: Sexual molestation. *Medical Aspects of Human Sexuality, 7(12)*:127-128, 1973.

Klingbeil, K.: Multi-disciplinary care of sexual assault victims. *Nurse Practitioner*, 21-25, July 1976.

Lambert, P.: Memo to child care workers: Management of sex and stealing. *Child Welfare, 55*:329-334, 1976.

Landis, J.: Experiences of 500 children with adult sexual deviation. *Psychiatric Quarterly Supplement, 30*:91-109, 1956.

Levine, M. and Selegmann, J.: *The Parents Encyclopedia*. New York, Crowell, 1973, pp. 429-430.

Lipton, G. and Roth, E.: Rape: A complex management problem in the pediatric emergency room. *Journal of Pediatrics,* 75:859-866, 1969.

Mac Farlane, K. and Lieber, L.: Parents Anonymous. *Child Abuse and Neglect*, June, 1978.

Massey, J. et al.: Management of the sexually assaulted female. *Obstetrics and Gynecology,* 38:29-36, 1971.

McCombie, S. et al.: Development of a medical center rape crisis program. *American Journal of Psychiatry, 133*:418-421, 1976.

McCubbin: Management of the alleged sex assault. *Texas Medicine, 69*:59-73, 1973.

McDonald, W.: *Criminal Justice and the Victim*. Beverly Hills, Ca., Sage, 1976, Chapter 6.

McGire, L. and Wagner, N.: Sex dysfunction in women who were molested as children. *Journal of Sex and Marital Therapy, 4(1)*:11-15, 1978.

Moore, W.: Promiscuity in a 13-year-old girl. *Psychoanalytic Study of The Child, 29*:301-318, 1974.

Motorola Teleprograms, Inc.: *Childhood Sexual Assault.*

16 mm., 48 min., 4825 N. Scott, Suite 23, Schiller Park, Il., 60076.

Motorola Teleprograms, Inc.: *Childhood Sexual Abuse: Four Case Studies*. 16 mm., 100 min., 1977. 4825 North Scott Street, Schiller Park, IL 60076.

Motorola Teleprograms, Inc.: *The Last Taboo*. 16 mm., 25 min., 1977. 4825 North Scott Street, Schiller Park, Il., 60076.

Motorola Teleprograms, Inc.: *The Reality of Rape*. 16 mm., 10 min. 4825 North Scott Street, Suite 23, Schiller Park, Il. 60076.

Murphy, L.: Coping, vulnerability and resilience in childhood. In G. Coelho et al.: *Coping and Adaptation*. New York, Basic Books, 1974, Chapter 4.

Murphy, L., and Moriarty, A.: *Vulnerability, Coping and Growth*. New Haven, Cn., Yale University Press, 1976.

My daughter was molested. *Good Housekeeping, 173*:14-15, September 1971.

My son was molested. *Good Housekeeping, 181*:14-15, August 1975.

National Center on Child Abuse and Neglect: *Sexual Abuse: The Family*. 16 mm., 30 min., 1977. Office of Human Development, P.O. Box 1182, Department of Health, Education and Welfare, Washington, DC 20013.

O'Connor, J. and Stern, L.: Developmental factors in sex disorders. *New York State Medical Journal, 72*:1838-1843, 1972.

Paul, J. et al.: *Child Advocacy within the System*. Syracuse, N.Y., Syracuse University Press, 1977.

Pollack, O. and Friedman, A.: *Family Dynamics and Female Sexual Delinquency*. Palo Alto, Ca., Science and Behavior Books, 1969.

Rebuilding families after sexual abuse of children. *Practice Digest. 1(2)*:22-25, 1978.

Roth, E.: Emergency treatment of raped children. *Medical Aspects of Sexual Behavior*, 88-91, August 1972.

Schmideburg, M.: Treating adolescent sex offenders. *Chittys Law Journal, 23(2)*:60-63, 1975.

Schmidt, B. and Kempe, C.: The pediatrician's role in child

abuse. *Current Problems in Pediatrics, 5(5)*:1-6, 1975.

Schultz, D.: Terrors of child molestation. *Parents Magazine, 52*: 44-45, 86-89, February 1977.

Schultz, L.: The emotional after-math of rape: Social work implications. *Journal of Humanics, 2(2)*:23-26, 1975.

Schultz, L.: Psychotherapeutic and legal approaches to the sexually victimized child. *International Journal of Child Psychotherapy, 1(1)*:115-128, 1972.

Schultz, L.: The social worker and the treatment of sex victims. In H. Gochros and L. Schultz: *Human Sexuality and Social Work.* New York, Association Press, 1972, pp. 174-185.

Seiden, A. and Grossman, M.: Proposed Additional Guidelines for Hospital Care of Child Victims or Alleged Rape. In *Recommendations and Report of the Citizens Advisory Council on Rape,* Cook County, Il, 1975.

Seligman, M.: *Helplessness,* San Francisco, Freeman, 1975.

Shalit, B.: Structural ambiguity and the limits of coping. *Journal of Human Stress, 3(4)*:32-45, 1977.

Sholevar, G.: A family therapist looks at incest. *Bulletin of the American Academy of Psychiatry and Law, 11.* 25-31, 1975.

Sierra, S.: Rx to check child molesting. *Illinois Medical Journal,* 731-735, June 1969.

Silverman, D.: Female rape victims and male counselors. *American Journal of Orthopsychiatry, 47*:91-96, 1977.

Splane, R.: Helping the child who is a victim of sex offenses, *Canadian Welfare, 36*:272-273, 1960.

Spock, B.: Can we protect children from molestation? *Redbook, 134*:46-47, November 1969.

Stein, E.: *Guilt: Theory and Therapy.* London, Allen and Unwin, 1969.

Texas Department of Public Welfare: *Sexual Abuse of Children.* Video Cassette, 51 minutes, Color 3/4", 1977. Reagan Building, Austin, Tx, 78701.

Twenty ways to prevent child molestation. *Harpers Bazaar, 109*: 123-124, October 1976.

Walters, D.: *Physical and Sexual Abuse of Children: Causes and Treatment.* Bloomington, Indiana University Press, 1975, pp. 111-154.

Ways to protect children from molestation. *Good Housekeeping,* *176*:165-166, February 1973.

Weeks, R.: Counseling parents of sexually abused children. *Medical Aspects of Human Sexuality,* 43-44, August 1976.

Westman, J.: Telling children about sexual molestation. *Medical Aspects of Human Sexuality,* 53-54, August 1975.

LEGAL ASPECTS

Andrews, M.: The evidence of children. *Criminal Law Review,* 769-774, 1964.

Applegath, L.: Sexual intercourse with the feeble-minded female: Problems of proof. *Criminal Law Quarterly,* 7:480-482, 1965.

Arthur, L. and Kalitowski, T.: Child vs. parent: Residence, education and dating. *Juvenile Justice,* 25:34-37, 1973.

Ashworth, A.: The doctrine of provocation. *Cambridge Law Journal,* 35:292-320, 1976.

Bernstein, B.: The social worker as a court room witness. *Social Casework,* 50:521-525, 1975.

Brazier, R.: Reform of sexual offenses. *Criminal Law Review,* 421-429, 1975.

Broeder, F.: Plaintiff's family status as affecting juror behavior. *Journal of Public Law,* 14:131-141, 1965.

Butler, O.: The value of bitemark evidence. *International Journal of Forensic Dentistry,* 1:23-24, 1973.

Fisher, J.: Obtaining and presenting evidence in sex cases. *Criminal Law Quarterly,* 4:150-152, 1961.

Foster, H. and Freed, A.: Offenses against the family. *University of Missouri K.C. Law Review,* 32:33-45, 1964.

Fraser, B.: Independent representation for the abused and neglected child. *California Western Law Review,* 13:16-45, 1977.

Glaister, J. and Rentoul, E.: *Medical Jurisprudence and Toxicology.* London, Livingstone, 1966, pp. 409-435.

Greenfield, D.: Prompt complaint: A developing rule of evidence. *Criminal Law Quarterly,* 9:286-290, 1967.

Grey, A.: The sexual law reform society's report. *Criminal Law Review,* 323-335, 1975.

Hunter, N. and Polikoffin, N.: Custody rights of lesbian mothers.

Buffalo Law Review, 25:691-733, 1976.

Huntington, K.: Forensic gynecology. *Practitioner, 216:*519-528, 1976.

Hughes, G.: Consent in sexual offenses. *Modern Law Review,* 25:672-686, 1967.

Kanowitz, L.: Law and the single girl. *St. Louis University Law Journal, 11:*293-330, 1967.

Koh, K.: Consent and responsibility in sex offenses. *Criminal Law Review,* 81-84, 1968.

Mathis, E. et al.: Clothing as nonverbal communication of sexual attitudes and behavior. *Perceptual Motor Skills, 42:*495-498, 1976.

Myers, L.: Reasonable mistake of age: Needed defense to statutory rape. *Michigan Law Review, 64:*105-136, 1966.

Newton, L.: The rule of law and the appeal to community standards. *American Journal of Jurisprudence, 21:*95-106, 1966.

Note: Children's evidence-corroboration. *Solicitors Journal, 117:* 608-612, 1973.

Note: Reasonable mistake of age: A defense to statutory rape. *Connecticut Law Review,* 2:43-45, 1969.

Reifen, D.: Court procedures in Israel to protect child victims of sex assaults. In I. Drapkin-E. Viano: *Victimology 3.* Lexington, Ma., Heath, 1976, Chapter 6.

Ryan, A.: Two kinds of morality. *New Society,* 23-25, April 3, 1975.

Schniffer, M.: Sex and the single defective. *University of Toronto Faculty Law Review, 34:*143-158, 1976.

Schultz, L.: The victim-offender relationship. *Crime and Delinquency,14:* 135-140, 1968.

Sex offenses, *Law and Contemporary Problems, 25(2):* 1960.

Solender, E. and E.: Minimizing the effect of the unattractive client on the jury, *Human Rights, 5:* 201-214,e1976.

Sussman, A.: *The Rights of Young People.* New York, Avon Press, 1977.

Thacker, G.: Mistake as to age: Statutory rape. *Journal of Family Law, 5:* 107-108, 1965.

Wald, M.: State intervention on behalf of neglected children.

Stanford Law Review, 27: 985-1040, 1975.

CHILD MOLESTATION

Anderson, C.: Molestation of children. *Journal of the American Medical Women's Association, 23:* 204-206, 1968.

Bender, L. and Blau, A.: The reaction of children to sexual relations with adults. *American Journal of Orthopsychiatry, 7:* 500-518, 1937.

Bender, L.: Offended and offender children. In R. Slovenko: *Sexual Behavior and the Law.* Springfield, Il., Charles C Thomas, 1965, pp. 687-703.

Berliner, L.: Child sexual abuse: What happens next? *Victimology, 2:* 327-331, 1977.

Blacker, R.: London's Homeless girls. *New Society, 36:* 289-291, 1976.

Blumberg, N.: Child sexual abuse. *New York State Journal of Medicine,* 612-616, 1978.

Brant, R. and Tisza, V. The sexually misused child. *American Journal of Orthopsychiatry, 47:* 80-90, 1977.

Burgess, A. and Lazare, A.: *Community Mental Health: Target Populations.* Englewood Cliffs, N.J., Prentice-Hall, 1976, pp. 239-263.

Burton, L.: *Vulnerable Children.* New York, Schocken, 1968, pp. 87-169.

Chapman, A.: *Sexual Maneuvers and Strategems.* New York, Putnam, 1969, pp. 141-167.

Elonen, A. and Zwarensteyn, S.: Sexual trauma in blind children. *New Outlook for the Blind, 69:* 440-445, 1975.

Finch, S.: Adult seduction of the child: Effects. *Medical Aspects of Human Sexuality, 7:* 170-187, 1973.

Finch, S.: Sexual abuse by mothers. *Medical Aspects of Human Sexuality,* 191, January 1973.

Forgione, A.: The use of mannequins in the behavioral assessment of child molesters: Two case reports. *Behavior Therapy, 7:* 678-685, 1976.

Freund, K.: Erotic preference in pedophilia. *Behavior Research and Therapy, 5:* 339-348, 1967.

Freund, K. et al.: The female child as surrogate object, *Archives of Sexual Behavior, 2:* 119-132, 1972.

Gagnon, J.: Female child victims of sex offenses, *Social Problems, 13:* 176-192, 1965.

Gagnon, J.: Sexual conduct and crime. In D. Glaser: *Handbook of Criminology.* Chicago, Rand McNally, 1974, pp. 233-272.

Gebhard, P. et al.: *Sex Offenders.* New York, Bantam Books, 1965, pp. 54-105.

Gibbens, T. and Prince, J.: *Child Victims of Sex Offenses.* London, Institute for the Study and Treatment of Delinquency, 1963.

Gorling, L.: *491.* New York, Grove, 1966, pp. 164-173.

Greene, N.: A view of family pathology involving child molesting: A juvenile probation perspective. *Juvenile Justice, 28:* 29-34, 1977.

Hartley, A.: Reporting child abuse. *Texas Medicine, 71(2):* 84-86, 1975.

Hollander, M. et al.: Genital exhibitionism in women. *American Journal of Psychiatry, 134:* 436-438, 1977.

Jaffe, A. et al.: Sexual abuse of children. *American Journal of the Disturbed Child, 129:* 689-692, 1975.

Kirchhoff, G. and Thelen, C.: Hidden victimization by sex offenders in Germany. In E. Viano (Ed.): *Victims and Society.* Washington, Visage, 1976, pp. 277-284.

Landis, J.: Experiences of 500 children with adult sexual deviation. *Psychiatric Quarterly,* Supplement, *30:* 91-109, 1956.

Lewis, M. and Sarrel, P.: Some psychological aspects of seduction, rape and incest in childhood. *Journal of the American Academy of Child Psychiatry.*

MacDonald, J.: *Indecent Exposure.* Springfield, Il., Charles C Thomas, 1973, Chapter 3.

MacFarlane, K.: Sexual abuse of children. In J. Chapman and M. Gates: *The Victimization of Women.* Beverly Hills, Ca., Sage, 1978, Chapter 4.

Marshall, M.: Early sexual trauma. *Sexual Behavior, 2:* 13-17, 1972.

Masters, R.: *Sex Driven People.* Los Angeles, Sherbourn, 1966, pp. 35-120.

McCaghy, C.: Child molestation. *Sexual Behavior, 1:* 16-20, 1971.

McCreary, C.: Personality differences among child molesters. *Journal of Personality Assessment, 39:* 591-593, 1975.

Meyer, G.: *Studies in Children.* New York, King's Crown Press, 1948.

Mohr, J.: A child is being molested. *Medical Aspects of Human Sexuality. 2:* 43-50, 1968.

Mohr, J. et al.: *Pedophilia and Exhibitionism.* Toronto, University of Toronto Press, 1964.

Peters, J.: Children who are victims of sexual assault. *American Journal of Psychotherapy, 30:* 398-421, 1976.

Queens Bench Foundation: *Sexual Abuse of Children.* San Francisco, QBF, 1976.

Quinsey, V.: The assessment and treatment of child molesters: A review. *Canadian Psychological Review, 18(3):* 204-220, 1977.

Radzinowicz, L.: *Sexual Offenses.* New York, Macmillan, 1957.

Rooth, G.: Exhibitionism, violence and pedophilia. *British Journal of Psychiatry, 122:* 705-110, 1973.

Rush, F.: The sexual abuse of children. *The Radical Therapist, 2(4):*December 1971.

Sagarin, E. and MacNamera, D.: The Homosexual as crime victim. In I. Drapkin and L. Viano: *Victimology,* Vol. 5. Lexington, Ma., Heath, 1975, Chapter 5.

Schultz, L.: The child as a sex victim. In L. Schultz: *Rape Victimology.* Springfield, Il., Charles C Thomas, 1975, Chapter 15.

Schultz, L.: The child sex victim. *Child Welfare,* 52:147-157, 1973.

Schultz, L.: The child sex victim. *Psychiatric Spectator, 7(11):* 14-18, 1972.

Schultz, L.: The sex victim. In H. Gochros and J. Gochros: *The Sexually Oppressed.* New York, Association Press, 1977, Chapter 8.

Sgroi, S.: Molestation of children: The last frontier. *Children Today,* 4:18-21, 1975.

Shoor, M. et al.: Syndrome of the adolescent child molester. *American Journal of Psychiatry, 122:*783-789, 1966.

Stokes, R.: A research approach to children's sexual offenses. *Canadian Journal of Corrections*, 6:87-94, 1964.

Swanson, D.: Adult sexual abuse of children. *Diseases of the Nervous System*, 29:20-28, 1968.

Swift, C.: Sex between adults and children—review essay. *Journal of Psychohistory*, 3:369-384, 1976.

Swift, C.: Sexual victimization of children: An urban mental health center survey. *Victimology*, 2:322-326, 1977.

Taylor, B.: Motives for guilt-free pederasty. *The Sociological Review*, 24:97-114, 1976.

Thompson, G.: The stepdaughter paraphilia neurosis. *Journal of Forensic Sciences*, 2:159-170, 1957.

Virkunen, M.: Victim-precipitated pedophilic offenses. *British Journal of Criminology*, 15:175-180, 1975.

Voight, J.: Sexual offenses in Copenhagen. *Forensic Sciences*, 67-76, 1972.

Walters, D.: *Physical and Sexual Abuse of Children*. Bloomington, Id., Indiana University Press, 1975.

Weiss, J. et al.: A study of girl sex victims. *Psychiatric Quarterly*, 29:1-27, 1955.

Williams, B.: *Jail Bait*, New York, Greenberg, 1949.

INCEST

Armstrong, L.: The crime nobody talks about. *Women's Day*, March 1, 1978.

Awad, C.: Father-son incest. *Journal of Nervous and Mental Disease*, 162:135-139, 1976.

Begley, C.: Incest behavior and incest taboos. *Social Problems*, 16:505-519, 1969.

Begley, C.: Varieties of incest. *New Society*, 14:280-282, 1969.

Bethschneider, J. et al.: A study of father-daughter incest in Harris County. *Criminal Justice Monograph*, 4(4):1-131, 1973.

Bischaf, N.: The biological foundations of the incest taboo. *Social Science Information*, 11(6):1972.

Browning, D. and Boatman, B.: Incest: Children at risk. *American Journal of Psychiatry*, 134:69-72, 1977.

Burgess, A. et al.: Child sexual assault by family member: Decisions following disclosure. *Victimology*, 2:236-250, 1977.

Burgess, A.: Divided loyalty in incest cases. In A. Burgess et al.: *Sexual Assaults of Children and Adolescents.* Lexington, Ma., Lexington Books, 1978, pp. 100-115.

Canepa, G. and Bandini, T.: The personality of incest victims. *International Criminal Police Review*, 22:140-145, 1967.

Carruthers, E.: Net of incest. *Yale Review*, 63:211-227, 1973.

Cavallin, H.: Incestuous fathers. *American Journal of Psychiatry*, 122:1132-1135, 1966.

Cepeda, M.: Incest without harmful repercussions. *Medical Aspects of Human Sexuality*, 131, January 1978.

Cohen, Y.: The disappearance of the incest taboo. *Human Behavior*, 1(7):72-79, 1978.

Colton, H.: Incest. *Coronet*, Vol. 14, January 1976, pp. 102-107.

Cormier, B. et al.: Psychodynamics of father-daughter incest. *Canadian Psychiatric Association Journal*, 7:203-209, 1962.

Coehler, R.: Incest: The secret sin against children. *Chatelaine*, 42:20-22, 1969.

Dynamics of incestuous families. *Response*, 1(2):8, 1976.

Farrell, W.: *The Last Taboo: The Three Faces of Incest.* In press, 1979.

Ferracuti, F.: Incest between father and daughter. In H. Resnik and N. Wolfgang: *Sexual Behaviors.* Boston, Ma., Little Brown, 1975, Chap. 7.

Fradkin, A.: Incest in middle-class differs from that processed by police. *Clinical Psychiatric Newsletter*, 2(3):1974.

Frankel, S. and Harrison, S.: Childrens' exposure to parental intercourse. *Medical Aspects of Human Sexuality*, 115-117, September, 1976.

Gentry, C.: Incestuous abuse of children: The need for an objective view. *Child Welfare*, 57:355-364, 1978.

Gowell, E.: Implications of the incest taboo for nursing practice. *Journal of Psychiatric Nursing*, 11:13-19, 1973.

Greenland, C.: Research and methodology: Incest. *British Journal of Delinquency*, 9:62-65, 1958.

Gutheil, T. and Avery, N.: Multiple overt incest as family defense against loss. *Family Process*, 16:105-116, 1977.

Harbert, T. et al.: Measurement and modification of incestuous behavior. *Psychological Reports, 34*:79-86, 1974.

Heims, L. and Kaufman, I.: Variations on a theme of incest. *American Journal of Orthopsychiatry, 33*:311-315, 1963.

Henderson, D.: Incest: Synthesis of data. *Canadian Psychiatric Association Journal, 17*:299-313, 1972.

Hermon, J. and Hirschman, L.: Incest between fathers and daughters. *Journal of Nursing Care,* 8-9, 25-26, May 1978.

Hersko, M. et al.: Incest: A three-way process. *Journal of Social Therapy, 7*:16-28, 1961.

Hoyt, M.: Primal scene experiences as recalled by college students. *Psychiatry, 41(2)*:1978.

Hughs, G.: The crime of incest. *Journal of Criminal Law. 55*:322-330, 1964.

Incest. *People, 7*:47-50, May 9, 1977.

Is incest really dull? *Time, 96*:40-42, August 24, 1970.

Landsley, D.: Father-son incest. *Comprehensive Psychiatry, 9*: 218-226, 1968.

Laury, G.: Effect of faulty sleeping arrangements on childrens' sexuality. *Medical Aspects of Human Sexuality,* 6-18, December 1976.

Laymen, W.: Pseudo-incest. *Comprehensive Psychiatry, 13*:385-89, 1972.

Levine, S.: Family relationship systems: A theoretical framework for understanding father-daughter incest. *Smith College Studies in Social Work, 45*:58-59, 1974.

Lukianowicz, N.: Paternal incest. *British Journal of Psychiatry, 12*:301-313, 1972.

Lustig, N.: Incest: A family survival pattern. *Archives of General Psychiatry, 14*:31-40, 1966.

Maisch, H.: *Incest.* New York, Stein and Day, 1972, Chap. 9.

Malle, L.: *Murmur of the Heart.* 16 mm., 90 min., 1971. Paris, France.

Manchotta, P. et al.: Incest as a family affair. *Family Process, 6*: 98-116, 1967.

Masters, R.: *Patterns of Incest.* New York, Basic Books, Inc., 1963.

Meiselman, K.: *Incest.* San Francisco, Jossey-Bass, 1978.

Miller, J. et al.: Recidivism among sex assault victims. *American*

Journal of Psychiatry, 135:1103-04, 1978.

Mitchell Gebhardt Film Co.: *Incest: The Victim Nobody Believes.* 16 mm., 20 min., 1976. 1380 Bush Street, San Francisco, Ca., 94109.

Molnar, G. and Cameron, P.: Incest syndrome: Observations in a psychiatric unit. *Canadian Psychiatric Association Journal, 20*:373-377, 1975.

New, J.: What's wrong with incest? *Inquiry, 19(9)*:22-40, 1976.

Owen, F.: Incest-taboo or over-familiarity? *Medical Aspects of Human Sexuality, 8(1)*:1974.

Ramsey, J.: My husband broke the ultimate taboo. *Family Circle,* March 8, 1977.

Rasconsky, M. and Rasconsky, A.: On consummated incest. *International Journal of Psychoanalysis, 31*:19-42, 1950.

Raybin, J.: Homosexual incest. *Journal of Nervous and Mental Disease, 148*:105-110, 1969.

Rosenfeld, A.: A case of sexual misuse. *Psychiatric Opinion,* 35-42, April 1976.

Rosenfeld, A. et al.: Incest and the sexual abuse of children. *Journal of the American Academy of Child Psychiatry, 16*:327-339, 1977.

Rosenfeld, A.: Sexual misuse and the family. *Victimology,2*:226-35, 1977.

Rosenfeld, A. et al.: The sexual misuse of children—A brief survey. *Psychiatric Opinion,* 6-12, April 1976.

Sagurin, E.: Incest: Problems of definition and frequency. *Journal of Sex Research, 13*:126-135, 1977.

Sagurin, E. and Ellis, A.: *The Origins of the Development of the Incest Taboo.* New York, Lyle Stuart, 1963.

Sarles, R.: Incest. *Pediatric Clinics of North America, 3*:633-42, 1975.

Schacter, A.: *Child Abuse Intevention,* Prescriptive Package. Washington, D.C., U.S. Government Printing Office, 1976.

Schecter, M. and Roberge, L.: Sexual exploitation. In R. Helfer and C. Kempe: *Child Abuse and Neglect.* Cambridge Ma., Ballinger, 1976, pp. 127-133.

Schultz, L.: *Incest: A Policy Perspective.* Morgantown, School of Social Work, West Virginia University, 1978.

Shelton, W.: A study of incest. *International Journal of Offender Therapy, 19*:153-193, 1975.

Sloane, P. and Karpinski, El: Effects of incest on participants. *American Journal of Orthopsychiatry, 24*:266-279, 1954.

Stein, R.: *Incest and Love.* New York, Third Press, 1973.

Summit, R. and Kryso, J.: Sexual abuse of children: A clinical spectrum. *American Journal of Orthopsychiatry, 48*:237-245, 1978.

Tuteur, W.: Further observations on incestuous fathers. *Psychiatric Annals, 2*:9-77, 1972.

Wahl, C.: Psychodynamics of consumated incest. *Archives of General Psychiatry, 3*:188-193, 1960.

Wathey, R. and Gerber, J.: Incest: Analysis of victim and aggressor. *Journal of Law and Psychiatry, 3*:1976.

Weber, E.: Incest: Sexual abuse begins at home. *Ms., 5*:64-67, April 1977.

Weiner, I.: On incest. *Excerpta Criminologica, 4*:135-155, 1966.

Weiner, I.: Father-daughter incest. *Psychiatric Quarterly, 36*: 607-632, 1962.

Weinberg, S.: *Incest Behavior.* New York, Citadel, 1st ed. 1955, 2nd ed. 1977.

Westermeyer, J.: Incest in psychiatric practice. *Journal of Clinical Psychiatry, 39*:643-648, 1978.

Williams, J. and Hall, J.: The neglect of incest. *Medicine, Science and Law, 14*:64-67, 1974.

Winston, C.: *The Closest Kin There Is.* New York, Paperback Library, 1952.

Wilson, P.: Incest: A case study. *Social and Economic Studies, 12*:200-209, 1961.

Wolf, A.: Childhood association and sexual attraction. *American Anthropologist, 72*:503-515, 1970.

Yorukoclu, A. and Kemph, J.: Children not severely damaged by incest. *Journal of the Academy of Child Psychiatry, 5*:111-124, 1966.

Young, J.: Incest. *Playgirl, 5(8)*:54-56, 66, 68, 1978.

Zellick, S.: Incest. *National Law Journal, 121*:715-717, 1971.

RAPE

Aims Instructional Media: *Rape: Problems of Proof I* and *Rape: Providing the Proof II.* 16 mm., 30 min. each. 626 Justin Avenue, Glendale, Ca., 91201.

Braen, G.: *Rape Examination.* 16 mm., 20 min., 1976. Abbot Motion Picture Library, Chicago, Il.

Burgess, A. and Holmstrom, L.: Complicating factors in rape: Adolescent case illustrations. In A. Burgess et al.: *Sexual Assault of Children and Adolescents.* Lexington, Ma., Lexington Books, 1978, pp. 61-84.

Burgess, A. and Holmstrom, L.: *Rape: Victims of Crisis.* Bowie, Md., Brady, 1974, Chapter 16.

Calhoun, L. et al.: Social perception of victims causal role in rape. *Human Relations, 29(6)*:517-526, 1976.

Camps, F.: *Legal Medicine.* Baltimore, Williams and Wilkins, 1968, pp. 424-431.

Cavallin, H.: Dangerous sex offenders. *Medical Aspects of Human Sexuality,* 134-148, June 1972.

DeRiver, P.: *The Sexual Criminal.* Springfield, Il., Charles C Thomas, 1951, pp. 75-86.

Feldman, S. and Linder, K.: Perceptions of victims and defendants in assault cases. *Criminal Justice and Behavior, 3*:135-149, 1976.

Fisher, G. and Rivilin, E.: Psychological needs of rapists. *British Journal of Criminology, 11*:182-185, 1971.

Furst, S.: *Psychic Trauma.* New York, Basic Books, 1967.

Gager, N. and Schur, C.: *Sexual Assault: Confronting Rape in America.* New York, Grosset and Dunlap, 1976, Chapter 2.

Garrett, T. and Wright, R.: Wives of rapists. *Journal of Sex Research, 11*:149-157, 1975.

Gibbens, T. et al.: Behavioral types of rape. *British Journal of Psychiatry, 130*:32-42, 1977.

Halleck, S.: Emotional effects of victimization. In R. Slovenko: *Sexual Behavior and the Law.* Springfield, Il, Charles C Thomas, 1965, pp. 673-686.

Hilberman, E.: *The Rape Victim.* Washington, American Psychiatric Association, 1976.

Huerd, D.: How a rape victim advocacy program works. *Hospital Progress, 58*:70-77, December 1977.

Katan, A.: Children who are raped. *Psychoanalytic Study of the Child, 28*:208-216, 1973.

Kaufman, A.: Follow-up of rape victims in family practice settings. *Southern Medical Journal, 69*:1569-1571, 1976.

Kinsey, A. et al.: *Sexual Behavior in the Human Female.* New York, Pocket Books, 1965, pp. 116-122.

Marie, L.: *I Must Not Rock.* New York, Daughters Publishing Co., 1978.

Meyers, S.: The child slayer—A twenty-five year survey. *Archives of General Psychiatry, 17*:211-213, 1967.

Mills, P.: *Rape Intervention Resource Manual.* Springfield, Il., Charles C Thomas, 1977.

Motorola Teleprograms, Inc.: *Investigation of Rape.* 16 mm., 20 min., 1976. 4825 North Scott Street, Schiller Park, IL, 60076.

Notman, M. and Nadelson, C.: The rape victim: Psychodynamic considerations. *American Journal of Psychiatry, 133*:408-413, 1976.

Peters, J.: Child rape: Defusing the time bomb. *Hospital Physician, 9*:46-47, 1973.

Peters, J.: The Philadelphia rape victim study. In I. Drapkin and E. Viano: *Victimology: A New Focus*, Lexington, Ma., 1975, pp. 181-199.

Ringrose, C.: Pelvic reflexes in rape complainents, *Canadian Journal of Public Health, 68*:31, 1977.

Ringrose, C.: Social, medical, and legal aspects of rape. *Criminal Law Quarterly, 17*:440-475, 1975.

Schiff, A.: The use and abuse of the rape treatment center. *Journal of Forensic Sciences, 22*:251-255, January 1977.

Selby, H.: *Last Exit to Brooklyn.* New York, Grove, 1961, pp. 93-114.

Selegman, C. et al.: Rape and physical attractiveness. *Journal of Personality, 45*:554-563, 1977.

Sloan, D.: Rape: The gynecologist's role. *Journal of Reproductive Medicine, 17*:324-326, 1976.

Smith, A. and Giles, J.: *An American Rape.* Washington, New Republic Press, 1975.

Soules, M. et al.: The spectrum of alleged rape. *Journal of Reproductive Medicine, 20*:33-39, 1978.

Spielmann, K.: *Outrage.* New York, Penthouse, 1976, pp. 75-84.

Sutherland, S. and Sheri, D.: Patterns of response among rape victims. *American Journal of Orthopsychiatry, 40*:503-511, 1970.

Swerdlow, H.: Trauma caused by anal intercourse. *Medical Aspects of Human Sexuality,* 93-98, July, 1976.

Symonds, M.: Victims of violence: Effects and after-effects. *American Journal of Psychoanalysis, 35*:19-26, 1975.

Taylor, S.: Aggression as a function of sex of victim and attitudes toward women. *Psychological Reports, 35*:763-770, 1974.

SEXUAL EXPLOITATION

A community alert on child prostitution. *Practice Digest, 1(1)*:12, 1978.

Baker, C.: Preying on playgrounds: The sex exploitation of children in pornography and prostitution. *Pepperdine Law Review, 5(3)*:809-846, 1978.

Bell, A.: Fate of the boys next door. *Esquire, 81*:96-99, March 1974.

Boys for sale. *Village Voice,* February 28, 1973.

Bridge, P.: What parents should know and do about kiddie porn. *Parents Magazine, 53*:42-43, 69, January 1978.

Campbell, B.: Help sought for children used in pornography. *New York Times,* 1, January 4, 1977.

C.B.S. T.V.: "Child Porn." *60 Minutes,* 1977.

Child's garden of perversity. *Time, 109*:55-56, April 4, 1977.

Drew, D., and Drake, J.: *Boys for Sale.* New York, Brown, 1964.

Dydar, H.: America discovers child pornography. *Ms.,*45-47, 80. August 1977.

Gerassi, J.: *The Boys of Boise.* New York, Macmillian, 1966.

Goodman, W., and Haag, E.: The coming of bold pornography. *Current, 190*:32-38, February 1977.

Gray, D.: Turning out: Teenage prostitution. *Urban Life and Culture, 1*:401-425, 1973.

Greller, J.: Baby pros: The child hustler. *Penthouse,* February 1975.

Greller, J.: *Young Hookers.* New York, Dell, 1976.

Harris, M.: *The Dilly Boys.* Rockville, Md., New Perspectives, 1974.

Haskell, M.: Sexy baby tùrn-on. *Vogue,* 128, 168, January 1978.

Lieberman, F.: Sex and the adolescent girl: Liberation or exploitation. *Clinical Social Work Journal, 1*:224-243, 1973.

Lloyd, R.: *For Love or Money.* New York, Vanguard, 1976.

Macpherson, M.: Children: The limits of porn. *Washington Post,* CI-5. January 30, 1977.

Malle, L.: *Pretty Baby.* 1 hour, 45 minutes, 1978. Hollywood, Paramount Pictures.

Morgan, Little ladies of the night: Runaways in New York. *New York Times Magazine,* November 16, 1975.

Murray, W.: A minor issue of major concern. *New West, 2*: November 7, 1977.

Olson, J.: *The Man with the Candy.* New York, Simon and Schuster, 1974.

Raven, S.: The male prostitute. *Encounter, 86*:7-11, 1960.

Riess, A.: The sexual integration of peers and queers. *Social Problems, 9*:102-120, 1961.

Rossman, G.: *Sexual Experiences Between Men and Boys.* New York, Association Press, 1976.

Rossman, G.: Literature on pederasty. *Journal of Sex Research, 9*:307-312, 1973.

Schorr, M.: Blood stewarts end. *New York, 11(13)*:53-58, 1978.

Schultz, L: *Kiddie Pornography: A Social Policy Analysis.* Morgantown, West Virginia University, School of Social Work, 1977.

Shea, R.: Kids in pornography. *Playboy, 24(8)*:54, 1977.

Weeks, R.: The sexually exploited child. *Southern Medical Journal, 69*:848-850, 1976.

Yes Virginia there is a P.I.E.: Paedophile Information Exchange. *National Review, 29*:1221-1222, 1977.

PREVENTION

Aptos Film Production Inc.: *Beware of Strangers.* 16 mm., 20 min., 729 Seward Street, Los Angeles, Ca., 90038.

Arnold, R.: *How to Protect Your Child Against Crime.* New York, Association Press, 1977, pp. 8-28, 115-130.

Balzerman, M.: Can the first pregnancy of young adolescents be prevented? *Journal of Youth and Adolescence, 6:*343-351, 1977.

Beauchamp, T.: *Ethics and Public Policy.* New Jersey, Prentice Hall, 1975, Chap. 5.

Beiser, H.: Sexual factors in antagonism between mothers and adolescent daughters. *Medical Aspects of Human Sexuality,* 32-47, April 1977.

BFA Educational Media: *Meeting Strangers: Red Light/Green Light.* 16 mm., 21 min., P.O. Box 1795, Santa Monica, CA 90406.

Briggs, D.: *Your Child's Self Esteem,* New York, Doubleday, 1970.

Caudill, W. and Platt, D.: Who sleeps by whom. *Psychiatry, 29:* 344-352, 1966.

Chess, S. et al.: *Your Child is a Person.* New York, Viking, 1972.

Cohen, M. et al.: The psychology of rapists. *Seminars in Psychiatry, 3:*307-327, 1971.

Comment: Civil liability for failure to report child abuse. *Detroit College Law Review,* 1977:135-165, 1977.

Court, J.: Pornography and sex crime. *International Journal of Criminology and Penology, 5:*129-157, 1977.

Dallas, D.: Kids view murder: Get mental health help. *Innovations, 4(3):*32-33, 1977.

Film Fair Communications: *Better Safe than Sorry.* 16 mm., 28 min., 10900 Ventura, P.O. Box 1728, Studio City, Ca.

Film Fair Communications: *No Exceptions.* 16 mm., 24 min. 10900 Ventura, P.O. Box 1728, Studio City, Ca.

Films, Inc.: *Not a Pretty Picture.* 16 mm., 83 min. 1144 Wilmette, Wilmette, Il., 60091.

Frankel, S. and Harrison, S.: Children's exposure to parental intercourse. *Medical Aspects of Human Sexuality.* 115-116, September 1976.

Gadpaille, W.: Sexual problems due to overdependence on parents. *Medical Aspects of Human Sexuality,* 32-55, May 1976.

Gardner, R.: Exposing children to parental nudity. *Medical As-*

pects of Human Sexuality. 99-100, June 1975.

Gibbs, J. et al.: Sex education for delinquent boys. *American Journal of Orthopsychiatry,* 311-315, March 1969.

Glucksberg, S.: The development of communication skills in children. *Review of Children's Developmental Research, 4:* 1975.

Hamilton, E.: *Sex with Love,* Boston, Beacon Press, 1978.

Hanks, C. and Rebelsky, F.: Mommy and the midnight visitor: A study of occasional co-sleeping. *Psychiatry, 40:*277-280, 1977.

Hartman, H. and Nicolay, R.: Sexually deviant behavior in expectant fathers. *Journal of Abnormal Psychology, 21:*232-235, 1967.

Kaplan, S. and Poznanski, El: Child patients who share a bed with parents. *Journal of the American Academy of Child Psychiatry.*

Kirkendall, L.: The arousal of fear: Does it have a place in sex education. *Family Coordinator, 13:*14-16, 1964.

Kolarsky, A. and Madlafousek, J.: Female behavior and sex arousal in offenders. *Journal of Nervous and Mental Disease, 155:*110-118, 1972.

Kutchinsky, B.: The effect of easy availibility of pornography and the incidence of sex crimes. *Journal of Social Issues, 29:*163-181, 1973.

Laury, G.: Effect of faulty sleeping arrangements on children's sexuality. *Medical Aspects of Human Sexuality,* 6-17, December 1976.

Monanan, J.: Toward a safe society: *Journal of Criminal Justice, 4:*1-7, 1976.

Motorola Teleprograms Inc.: *Street Crime: What to do About It?* 16 mm., 20 min. 4825 N. Scott, Suite 23, Schiller Park, Il., 60176.

Mumford, D. et al.: An attempt to detect pregnancy susceptibility in indigent adolescent girls. *Journal of Youth and Adolescence, 6:*127-144, 1977.

Pettit, P. and Eike, C.: *Rape Prevention: No Pat Answer.* 16 mm., 16 min. 2164 West 15th., Lawrence, Ka., 66044.

Rada, R.: Alcoholism and the child molester. *Annals of the New*

York Academy of Science, 273:492-496, 1976.

Rechy, J.: *The Sexual Outlaw*. New York, Grove Press, 1977, pp. 120-125.

Salk, L.: *What Every Child Would Like His Parents to Know*. New York, Warner, 1973.

Sanctuary, G.: Sex education for children in foster homes. *Child Welfare, 50*:154-59, 1971.

Sefeik, T. and Ormsby, N.: Establishing a rural child abuse neglect treatment program. *Child Welfare, 57(3)*:189-195, 1978.

Sex education and residential child care. *Child Care Quarterly, 6(3)*:204-230, 1977.

Wirt, R.: Enhancing of maturity of moral judgment by parent education. *Journal of Abnormal Child Psychiatry*, 5:177-186, 1977.

W.D.A.R.: *Discussing Rape with Children*, Philadelphia, Women Organized Against Rape, 1977.

Women Make Movies, Inc.: *Fear*. 16 mm., 7 min. 257 West 19th Street, New York, N.Y. 10011.

Yates, A.: *Sex Without Shame*. New York, Morrow, 1978.

SEXUAL CONTROL VERSUS FREEDOM

Bennett, W. and McDonald, L: Rights of children. *The Family Coordinator*, 333-337, October 1977.

Brant, J.: The child's right to privacy. *Harvard Law School Bulletin*, 28:41-44, 1977.

Burt, R.: Developing constitutional rights of, in and for children. In M. Rosenheim: *Pursuing Justice for the Child*. Chicago, University of Chicago Press, 1976, pp. 225-245.

Burt, R.: The therapeutic use and abuse of state power over adolescent. In J. Schooler: *Current Issues in Adolescent Psychiatry*. 1973, pp. 243-251.

Card, R.: Sexual relations with minors. *Criminal Law Review*, 370-380, 1975.

Comment: Do children have the legal right to be incorrigible? *Brigham Young University Law Review*, 659-691, 1976.

Farson, R.: *Birthrights*. New York, McMillan, 1974, pp. 129-153.

Fox, G.: Nice girl: Social control of women through a value construct. *Signs: Journal of Women in Culture and Society, 2*: 805-817, 1977.

Geiser, R.: The rights of children. *Hastings Law Journal, 28*: 1027-51, 1977.

Gold, S.: Equal protection for the juvenile girl in need of supervision in New York. *New York Law Review Forum, 17*:570-598, 1971.

Gough, A. and Grilli, M.: The unruly child and the law. *Juvenile Justice, 23*:9-12, 1972.

Greene, N. and Esselstyn, T.: The beyond control girl. *Juvenile Justice, 23*:13-19, 1972.

Grey, A.: Civilizing our sex laws. *Journal of the Society of Teachers of Law, 13*:106-112, 1975.

Hafen, B.: Children's liberation and the new egalitarianism: Reservations about abandoning youth to their rights. *Brigham Young University Law Review*, 605-658, 1976.

Kerscher, K.: *Emancipatory Sexual Education and Criminal Law.* Neuwied am Rhein, Germany, Herman Verlog, Publisher, 1973.

Kohlberg, L. and Gilligan, C.: The adolescent as philosopher. *Daedelus, 100*:1051-86, 1971.

Konopka, G.: The needs, rights, and responsibilities of youth. *Child Welfare, 55*:173-182, 1976.

Lewis, D. and Balla, D.: Sociopathy and its synonyms: Inappropriate diagnosis in child psychiatry. *American Journal of Psychiatry, 132*:720-722, 1975.

Mnookin, R.: Children's rights, legal and ethical dilemmas. *Pharos, 41(4)*:2-7, 1978.

Note: Parens patriae and statutory vagueness in the juvenile court. *Yale Law Review, 82*:745-771, 1973.

Note: Ungovernability: The unjustified jurisdiction. *Yale Law Review, 83*:1383-1409, 1974.

Reiss, A.: Sex offenses: The marginal status of the adolescent. *Law and Contemporary Problems, 25*:278-312, 1960.

Riback, L.: Juvenile delinquency: Juvenile women and the double standard of morality. *University of California (Los Angeles) Law Review, 19*:313-342, 1971.

Rodham, H.: Children under the law. *Harvard Educational Review, 43*:487-514, 1973.

Rosenheim, M.: Notes on helping juvenile nuisances. *Social Service Review, 50*:177-194, 1976.

Parker, H.: *View from the Boys.* Devon, Great Britain, David and Charles, 1974.

Prevost, S.: Statutory rape: A growing liberalization. *South Carolina Law Review, 18*:254-264, 1966.

Schrag, F.: The child in the moral order. *Philosophy, 52*:126-135, 1977.

Sheehy, G.: Nice girls don't get in trouble. *New York 4(26)*: Feb. 15, 1971.

Shopper, M.: Psychiatric and legal aspects of statutory rape. *Journal of Psychiatry and Law, 1*:275-295, 1973.

Stafford, A.: *The Age of Consent.* London, Hodder and Stoughton, 1964.

Strouse, J.: To be minor and female. *Ms.,* 70-75, August 1972.

Tallent, N.: Sexual deviation as a diagnostic entity: A confused and sinister concept. *Bulletin of the Menninger Clinic, 41*:40-60, 1977.

Teitelbaum, A. and Gough, A.: *Beyond Control.* Cambridge, Ma., Ballinger, 1978.

Wald, R.: Making sense out of the rights of youth. *Child Welfare, 55*:379-394, 1976.

West, D.: Thoughts on sex law reform. In R. Hood: *Crime, Criminology and Public Policy.* New York, Free Press, 1974, pp. 469-488.

Winslade, W.: The juvenile court: From idealism to hypocracy. *Social Theory and Practice, 3*:181-200, 1974.

Young people, sex and the law, Parts I and II. *Children's Rights Report, 2*: 1978.

THE FUTURE

American Film Advertising: *Development of a Community Response System to Sexual Abuse.* audio-tape, 1978. Six 11th Street N.E. Atlanta, Ga., 30309.

Bernard, F.: An enquiry among a group of pedophiles. *Journal of Sex Research, 11*:242-255, 1975.

Boulding, E.: Children's Rights. *Society, 15(1)*:39-43, 1977.

Bronfenbrenner, U.: Developmental research and public policy. In J. Romanshyn: *Social Science and Social Welfare.* New York, Council on Social Work Education, 1972.

Card, R.: Sexual relations with minors. *Criminal Law Review,* 370-380, 1975.

CSC Newsletter (since 1975): *Childhood Sensuality Circle.* POB 20163, El Cajon, Ca., 92021.

Duersted, Y.: *Green Fruit.* New York, Grove Press, 1974.

Farson, R.: *Birthrights.* New York, Macmillan, 1974, pp. 129-153.

Francoeur, R. and A.: The aesthetics of social sex: A revolution in values. *Journal of Operational Psychiatry. 6*:152-161, 1975.

Grey, A.: Civilizing our sex laws. *Journal of the Society of Teachers of Law, 13*:106-112, 1975.

Hamilton, D.: *Dreams of a Young Girl.* New York, Morrow, 1971.

Hofman, A. and Pilpel, H.: The legal rights of minors. *Pediatric Clinics of North America, 20*:989-1004, 1973.

Hunt, M.: *Gay.* New York, Farrar, Strous, and Grioux, 1977.

Kerscher, K.: *Emancipatory Sexual Education and Criminal Law.* Neuwied am Rhein, Germany, Herman Verlog, Publishers, 1973.

Marwell, G.: Adolescent powerlessness and delinquent behavior. *Social Problems, 14*:35-47, 1966.

Michalowski, R.: Legality vs. morality: Toward a science of social harms. Presented at the American Society of Criminology, Annual Meeting, Tuscon, Az., November 1976.

Mundel, D.: Some more thoughts on the direction of children's policy. In N. Talbot: *Raising Children in Modern America.* Boston, Ma., Little Brown, 1976, pp. 454-470.

National Council on Crime and Delinquency: Jurisdiction over status offenses should be removed from the court. *Crime and Delinquency, 21*:97-99, 1975.

Noble, P.: Incest: The last taboo. *Penthouse, 9(4)*:116-118, 126, 157-158, 1977.

Note: Ungovernability: The unjustified jurisdiction. *Yale Law Review, 83*:1282-1409, 1974.

Oates, J.: *Childwold.* Greenwich, Cn., Fawcett, 1976.

Ollendorff, R.: The rights of adolescents. In P. Adams et al.: *Children's Rights*, New York, Pralger, 1971, pp. 91-126.

Patrikios, T.: Age 16, civil majority 18, voting age 21, why? *UNESCO COURIER*, 26:24-31, October 1973.

Polier, J.: External and internal roadblocks to effective child advocacy. *Child Welfare*, 56:497-508, 1977.

Polier, J.: The myth that our society is child centered. *New York Times*, January 25, 1972.

Pomeroy, W.: Incest: A new look. *Forum*, November 1976.

Quinney, R.: Who is the victim? *Criminology*, 10:1972.

Schrag, F.: The child in the moral order. *Philosophy*, 52:126-135, 1977.

Schrag, F.: Rights over children. *Journal of Value Inquiry*, 7: 96-105, 1973.

Sexual Freedom League: *Statement of Position*. Berkely, Ca., n.d. p. 3.

Sexual Law Reform Society: *Report of the Working Party on Law in Relation to Sexual Behavior*. London, SLRS, 1974.

Terayama, S.: *Emperor Tomato Ketchup*. 16 mm., 1972. Japan.

Ullerstam, L.: *The Exotic Minorities*. New York, Grove, 1966.

Vaupel, J. and Cook, P.: Life, liberty, and the pursuit of self-hazardous behavior. Paper 8781, Institute of Policy Science and Public Affairs, Duke University, Durham, N.C., 1978.

Wald, G.: Making sense of the rights of children. *Human Rights*, 4:13-29, 1974.

Watman, F.: Sex offenses against children and minors: Proposals for legal reform. In L. Drapkin and E. Viano: *Victimology*, Vol. 3, Lexington, Ma., Heath, 1974, Chapter 22.

Wells, H.: *Your Child's Right to Sex*. New York, Stein and Day, 1976.

West, D.: Thoughts on sex law reform. In R. Hood: *Crime, Criminology, and Public Policy*, New York, Free Press, 1974, pp. 469-488.

Yudof, M.: The dilemma of children's autonomy. *Policy Analysis*, 2:371-385, 1976.

Zuckerman, M.: Children's rights: The failure of reform. *Policy Analysis*, 2:371-383, 1976.